Magnesium and Microelements in
Older Persons

Magnesium and Microelements in Older Persons

Editors

Nicola Veronese
Mario Barbagallo

MDPI • Basel • Beijing • Wuhan • Barcelona • Belgrade • Manchester • Tokyo • Cluj • Tianjin

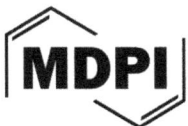

Editors
Nicola Veronese
Dipartimento PROMISE-UOC
Geriatria
University of Palermo
Palermo
Italy

Mario Barbagallo
Dipartimento PROMISE-UOC
Geriatria
University of Palermo
Palermo
Italy

Editorial Office
MDPI
St. Alban-Anlage 66
4052 Basel, Switzerland

This is a reprint of articles from the Special Issue published online in the open access journal *Nutrients* (ISSN 2072-6643) (available at: www.mdpi.com/journal/nutrients/special_issues/Microelements_Elderly).

For citation purposes, cite each article independently as indicated on the article page online and as indicated below:

LastName, A.A.; LastName, B.B.; LastName, C.C. Article Title. *Journal Name* **Year**, *Volume Number*, Page Range.

ISBN 978-3-0365-1412-3 (Hbk)
ISBN 978-3-0365-1411-6 (PDF)

© 2021 by the authors. Articles in this book are Open Access and distributed under the Creative Commons Attribution (CC BY) license, which allows users to download, copy and build upon published articles, as long as the author and publisher are properly credited, which ensures maximum dissemination and a wider impact of our publications.

The book as a whole is distributed by MDPI under the terms and conditions of the Creative Commons license CC BY-NC-ND.

Contents

Nicola Veronese and Mario Barbagallo
Magnesium and Micro-Elements in Older Persons
Reprinted from: *Nutrients* **2021**, *13*, 847, doi:10.3390/nu13030847 1

Ligia J. Dominguez, Nicola Veronese, Fernando Guerrero-Romero and Mario Barbagallo
Magnesium in Infectious Diseases in Older People
Reprinted from: *Nutrients* **2021**, *13*, 180, doi:10.3390/nu13010180 5

Aniqa B. Alam, Pamela L. Lutsey, Rebecca F. Gottesman, Adrienne Tin and Alvaro Alonso
Low Serum Magnesium is Associated with Incident Dementia in the ARIC-NCS Cohort
Reprinted from: *Nutrients* **2020**, *12*, 3074, doi:10.3390/nu12103074 29

Ligia J. Dominguez, Nicola Veronese and Mario Barbagallo
Magnesium and Hypertension in Old Age
Reprinted from: *Nutrients* **2020**, *13*, 139, doi:10.3390/nu13010139 41

Alvaro Alonso, Lin Y. Chen, Kyle D. Rudser, Faye L. Norby, Mary R. Rooney and Pamela L. Lutsey
Effect of Magnesium Supplementation on Circulating Biomarkers of Cardiovascular Disease
Reprinted from: *Nutrients* **2020**, *12*, 1697, doi:10.3390/nu12061697 73

Héctor Vázquez-Lorente, Lourdes Herrera-Quintana, Jorge Molina-López, Yenifer Gamarra-Morales, Beatriz López-González, Claudia Miralles-Adell and Elena Planells
Response of Vitamin D after Magnesium Intervention in a Postmenopausal Population from the Province of Granada, Spain
Reprinted from: *Nutrients* **2020**, *12*, 2283, doi:10.3390/nu12082283 83

Laetitia Lengelé, Pauline Moehlinger, Olivier Bruyère, Médéa Locquet, Jean-Yves Reginster and Charlotte Beaudart
Association between Changes in Nutrient Intake and Changes in Muscle Strength and Physical Performance in the SarcoPhAge Cohort
Reprinted from: *Nutrients* **2020**, *12*, 3485, doi:10.3390/nu12113485 97

Carla Gonçalves and Sandra Abreu
Sodium and Potassium Intake and Cardiovascular Disease in Older People: A Systematic Review
Reprinted from: *Nutrients* **2020**, *12*, 3447, doi:10.3390/nu12113447 113

Tanja Grubić Kezele and Božena Ćurko-Cofek
Age-Related Changes and Sex-Related Differences in Brain Iron Metabolism
Reprinted from: *Nutrients* **2020**, *12*, 2601, doi:10.3390/nu12092601 129

Editorial
Magnesium and Micro-Elements in Older Persons

Nicola Veronese * and Mario Barbagallo

Geriatrics Section, Department of Internal Medicine, University of Palermo, 90127 Palermo, Italy; mario.barbagallo@unipa.it
* Correspondence: nicola.veronese@unipa.it

Macro- and micro-element deficiencies are widely diffused in older people. The deficiency of these elements in older people is often attributable to malnutrition, even if other medical conditions (such as gastrointestinal problem) or non-medical conditions (such as polypharmacy) can lead to these deficiencies [1]. It is estimated that malnutrition is present in 1.3–47.8% of older people living in the community, being higher in other settings and in low-middle income countries [2].

Malnutrition is often followed by deficiency in both macro-elements (i.e., minerals with a requested amount of at least 100 mg, e.g., calcium (Ca), sodium (Na) or Magnesium (Mg) and micro-elements (<100 mg/day, such as iron (Fe), Zinc (Zn) or Selenio (Se). Moreover, the scarcity of trace elements, such as Chromium (Cr+++), Silicium (Si), or Vanadium (V), could be present in malnourished older people.

At the same time, for several years, it was assumed that malabsorption of both macro- and micro-elements was a common problem among older people [3], but increasing literature has suggested that it is not ever true, since older persons who malabsorb macronutrients often do so because of a disease (such as cancer or gastrointestinal problems), not because of age itself [3].

From an epidemiological point of view, the limited introduction of macro- and micro-elements is traditionally associated with a wide spectrum of medical conditions common in geriatric medicine, especially metabolic and cardiovascular diseases [4], dementia [5], frailty [6], sarcopenia [7] and, finally, mortality [8].

For these reasons, in this Special Issue entitled Magnesium and Micro-Elements in Older Persons and published in Nutrients, we decided to report the state-of-the-art regarding the deficiency of both Mg and micro-elements and the consequences in terms of higher risk of certain diseases in geriatric medicine.

In particular, the interest in Mg is due to several reasons. First, Mg is sometimes defined as "the forgotten electrolyte" [9], since it is less frequently required in our patients than other similar elements. Despite this, as also shown in our Special Issue, poor Mg status is associated with several negative outcomes in older people. For example, novel data on Mg and dementia in more than 10,000 older participants followed-up for about 25 years were reported, showing that low midlife serum Mg is associated with increased risk of incident dementia, independently from several confounder factors [10]. Other authors have explored the importance to supplement Mg for increasing vitamin D levels in post-menopausal women [11] and for improving several cardiovascular biomarkers [12]. These novel findings could partly explain the role of Mg in improving outcomes in infectious diseases [13] and for improving hypertension [14], one of the most common condition in older subjects, as discussed in two reviews. Furthermore, the correct assessment of Mg status, particularly in older people, is often problematic. Serum Mg, in fact, could be not considered as a good proxy of Mg deposits in human bodies, since it is poorly correlating with intracellular Mg [15]. Other laboratory assessments are expensive and difficult to realize in daily clinical practice, particularly in older subjects [16]. It is important to note that about 2/3 of older people did not consume enough amounts of this micronutrient [17] and as previously mentioned, Mg deficiency is associated with several conditions in geriatric medicine.

In our Special Issue, we have also collected data regarding micro-elements. In our opinion, this aspect better completes the scenario of poor nutritional status in older people. Cardiovascular aspects are also covered by a systematic review that shows the importance of low sodium intake and a high potassium/sodium intake for preventing cardiovascular conditions in older people [18]. These topics are of critical importance since cardiovascular diseases are the leading cause of mortality in aged people. Furthermore, our Special Issue is completed by other studies regarding the importance of some micro-elements in sarcopenia, such as omega-3 fatty acids, and vitamins D, A, and K [19]. Finally, an interesting Review regarding iron metabolism is presented [20]. Iron deposits, in fact, can contribute to the development of inflammation, abnormal protein aggregation, and degeneration in the central nervous system that may increase the risk of several neurological disorders such as multiple sclerosis, Parkinson's disease, Alzheimer's disease, or stroke [20].

We hope that with this Special Issue the Reader can better understand the importance of Mg and micro-elements in healthy aging and in some medical conditions in older people, further highlighting the impelling necessity to frequently monitor the nutritional status of aged subjects, a topic often forgotten in actual geriatric medicine.

Author Contributions: Writing—original draft preparation, N.V.; writing—review and editing, M.B. All authors have read and agreed to the published version of the manuscript.

Funding: This research received no external funding.

Institutional Review Board Statement: Not applicable.

Informed Consent Statement: Not applicable.

Data Availability Statement: Not applicable.

Conflicts of Interest: The authors declare no conflict of interest.

References

1. Guyonnet, S.; Rolland, Y. Screening for malnutrition in older people. *Clin. Geriatr. Med.* **2015**, *31*, 429–437. [CrossRef] [PubMed]
2. World Health Organization. *Integrated Care for Older People: Guidelines on Community-Level Interventions to Manage Declines in Intrinsic Capacity*; World Health Organization: Geneva, Switzerland, 2017.
3. Russell, R.M. Factors in aging that effect the bioavailability of nutrients. *J. Nutr.* **2001**, *131*, 1359S–1361S. [CrossRef] [PubMed]
4. Tang, Y.-R.; Zhang, S.-Q.; Xiong, Y.; Zhao, Y.; Fu, H.; Zhang, H.-P.; Xiong, K.-M. Studies of five microelement contents in human serum, hair, and fingernails correlated with aged hypertension and coronary heart disease. *Biol. Trace Elem. Res.* **2003**, *92*, 97–103. [CrossRef]
5. Kieboom, B.C.; Licher, S.; Wolters, F.J.; Ikram, M.K.; Hoorn, E.J.; Zietse, R.; Stricker, B.H.; Ikram, M.A. Serum magnesium is associated with the risk of dementia. *Neurology* **2017**, *89*, 1716–1722. [CrossRef] [PubMed]
6. Gimeno-Mallench, L.; Sanchez-Morate, E.; Parejo-Pedrajas, S.; Mas-Bargues, C.; Inglés, M.; Sanz-Ros, J.; Román-Domínguez, A.; Olaso, G.; Stromsnes, K.; Gambini, J. The Relationship between Diet and Frailty in Aging. *Endocr. Metab. Immune Disord. Drug Targets (Former. Curr. Drug Targets Immun. Metab. Disord.)* **2020**, *20*, 1373–1382. [CrossRef] [PubMed]
7. Giglio, J.; Kamimura, M.A.; Lamarca, F.; Rodrigues, J.; Santin, F.; Avesani, C.M. Association of sarcopenia with nutritional parameters, quality of life, hospitalization, and mortality rates of elderly patients on hemodialysis. *J. Ren. Nutr.* **2018**, *28*, 197–207. [CrossRef] [PubMed]
8. Black, R. *Micronutrient Deficiency: An Underlying Cause of Morbidity and Mortality*; SciELO Public Health: Baltimore, MA, USA, 2003.
9. Ahmed, F.; Mohammed, A. Magnesium: The forgotten electrolyte—A review on hypomagnesemia. *Med. Sci.* **2019**, *7*, 56. [CrossRef] [PubMed]
10. Alam, A.B.; Lutsey, P.L.; Gottesman, R.F.; Tin, A.; Alonso, A. Low serum magnesium is associated with incident dementia in the ARIC-NCS cohort. *Nutrients* **2020**, *12*, 3074. [CrossRef]
11. Vázquez-Lorente, H.; Herrera-Quintana, L.; Molina-López, J.; Gamarra-Morales, Y.; López-González, B.; Miralles-Adell, C.; Planells, E. Response of vitamin D after magnesium intervention in a postmenopausal population from the province of Granada, Spain. *Nutrients* **2020**, *12*, 2283. [CrossRef] [PubMed]
12. Alonso, A.; Chen, L.Y.; Rudser, K.D.; Norby, F.L.; Rooney, M.R.; Lutsey, P.L. Effect of magnesium supplementation on circulating biomarkers of cardiovascular disease. *Nutrients* **2020**, *12*, 1697. [CrossRef] [PubMed]
13. Dominguez, L.J.; Veronese, N.; Guerrero-Romero, F.; Barbagallo, M. Magnesium in Infectious Diseases in Older People. *Nutrients* **2021**, *13*, 180. [CrossRef] [PubMed]

14. Dominguez, L.; Veronese, N.; Barbagallo, M. Magnesium and Hypertension in Old Age. *Nutrients* **2021**, *13*, 139. [CrossRef] [PubMed]
15. Veronese, N.; Zanforlini, B.M.; Manzato, E.; Sergi, G. Magnesium and healthy aging. *Magnes. Res.* **2015**, *28*, 112–115. [CrossRef] [PubMed]
16. Barbagallo, M.; Belvedere, M.; Dominguez, L.J. Magnesium homeostasis and aging. *Magnes. Res.* **2009**, *22*, 235–246. [CrossRef] [PubMed]
17. Wood, R.J.; Suter, P.M.; Russell, R.M. Mineral requirements of elderly people. *Am. J. Clin. Nutr.* **1995**, *62*, 493–505. [CrossRef] [PubMed]
18. Gonçalves, C.; Abreu, S. Sodium and Potassium Intake and Cardiovascular Disease in Older People: A Systematic Review. *Nutrients* **2020**, *12*, 3447. [CrossRef]
19. Lengelé, L.; Moehlinger, P.; Bruyère, O.; Locquet, M.; Reginster, J.-Y.; Beaudart, C. Association between Changes in Nutrient Intake and Changes in Muscle Strength and Physical Performance in the SarcoPhAge Cohort. *Nutrients* **2020**, *12*, 3485. [CrossRef] [PubMed]
20. Grubić Kezele, T.; Ćurko-Cofek, B. Age-Related Changes and Sex-Related Differences in Brain Iron Metabolism. *Nutrients* **2020**, *12*, 2601. [CrossRef] [PubMed]

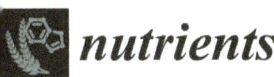

Review

Magnesium in Infectious Diseases in Older People

Ligia J. Dominguez [1], Nicola Veronese [1,*], Fernando Guerrero-Romero [2] and Mario Barbagallo [1]

1. Geriatric Unit, Department of Internal Medicine and Geriatrics, University of Palermo, 90100 Palermo, Italy; ligia.dominguez@unipa.it (L.J.D.); mario.barbagallo@unipa.it (M.B.)
2. Mexican Institute of Social Security IMSS, Biomedical Research Unit, Durango, ZC 34067, Mexico; guerrero.romero@gmail.com
* Correspondence: nicola.veronese@unipa.it; Tel.: +39-0916554828; Fax: +39-0916552952

Abstract: Reduced magnesium (Mg) intake is a frequent cause of deficiency with age together with reduced absorption, renal wasting, and polypharmacotherapy. Chronic Mg deficiency may result in increased oxidative stress and low-grade inflammation, which may be linked to several age-related diseases, including higher predisposition to infectious diseases. Mg might play a role in the immune response being a cofactor for immunoglobulin synthesis and other processes strictly associated with the function of T and B cells. Mg is necessary for the biosynthesis, transport, and activation of vitamin D, another key factor in the pathogenesis of infectious diseases. The regulation of cytosolic free Mg in immune cells involves Mg transport systems, such as the melastatin-like transient receptor potential 7 channel, the solute carrier family, and the magnesium transporter 1 (MAGT1). The functional importance of Mg transport in immunity was unknown until the description of the primary immunodeficiency XMEN (X-linked immunodeficiency with Mg defect, Epstein–Barr virus infection, and neoplasia) due to a genetic deficiency of MAGT1 characterized by chronic Epstein–Barr virus infection. This and other research reporting associations of Mg deficit with viral and bacterial infections indicate a possible role of Mg deficit in the recent coronavirus disease 2019 (COVID-19) and its complications. In this review, we will discuss the importance of Mg for the immune system and for infectious diseases, including the recent pandemic of COVID-19.

Keywords: magnesium; oxidative stress; inflammation; aging; infectious diseases; vitamin D; COVID-19

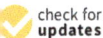

Citation: Dominguez, L.J.; Veronese, N.; Guerrero-Romero, F.; Barbagallo, M. Magnesium in Infectious Diseases in Older People. *Nutrients* **2021**, *13*, 180. https://doi.org/10.3390/nu13010180

Received: 16 December 2020
Accepted: 4 January 2021
Published: 8 January 2021

Publisher's Note: MDPI stays neutral with regard to jurisdictional claims in published maps and institutional affiliations.

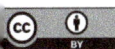

Copyright: © 2021 by the authors. Licensee MDPI, Basel, Switzerland. This article is an open access article distributed under the terms and conditions of the Creative Commons Attribution (CC BY) license (https://creativecommons.org/licenses/by/4.0/).

1. Introduction

About eleven thousand years ago, with the introduction of agriculture, the human beings radically modified their way of living from the remote and primitive hunter–gatherer organization towards a new form of more sedentary cohabitation, which also included the domestication of animals. The new epidemiological scenario allowed the coexistence of microorganisms, wild and domestic animals, and the human beings, which is now recognized as the origin of the most important human infectious diseases [1]. These diseases can only be sustained in large dense human populations that did not exist anywhere in the world before agriculture. Despite the fact that this story began so long ago and notwithstanding the advances in the development of vaccines and antibiotics, infectious diseases continue to be a major burden in global public health [2]. Furthermore, new emerging infectious diseases continue to be described and can lead, as at the present time, to pandemics that reveal our unpreparedness to face new infectious noxae. In fact, overcrowding and population movements can make a local infectious problem turn into a serious and feared pandemic attack in a short period of time as a consequence of globalization.

Historians increasingly recognize that infectious diseases have shaped the course of history as in the emblematic example of how more Native Americans died from microbes brought by the European conquerors rather than by their swords and guns allowing the relatively easy conquest of the new discovered territories [1]. Humanity today is again witnessing the profound changes that infectious diseases can produce in history with the tragic mortality toll and economic hardship caused by the coronavirus disease 2019 (COVID-19) pandemic.

Infections are more frequent in vulnerable populations such as older adults for a number of reasons, including the physiologic changes that accompany "normal" aging and the multimorbidity frequent in older populations with various simultaneously occurring chronic diseases as well as the medical, diagnostic, and surgical interventions that accompany them. Not only are infections more frequent in older adults, but they can be more injurious generating a cascade of complications that result in substantial human and financial costs [3].

Magnesium (Mg), a mineral of primary physiological importance, is the most abundant divalent cation in living cells. In the human body, Mg is the second most abundant intracellular cation after potassium and the fourth most common mineral in the whole body after calcium, sodium, and potassium. Mg is an essential cofactor for numerous biological processes (estimated at over 600) acting both on the enzymes as a structural or catalytic component and on the substrates [4] and it is required for oxidative phosphorylation, energy production, protein synthesis, glycolysis, and nucleic acid synthesis and stability [5,6]. This fundamental ion also plays an essential role in the active transport of other ions across cell membranes, therefore modulating neuron excitability, muscle contraction, and normal heart rhythm [7]. In the serum, Mg exists in three forms: a protein-bound fraction (25% bound to albumin and 8% bound to globulins), a chelated fraction (12%), and the metabolically active ionized fraction (55%) [5,6].

For all these reasons, Mg is a critical factor for normal cellular and body homeostasis, including the processes involving the immune system. In particular, Mg has a strong relationship with both innate and acquired immune responses, playing a key role in the signaling pathways that regulate the development, homeostasis, and activation of immune cells [8]. Mg deficiency, frequent in old age, can cause inflammation by diverse mechanisms, including activation of phagocytic cells, opening of calcium channels, activation of the N-methyl-d-aspartate (NMDA) receptor and of nuclear factor kappa-light-chain-enhancer of activated B cells (NF-κB) [9], while it can also increase oxidative stress [10,11]. The discovery of a genetic disease, X-linked immunodeficiency with magnesium defect (XMEN), that can lead to severe and chronic Epstein–Barr virus infections and neoplasia confirmed the important role of Mg as a second messenger in immunity [12–14].

Over the past decades, the clinical relevance and biological significance of Mg have been documented, as well as the impact of Mg on molecular and physiological processes of aging, especially those regarding the immune system and infectious diseases [11,15]. Older adults, together with the frequent magnesium deficiency due to a variety of reasons [15], undergo modifications of the immune response that can make them particularly susceptible to infections and their complications [3].

In this review, we will discuss the importance of Mg for the immune system and for infectious diseases, including the recent pandemic of COVID-19, with particular focus on older populations.

2. Mg and the Immune Responses

Previous and also subsequent studies have shown that Mg plays a role in the immune response as a cofactor for immunoglobulin (Ig) synthesis, C3 convertase, immune cell adherence, antibody-dependent cytolysis, IgM lymphocyte binding, macrophage response to lymphokines, and T helper–B cell adherence [8,16]. Mg reduces the expression and release of substance P and other proinflammatory molecules by controlling NF-κB activity under physiological Mg conditions and leads to increased NF-κB activation and cytokine production when in suboptimal concentrations [17]. Mg also affects acquired immunity by regulating the proliferation and development of lymphocytes [18]. Most of these studies have been carried out on experimental animals fed Mg-deficient diets. These animals also exhibited altered polymorphonuclear cell number and function together with an increased number of neutrophils, which was related to increased phagocytosis [19]. Mg deficiency also alters mast cell proliferation and function (histamine storing and secretion) and might be involved in mast cell-dependent hepatic fibrosis and steatosis [20,21]. This cation participates in human cell apoptosis, because Fas-induced B cell apoptosis is a Mg-dependent process. Elevation of intracellular free Mg concentrations are needed for Fas molecule binding expression on the B cell surface to trigger signaling pathways that cause apoptosis and cellular death [22]. Other studies confirm the importance of Mg in immunoinflammatory processes with the evidence that Mg-deficient experimental animals exhibit increased inflammation, exacerbated immune stress responses, and decreased specific immune responses [23–26].

A remarkable effect observed in Mg-deficient animals is the accelerated thymus involution even at early stages of Mg deficiency. Malpuech–Brugere et al. showed a higher level of apoptosis in thymuses from Mg-deficient rats compared to the control normally Mg-fed group starting from the second day of deficiency and accompanied by the presence of inflammatory cells. Later on, after eight days, they observed an increased proportion of epithelial reticular cells in the cortex, indicative of a remodeling process [27]. Altogether, these findings suggest that Mg deficiency can be associated with a significant impaired function in T cells.

The regulation of cytosolic free Mg in the immune cells involves Mg transporters, channels, and exchangers, such as the Mg/Na exchanger and the melastatin-like transient receptor potential 7 (TRPM7) channel [28]. TRPM7 is a non-selective Mg channel (also conducts Ca, Zn, and Na) that is expressed ubiquitously [28–32]. TRPM7 has a serine/threonine kinase domain, whose activity can modulate the gating of TRPM7 [33]. TRPM7 is fundamental for Mg homeostasis in immune cells. This is illustrated by the fall in cytosolic free Mg and cell cycle arrest in TRPM7-deficient B cell lines, which was partially rescued by culturing the cells in a high Mg-containing medium and by the impaired development of T cells in TRPM7 conditional knockout mice [33]. In a mouse model with a specific T cell deletion of TRPM7, T lymphocyte development was blocked at the CD4CD8 stage, resulting in decreased CD4 and CD4CD8 cells in the thymus [34]. In addition, TRPM7-deficient T cells seemed to be protected from Fas receptor-induced apoptosis [35]. Other regulators of free Mg homeostasis in immune cells include members of the solute carrier (SLC) family SLC41A1 and SLC41A2, which are homologous to the bacterial Mg transporter and expressed quite ubiquitously [29,31]. The role of SLC41A1/2 in Mg homeostasis in immune cells has been confirmed by their ectopic expression in a B cell line deficient in TRPM7, which was able to restore the reduced intracellular Mg concentrations and defective proliferation [36,37]. The third type of Mg transporter, MAGT1, is crucial in immune signaling [38,39]. With respect to the other transporters, MAGT1 is expressed at higher levels in immune and epithelial cells [40,41]. The functional importance of Mg transport in immunity was unknown until the description of a new primary immunodeficiency named XMEN (X-linked immunodeficiency with Mg defect, Epstein–Barr virus infection, and neoplasia) due to a genetic deficiency of MAGT1 [12–14] suggesting that Mg could function as a second messenger in cellular signaling. Patients with XMEN Patients with chronic Epstein–Barr virus infections, low CD4+ T cell counts, and defective T lymphocyte activation. These effects are hypothesized to result from a loss of phospholipase C (PLC)-g1 activation due to reduced Mg influx via MAGT1. Indeed, XMEN patients display impaired PLC signaling with reduced Ca/Mgresponses after T cell receptor stimulation and abolished expression of the natural killer activating receptor NKG2D in natural killer and CD8T cells [12–14]. The MAGT1-dependent Mg flux is essential for the optimal activation of PLC-g1, inositol triphosphate (IP3) generation, protein kinase Cu phosphorylation, and calcium mobilization via store-operated calcium entry [12]. MAGT1 deficiency also leads to decreased cytosolic free Mg and decreased Mg uptake in T cells and B cells [12,13]. Furthermore, it was shown that in some patients, oral Mg supplementation restored the concentration of intracellular free Mg in XMEN patients [13]. After the discovery of the XMEN disease [12–14], new variants of the XMEN disease have been described [42], as well as new mechanisms explaining the immunodeficiency, such as the glycosylation defects of a specific subset of N-glycoproteins and reduced killing function of cytotoxic immune cells in cells from XMEN patients [43,44].

In patients with asthma, Mg administration has been shown to promote bronchodilation and improve lung function [45–47]. In addition to its bronchodilating effects, one study showed that Mg supplementation was able to modulate the immune responses of acute asthmatic CD4+ T cells and decrease the secretion of type 2 CD4+ T lymphocyte cytokines [48].

3. Magnesium, Inflammation, and Oxidative Stress

3.1. Inflammation

Poor Mg diets are associated with a low-grade chronic inflammatory state, a condition associated with several chronic diseases in older people [49]. The Mg-associated low-grade chronic inflammation might be explained in in vitro studies by initiating excessive production and release of interleukin (IL)-1β and tumor necrosis factor (TNF)-α and by activating phagocytic cells, opening calcium channels, activating the NMDA receptor, and NF-κB signaling, as well as by stimulating the synthesis of nitric oxide and inflammatory markers [9,50]. Mg deficit also increases platelet aggregation and adhesiveness and inhibits growth and migration of endothelial cells, potentially altering microvascular functions [9]. Moreover, some evidence has shown that Mg concentration in acutely inflamed tissues is reduced through the activation of the IL-33/ST2 axis, further indicating the importance of Mg in inflammatory pathways [51].

In animal models, it was reported that Mg deprivation may cause several consequences that finally lead to increased inflammatory parameters and in particular to (i) marked elevation of proinflammatory molecules TNF-α, IL-1-β, IL-6, vascular cell adhesion molecules, and plasminogen activator inhibitor-1 [24]; (ii) increased number of circulating inflammatory cells [16]; and (iii) increased hepatic production and release of acute phase proteins (i.e., complement, α2-macroblobulin, fibrinogen) [9,19]. Endothelial dysfunction associated with low magnesium exposure has also been linked to the release of inflammatory mediators [52]. Conversely, magnesium sulfate supplementation was shown to mediate anti-inflammatory effects in stimulated murine macrophages via attenuation of endotoxin-induced upregulation of inflammatory mediators and NF-κB, as well as by activation of phosphoinositide 3-kinase and inhibition of L-type ion channels [53]. The calcium channel-blocking effects of Mg lead to the downstream suppression of NF-κB, IL-6, and CRP [54].

In human beings, it has been reported that low serum Mg concentrations as well as inadequate dietary Mg intake are associated with low-grade systemic inflammation [55–57]. Other studies have confirmed an inverse relationship between Mg intake, serum Mg, and inflammation markers [58–60]. Probably one of the most important contributions was made by the Women's Health Study, in which Mg intake was found to be inversely related to systemic inflammation, as measured by serum CRP concentrations, partly justifying a higher prevalence of metabolic syndrome in those with lower Mg intake [58]. Similar results were evident using the 1999–2002 National Health and Nutrition Examination Survey (NHANES) databases [55]. Of interest, in the study by King et al. conducted in 70% of the NHANES population not taking supplements, Mg intake below the recommended daily allowance (RDA) was significantly associated with elevated CRP [55]. Recently, a study performed in a large Finish population confirmed once more the inverse relationship between low dietary magnesium intake and serum hs-CRP concentrations [60]. A meta-analysis of eight randomized controlled trials (RCTs) evaluating the impact of Mg supplementation on CRP found a significant reduction in serum CRP concentrations following Mg supplementation, which was independent of the dosage of Mg supplementation or the duration of follow-up. [61]. Nevertheless, these results in small RCTs should be confirmed by larger and longer future investigations.

3.2. Oxidative Stress

Mg deficiency has been associated with increased oxidative stress and decreased antioxidant defense barriers. Previous in vitro studies have shown that Mg deficiency results in an increased production of oxygen-derived free radicals in various tissues [9,10], increased free radical-elicited oxidative tissue damage [10], increased production of superoxide anion by inflammatory cells [62], decreased antioxidant enzyme expression and activity [63], decreased cellular and tissue antioxidant concentrations [63], and increased oxygen peroxide production [64].

In animal models, Mg deficiency has been shown to increase lipid peroxidation and malondialdehyde and to decrease hepatic glutathione, superoxide dismutase, and vitamin E [65]; therefore, increasing oxidative stress concentrations. In this regard, our group has suggested an association between the action of Mg deficit in altering the antioxidant capacity and in activating oxidative stress, inflammation, and lipid oxidation that justify a high presence of metabolic conditions in people with low Mg intake or low serum Mg concentrations [7]. Mg itself seems to have antioxidant properties scavenging oxygen radicals, possibly by affecting the rate of spontaneous dismutation of the superoxide ion [64].

It has been shown that low serum Mg concentrations can stimulate Mg transporters such as TRPM7 and SLC41A [66], provoking the outflow of Mg from cells in order to increase serum Mg concentrations. As a consequence, intracellular Mg concentrations may decrease leading to modifications in cellular signaling functions depending on Mg and ATP. The reduction of intracellular Mg may elicit Mg stores in the mitochondria to release Mg [67] through SLC41A3 [68]. This drop in mitochondrial Mg content may further alter Mg- and ATP-linked mitochondrial signaling and functions, which may help explain the mitochondrial overproduction of free radicals, also called reactive oxygen species (ROS), and the reduction in ATP observed in Mg-deficient animal models [69,70].

Recently, it was shown that diabetic mice with Mg deficiency had increased mitochondrial oxidative stress, which contributed to cardiac diastolic dysfunction reversed after Mg supplementation [69]. This confirms that Mg can act as a mitochondrial antioxidant. According to a number of experimental studies, Mg deficiency disrupts mitochondrial function by diverse mechanisms, including alterations in coupled respiration [71–73], increased mitochondrial ROS production [9,10,69,70,74], suppression of the antioxidant defense system (e.g., superoxide dismutase, glutathione, catalase, vitamin E) [63–65,75–77], induction of calcium overload via the mitochondrial calcium uniporter [69,78,79], attenuation of pro-survival signaling [80–82], as well as by promoting the opening of the mitochondrial ATP-sensitive potassium channel [83], the inner membrane anion channel [84], and the mitochondrial permeability transition pore [85]. All these actions lead to the depolarization of the mitochondrial membrane potential [78]. Contrariwise, there are studies showing that Mg repletion improves mitochondrial function by diverse mechanisms, including the suppression of mitochondrial ROS overproduction [69,70], inhibition of the mitochondrial permeability transition pore opening and cytochrome C release [86–88], preservation of the mitochondrial membrane potential [89,90], reduction of the mitochondrial calcium accumulation [91–93], increase in protein expression of the anti-apoptotic B cell lymphoma 2 (Bcl-2) family and concurrent decrease of pro-apoptotic protein expression (such as of the Bcl-2-associated X protein) [80,90], decreasing apoptosis by quenching the activation of hypoxia-inducible factor 1-alpha and p38 mitogen-activated protein kinase/c-Jun N-terminal kinase (p38/JNK) signaling [90], and downregulating autophagy [93].

As mentioned, aging is characterized by a chronic low-grade inflammatory state that involves several tissues and organs frequently associated with multiple chronic diseases, and that has been named "inflammaging" [49]. Franceschi et al. [94] propose that the major source of inflammatory stimuli and oxidative stress is represented by endogenous/self, misplaced, or altered molecules resulting from damaged and/or dead cells and organelles (cell debris) recognized by receptors of the innate immune system, which are increased in old age due to a progressive decline in their disposal by the proteasome via autophagy and/or mitophagy.

Given all the abovementioned background, we proposed that the Mg deficiency, through its role in facilitating an impairment of the redox status and low-grade inflammation, might be considered a link to several age-related diseases and/or accelerated aging including a major predisposition to infectious diseases [11,15].

4. Mg and Vitamin D in Infectious Diseases

The study of vitamin/hormone D has undergone an enormous boost in the past decade, while its role as a hormone has been confirmed in various enzymatic, metabolic, physiological, and pathophysiological processes related to many organs and systems of the human body [95]. This growing interest is mostly due to the evidence that modest to severe vitamin D deficiency is widely prevalent around the world [96]. There is extensive agreement that an optimal vitamin D status is necessary not only for bone and muscle, but also for general health due to its association with multiple disorders including infectious diseases, primarily respiratory infections [95–97]. There is convincing evidence that vitamin D is an immunomodulatory hormone with significant biologic effects on the innate and adaptive immune systems [97].

4.1. Interaction between Mg and Vitamin D

The overall metabolism and effects of vitamin D in numerous organs are well known [96]. Several steps in the metabolism of vitamin D, such as the binding of vitamin D and 25-hydroxyvitamin D —25(OH)D or calcifediol— to their transport protein and the conversion of vitamin D into the active hormonal form 1,25-dihydroxyvitamin D (calcitriol) by hepatic and renal hydroxylation, depend on Mg as a cofactor [98–102]; therefore, in the presence of Mg deficit, these actions would be blunted (Figure 1). Magnesium also plays a critical role in the synthesis and metabolism of parathyroid hormone (PTH), hence Mg deficiency inhibits PTH secretion or synthesis [103–106]. Mg-depleted patients with hypocalcemia despite high PTH levels suggest bone and kidney resistance to PTH [107]. Mg deficit-related hypocalcemia secondary to peripheral PTH resistance or decreased PTH secretion is further complicated by the loss of PTH stimulation of renal 1-alpha-hydroxylation with worsening vitamin D deficit [98]. Mg deficiency leading to reduced calcitriol and impaired PTH response [98] has been implicated in "Mg-dependent vitamin D-resistant rickets" [99,108]. Two studies in patients with Mg deficiency [98,109] showed that Mg infusion alone resulted in a non-significant increase in calcitriol and in 25(OH)D [98], while Mg infusion added to oral vitamin D markedly increased both serum calcitriol and 25(OH)D [109], confirming the interaction between Mg and vitamin D. These findings should be tested in larger clinical trials. Of note, vitamin D, in turn, plays a key role in the metabolism of Mg both by stimulating intestinal Mg absorption and by preventing renal Mg excretion [110]. Thus, it appears that the deficit of each of these compounds, Mg and vitamin D, feeds the deficit of the other, which may lead to a perverse cycle with further worsening of both deficits. The combined effects of Mg and vitamin D deficiency may lead to clinically relevant outcomes, such as a higher risk of fragility fractures, particularly in women [111]. It is plausible that similar harmful effects of this detrimental combination could be observed in other major clinical outcomes, such as infections.

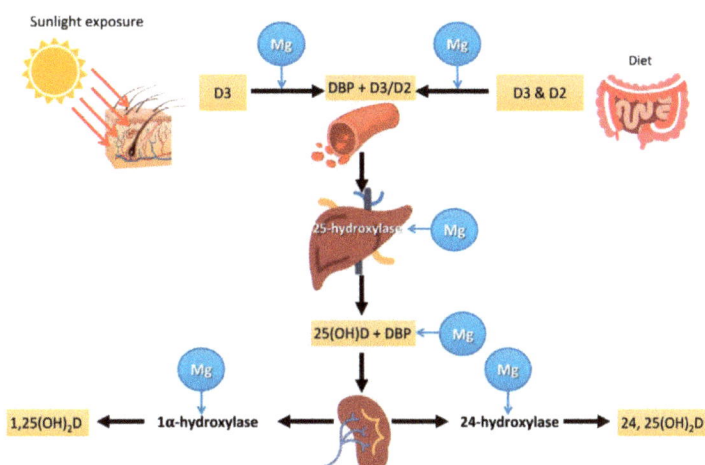

Figure 1. Mg and vitamin D metabolism. Vitamin D3 is produced in the skin through the action of UVB radiation reaching 7-dehydrocholesterol in the skin, followed by a thermal reaction. That vitamin D3 or oral vitamin D (D2 (ergocholecalciferol) or D3 (cholecalciferol) are converted to 25(OH)D in the liver and then to the active hormonal metabolite 1,25(OH)$_2$D (calcitriol) in the kidneys or other organs as needed. As shown in the graph, Mg is a cofactor that is required for the binding of vitamin D to its transport protein, for the conversion of vitamin D by hepatic 25-hydroxlation, for the transport of 25(OH)D, and for renal 1α-hydroxylation into the active hormonal form. Therefore, all these steps are Mg-dependent. DBP: vitamin D-binding protein.

A study by Deng et al. [112] investigated potential interactions between Mg intake, vitamin D status, and mortality. They analyzed data from NHANES 2001 to 2006 and NHANES III reporting that 12% of participants had a severe 25(OH)D deficit (<12 ng/mL) and 30% had an insufficient level of vitamin D (12 to 20 ng/mL). High total Mg intake (dietary or supplemental) was independently associated with reduced risk of vitamin D deficit or insufficiency. They also found an inverse association of serum 25(OH)D with mortality (particularly due to cardiovascular disease and colorectal cancer) that was modified by high Mg intake (i.e., the inverse association was primarily present among those with Mg intake above the median). Thus, Mg intake alone or its interaction with vitamin D intake may contribute to vitamin D status and the association of 25(OH)D with mortality risk may be modified by the level of Mg intake. A recent nested RCT within the Personalized Prevention of Colorectal Cancer Trial tested whether Mg supplementation affects vitamin D metabolism, evaluating 180 participants in a double-blind 2 × 2 factorial RCT and measuring plasma vitamin D metabolites by liquid chromatography–mass spectrometry. The analyses showed that an optimal Mg status was related to improvement of the 25(OH)D status [113].

4.2. Vitamin D and Infections

In addition to its musculoskeletal actions, vitamin D seems to have an important role in infectious diseases. One of the first evidences regards the impact of vitamin D on *Mycobacterium tuberculosis* infection. In this specific condition, the crucial role played by vitamin D in the immune response consists in promoting phagolysosome formation, as well as the production of the human antimicrobial peptides cathelicidin LL-37 and defensins [114,115]. The effects of vitamin D supplementation and tuberculosis have been subsequently extensively studied [116]. Furthermore, it was reported that vitamin D concentrations are associated with other infectious diseases, including acquired immunedeficiency syndrome, and respiratory diseases, particularly pneumonia [117], even if measurement of serum vitamin D concentrations may be profoundly perturbed [118].

In fact, it is still debated whether low vitamin D levels are a cause or a consequence of disease. However, it could be considered that during the course of a severe infection, the increase in energy consumption and in the demand for ATP and Mg closely related to it may decrease the efficacy of the immunomodulatory actions of vitamin D. As discussed above, low Mg can further decrease the activation of vitamin D, initiating a vicious cycle that may lead to even worse deficiencies, which are difficult to correct if they are not taken into account and detected early.

As mentioned, compelling evidence shows that vitamin D is an immunomodulatory hormone [97], while vitamin D deficit has been linked to various infective diseases, including upper respiratory and enteric infections, pneumonia, otitis media, *Clostridium* infections, vaginosis, urinary tract infections, sepsis, influenza, dengue, hepatitis B, hepatitis C, and HIV infections [119,120]. The protective properties that vitamin D exerts during infections have been attributed to upregulation of the expression of cathelicidin and beta-defensin 2 in phagocytes and epithelial cells [119]. Particular attention has been given to respiratory infections and the mechanisms of the protection given by vitamin D. This includes the maintenance of tight junctions, gap junctions, and adherens junctions, as well as induction of antiviral cytokines to interfere with the viral replicative cycle, in addition to the mentioned effects on cellular innate immunity partly through the induction of antimicrobial peptides, i.e., human cathelicidin LL-37 and defensins [120,121].

We cited the frequent association of low vitamin D status with a number of chronic diseases [95–97]. Intervention trials have rarely shown benefits of vitamin D supplementation as treatments or preventive measures, except for mortality in older adults [122]. Nevertheless, another important exception to the general trend is for upper respiratory tract infections: a recent meta-analysis involving 25 RCTs and data from 10,933 participants aged 0 to 95 years showed that vitamin D supplementation reduced the risk of acute respiratory tract infection among all participants. In subgroup analyses, the protective effects were better for those receiving daily or weekly doses compared to those receiving boluses and stronger for those with baseline 25(OH)D below 25 nmol/L (10 ng/mL), in whom there was a remarkable 70% lower incidence of acute respiratory infections [123].

4.3. Mg and Infectious Diseases

The close relationship of Mg and vitamin D and the necessity of an optimal Mg status for the synthesis, transport, and activation of vitamin D discussed in the previous subsection suggest that the higher incidence of infectious diseases associated with vitamin D deficiency can be at least in part explained by a deficit of Mg. Even if most studies regarding the direct association between poor Mg status and poor immune system function are derived from animal models (see above section on "Mg and the Immune Responses"), in human beings, Mg deficiency seems to be associated with a higher rate of infectious diseases, particularly when considering older people. As mentioned, the functional importance of Mg transport in immunity was put in evidence with the discovery of the XMEN disease that presents with defective T lymphocyte activation and chronic Epstein–Barr virus infection due to a genetic deficiency of MAGT1 and showing for the first time that Mg could function as a second messenger in cellular signaling [12–14]. Recent studies have added new mechanisms explaining the immunodeficiency and the development of chronic Epstein–Barr virus infection [43,44].

It has been suggested that Mg deficiency may play a role in liver diseases, especially in their progression due to a disruption in mitochondrial function, defective protein C translocation, inflammatory responses, oxidative stress, or metabolic disorders [124]. Mg may play a vital role in inhibiting the progression of HBV infection to hepatocellular cancer (HCC) [125]. Once HBV infection is established, the viral regulatory protein hepatitis B virus X amplifies the transforming growth factor (TGF)-β signal, which functions as a tumor promoter enhancing cancer metastasis and invasion by HCC. Mg administration can increase the expression of protein phosphatase Mg-dependent 1A, blocking TGF-β signaling by dephosphorylating p-Smad2/3 and thus preventing the transcription of specific genes needed for HCC growth [125].

A recent study showed that altered Mg status seems to have a prognostic role in older people affected by bacterial pneumonia. Of interest, hypomagnesemia and hypermagnesemia were both associated with excessive short-term mortality, 18.4% and 50%, respectively, compared to normal values of serum Mg [126]. Moreover, low serum Mg status was a significant predictor of frequent readmissions for acute exacerbation of chronic obstructive pulmonary disease (COPD) in a retrospective study of older adults [127].

5. Infectious Diseases in Old Age

Infections are a common cause of increased morbidity and mortality in older adults due to the various physiological modifications and progressive deterioration of homeostatic mechanisms, which lead to organ alterations, functional decline, multimorbidity, frailty, disability, and associated medical interventions [128], as well as to alterations in the immune response with aging [129]. Infectious diseases in older adults are usually more injurious than in younger populations and frequently generate a series of complications that result in substantial human and financial burden [3]. This is particularly true for residents in long term care facilities [130].

Data from the first-listed infectious disease (ID) hospitalizations in the USA using the Nationwide Inpatient Sample for 1998–2006 indicated that the mortality caused by acute infections was more than fifty-fold higher in persons aged over 65 years compared to that of persons aged 30–50 years [131]; older adults have a four times higher risk of being admitted to hospital for an acute infection compared to the general population [132]. In fact, infections are a frequent cause of hospitalization in older adults and hospitalization itself may lead to life-threatening nosocomial infections often caused by invasive diagnostic procedures and inappropriate use of urinary and venous catheters [133]. Older adults who survive a serious infection may afterwards have a functional deterioration that later leads to loss of self-sufficiency [134,135]. For example, pneumonia carries elevated long-term morbidity and mortality after hospitalization; over 70% of the surviving patients were reported to be readmitted to hospital at least once within the next 3 years of being hospitalized for pneumonia [136].

In the past century, there was a conspicuous decreasing trend of infectious diseases in developed countries, such as the USA, where infectious diseases went from 797:100,000 population in 1900 to 97:100,000 population in 1996 [131,137]. Conversely, taking into account only older adults, the hospital admission rate for infectious diseases increased by 13% from 1990 to 2002 [137].

The modifications in the immune system during aging, described with the term "immunosenescence" (Table 1), alter the organism's capacity to overcome external noxae. All older adults exhibit the features of immunosenescence with variable severity; nevertheless, the degree of frailty is associated with the degree of immunocompetence [138]. As people grow old, the immune system loses the normal ability to fight infections, there is an increased susceptibility to get infections, to develop neoplasms and autoimmunity, and a reduced ability to heal skin lesions [129,139]. In general, older adults have a mild degree of immunosuppression consequent to immunosenescence in addition to the age-associated organ decline, multimorbidity, malnutrition, frailty, functional failure, geriatric syndromes, and polypharmacotherapy. All these factors together worsen the prognosis of older adults with infections [128,138].

Table 1. Immunosenescence: modifications of the immune response with aging.

	Decreased	Increased
	Innate immune system	
	• Anatomical and biochemical barriers: - Regeneration, sweat production, and barrier function of the skin and mucus • Hematopoietic tissue: - Total number of HSCs and hematopoietic tissue in the bone marrow, proliferative capacity of HSCs • Macrophages: - Bone marrow precursors, phagocytic capacity, and oxidative killing activity of macrophages • Neutrophils: - Chemotactic responses, migration capacity, phagocytic capacity, and superoxide generation • NK cells: - $CD56^{bright}$ NK cell number	• NK cells: - $CD56^{dim}$ - NK cell number
	Adaptive immune system	
T cells	• Thymus gland involution • Number of thymic precursors • Number of naïve T cells T cell repertoire • Functional activity of regulatory T cells (Treg) • Number of CD4+ T cells • Number of CD28+ T cells	• Number of CD8+ T cells
B cells	• B cell precursors in the bone marrow • Number of B cells • Plasma cell differentiation • Specific antibody production • B cell response to antigen exposure • Diversity of the B cell repertoire • Opsonizing capacity of immunglobulins	• Autoreactive serum antibodies

HSCs: hematopoietic stem cells; NK: natural killer; CD: cluster of differentiation; CD4+: T helper cell; CD8+: cytotoxic T cell.

Functional decline and deterioration of the immune system competence are linked to disease burden rather than chronological age. Older adults with chronic diseases (e.g., COPD, heart failure, diabetes) are more susceptible to common infections and exhibit reduced responses to vaccines when compared to those without comorbidity [140]. Thus, not all older adults exhibit hyporesponsiveness towards vaccination and some are able to maintain a fully functional immune system during old age. However, due to the deterioration of the immune response, any infection may be associated with a high risk of complications or mortality in frail older adults. For example, an influenza infection may be benign and self-limiting, but it can as well lead to complications and death or require hospital admission in a more vulnerable older patient. In the current COVID-19 pandemic, older adults and patients with pre-existing comorbidities (i.e., cardio- and cerebrovascular disease, diabetes, COPD, malignancy, chronic kidney disease, dementia) are those bearing the highest fatality rate of the disease, which is affecting the frailest groups of the population [141,142].

6. Magnesium and COVID-19 Pandemic

The outbreak of COVID-19 caused by severe acute respiratory syndrome coronavirus 2 (SARS-CoV2), a variant of coronavirus thought to originate in the Wuhan province in China [143], was declared a pandemic by the World Health Organization (WHO) in March 2020. According to the WHO, the confirmed cases reported worldwide at the time this review was written (14 December 2020) are over 70 million with 1,605,091 related deaths [144].

A portion of these patients develop interstitial pneumonia, which can evolve into acute respiratory distress syndrome (ARDS), requiring active hyperoxic ventilation with possible fatal outcomes [145]. COVID-19 not only affects lungs, but the virus can extend and impact profoundly many other organs and systems, including the cardiovascular system, the kidneys, the intestines, the liver, and the brain; hence, now it is considered a systemic disease. COVID-19 is characterized by a heterogeneous clinical presentation ranging from mild influenza-like symptoms to life-threatening pneumonia, cytokine storm, and multiple organ failure. Older adults are more susceptible to severe illness, to be admitted to the ICU, and to die from this disease [146,147]. This trend has been persistently present since the onset of the disease, and it is particularly high for older adults living in long-term care homes [148] due to their advanced age, poor health, multiple chronic diseases, living environment, immunosenescence, and exposure to potentially asymptomatic care providers. So far, there is no effective therapy available against COVID-19; therefore, supportive care is used currently as the mainstay of management of patient with the disease [149]. Although the mechanisms of respiratory involvement and multiple organ failure in COVID-19 are not completely clear and under investigation, cytokine storm seems to significantly contribute to the pathogenesis of the most severe manifestation of the disease [145].

Nutritional issues seem to be important in COVID-19 pathogenesis and prognosis. For example, obesity, a condition associated with low Mg intake [150,151], seems to be a negative factor for increasing mortality and hospitalizations in people affected by COVID-19 [152,153]. Moreover, as mentioned before and shown in Figure 1, Mg is a cofactor necessary for vitamin D biosynthesis, transport, and activation, while both Mg and vitamin D deficiencies have been associated with several chronic diseases. Both Mg and vitamin D deficiencies seem to be important in the pathogenesis of COVID-19 as reported by some investigations [121,154–159]. COVID-19 is associated with relevant lung [160] and cardiac impairment [161]. Again, the literature suggests that Mg plays an important role in lung and heart function [11,15,45–47,162]. In addition to obesity, other coexisting conditions such as hypertension [163], diabetes [164], and primarily old age [165] are associated with increased severity of COVID-19, plausibly because of an underlying chronic inflammatory state or a lower threshold for the development of organ dysfunction from the immune response. All these conditions, including old age and a chronic inflammatory state discussed above, have been associated with a low Mg status [7,11,15,166].

Patients with severe manifestations of COVID-19 may need hospitalization in intensive care units (ICU). Interestingly, up to 60% of critically ill patients in ICU have been reported to present some degree of Mg deficiency [167–169], predisposing these patients to serious, even life-threatening effects, also because of the consequent hypokalemia and hypocalcemia. Unfortunately, so far, no direct data regarding the importance of Mg in COVID-19 is available, probably because Mg is not measured routinely in major databases and studies [154]. In addition, serum concentrations representing only 1% of total body Mg do not accurately reflect intracellular concentrations and, finally, total body status [15]. In a thoughtful review, Wallace reported that constant monitoring of ionized Mg status with repletion, when appropriate, might be an effective strategy to influence disease contraction and progression [155]. In this regard, the literature supports several aspects of Mg as an anti-COVID-19 nutrient, including its "calcium channel-blocking" effects that lead to downstream suppression of NF-κB, IL-6, CRP [54], and other related endocrine disrupters; its role in regulating renal potassium loss; and its ability to activate and enhance the functionality of vitamin D [158], among others [155]. In a cohort observational study by Tan et al., among 43 consecutive hospitalized patients with COVID-19 aged ≥ 50 years and not requiring oxygen therapy at admission, 17 patients received a combined daily oral supplementation with 1000 IU of vitamin D3, 150 mg of Mg, and 500 mcg of vitamin B12, while 26 patients did not receive the supplementation. They found significant differences in the clinical course with fewer treated patients than controls requiring oxygen therapy (17.6 vs. 61.5%) and/or intensive care support (6 vs. 32%) during hospitalization. This small but significant study illustrates the importance of providing sufficient supplementation of these nutrients in circumstances where the requirements are most likely higher while fighting COVID-19 [156]. Other authors reviewing potential actions of Mg on SARS-Cov2 infection point toward Mg as a possible supporting treatment of COVID-19 patients, especially those critically ill and/or at highest risk of complications [154,157], including also pregnant women [157].

The hypothesis that COVID-19 pneumonia may have a vascular basis is strong [170, 171]. Again, Mg has robust anti-thrombotic effects [52], while low Mg concentrations have been associated with endothelial dysfunction [172,173]. A recent systematic review and meta-analysis summarized the effects of oral Mg supplementation on vascular function in RCTs. Even if few studies were available and heterogeneity was high among the studies, in subgroup analyses, oral Mg significantly improved flow-mediated dilation in studies longer than 6 months, including unhealthy persons, persons older than 50 years, or with the BMI higher than 25 kg/m^2 [174]. Therefore, it is possible that a chronic Mg deficiency, very frequently seen in old age [15], might create a favorable microenvironment for the virus to promote thromboembolism [154], the main feature of COVID-19.

Because no vaccinations (or definitive therapies) are available against COVID-19, we encourage specific research regarding the role of Mg in this infection, since the role of Mg in inflammation, oxidative stress, endothelial dysfunction, and immune response in infectious diseases, particularly in viral infections, is largely supported by preclinical and clinical evidence.

We discuss below some salient points intensely studied in COVID-19, which have been shown to be related to Mg in previous investigations. Below we discuss some salient points and those most studied with respect to Covid-19 and which have also been shown to be related to Mg.

They are plausible mechanisms that support the indication of maintaining an optimal Mg status to combat the severity and complications of COVID-19.

6.1. Cytokine Storm in COVID-19

Even if there are still many unresolved questions regarding the pathogenesis and the extreme variability in the clinical course of COVID-19, the available evidence indicate that the so called "cytokine storm", which refers to uncontrolled overproduction of soluble markers of inflammation and which, in turn, maintains an aberrant systemic inflammatory response, is a major contributor to the occurrence of ARDS [145].

It appears that the collateral damage caused by excessive production of inflammatory mediators as the immune response attempts to clear the pathogen can be more injurious than the pathogen itself. This exuberant inflammatory response may be initially appropriate to control the infection, but if uncontrolled and continuous, the secondary multiple organ dysfunction can follow. The cascade of inflammatory mediators released during cytokine storm includes many immunoactive molecules, such as interferons, interleukins, chemokines, colony-stimulating factors, and TNF-α [175]. As we have discussed above, there is extensive evidence in experimental animals and in observational studies in humans confirming that low Mg status is associated with a chronic inflammatory state with increased levels of inflammation markers, particularly IL-6, TNF-α, and IL-33/ST2 axis (see subsection "Magnesium, Inflammation, and Oxidative Stress"). Hence, the preceding deficient Mg status associated with conditions that favor a detrimental course of COVID-19, such as aging, hypertension, and diabetes [7,11,15,166] and the Mg deficiency frequently seen in critical patients [167–169] may exacerbate the inflammatory response induced by SARS-CoV2, which in turn may determine increased Mg consumption resulting in further decreased intracellular levels, maintaining and propagating the uncontrolled inflammatory reaction, or cytokine storm.

Another well-known action of Mg relates to its calcium channel antagonist properties [176,177]. Indeed, Mg counteracts calcium as a physiological calcium blocker, similarly to synthetic calcium antagonists [178]. Interestingly, the calcium channel-blocking effects of Mg lead to the downstream suppression of NF-κB, IL-6, and CRP [54], which may limit systemic inflammation (Figure 2).

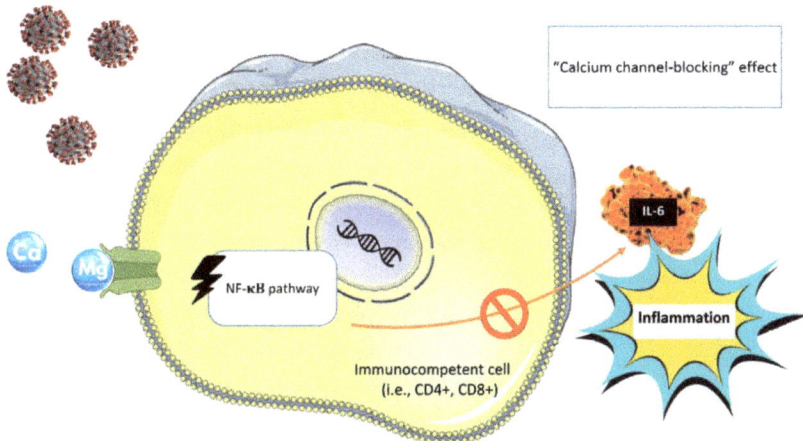

Figure 2. Mg's "calcium channel-blocking" effect, which can lead to the downstream suppression of NF-κB, IL-6 and may limit systemic inflammation. NF-kB: nuclear factor 70 kappa-light-chain-enhancer of activated B cells; IL-6: interleukin 6; CD4+: T helper cell; CD8+: cytotoxic T cell.

6.2. COVID-19 and Endothelial Dysfunction

Another pathophysiological mechanism that has been invoked and discussed extensively in the medical literature to explain the protean manifestations of COVID-19 and its multiorgan involvement is endothelial dysfunction [171]. The vascular endothelium is crucial for the maintenance of homeostasis, controlling fibrinolysis, vasomotion, inflammation, oxidative stress, vascular permeability, and structure. All these functions, acting in a concerted manner, regulate many host defense mechanisms against external noxae, but they can also contribute to disease at multiple levels when their usual homeostatic functions overreach and turn against the host, as has been reported in COVID-19 [179].

SARS-CoV-2 infects the host through the angiotensin-converting enzyme (ACE2) receptor, which is expressed in several organs, including the lung, heart, kidneys, and intestines. ACE2 receptors are also expressed by endothelial cells [179]. It is uncertain whether vascular alterations in COVID-19 are due to endothelial cell involvement by the virus. However, the endothelial cell involvement across vascular beds of different organs has been reported in a series of patients with COVID-19 [180] and anticoagulant treatment (i.e., heparin) is considered for the prevention of thromboembolic complications [181].

Mg is key for the preservation of endothelial function and vascular integrity. Low concentrations of extracellular Mg reduce endothelial cell proliferation, stimulate monocyte adhesion, and impairs vasoactive molecules, such as nitric oxide and prostacyclin [182]. Mg deficiency promotes platelet aggregation and the release of beta-thromboglobulin and thromboxanes [183]. In humans, oral Mg supplementation is significantly associated with improvement in the brachial artery's endothelial function and exercise tolerance in patients with coronary artery disease [173] and in diabetic older adults [172]. A recent systematic review and meta-analysis reported a significantly improved flow-mediated dilation in studies with Mg supplementation for over 6 months of the follow-up, including unhealthy persons, persons older than 50 years, or with BMI > 25 kg/m^2 [174].

6.3. COVID-19 and Vitamin D

As mentioned, there is convincing evidence showing that vitamin D is an immunomodulatory hormone and that its deficit has been linked to various infective diseases (see subsection "Vitamin D and Infections"). In a recent review, Grant et al. argued that vitamin D supports innate immunity, keeps the integrity of the tight junctions and the pulmonary barrier, provides immunoregulatory activity, and modulates the renin–angiotensin system, all factors of potential relevance for acute pneumonia and hyperinflammation observed in patients with COVID-19 [121](Figures 3 and 4).

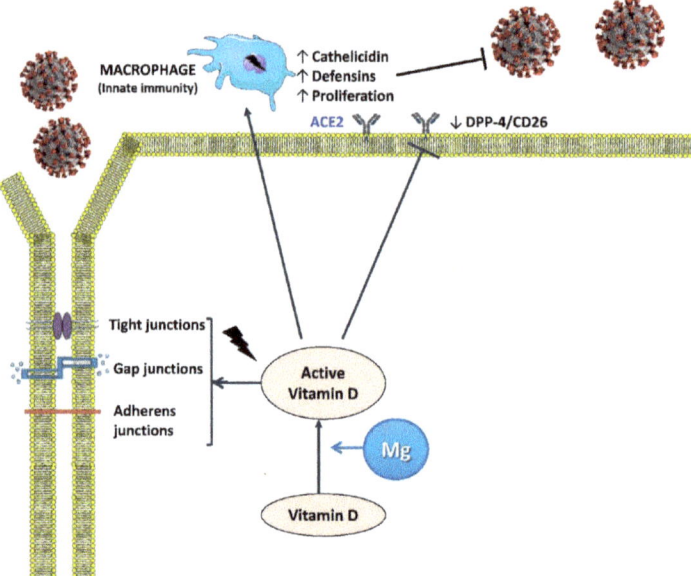

Figure 3. Active vitamin D (calcitriol or dihydroxycholecalciferol) helps maintain tight junctions, gap junctions, and adherens junctions in order to prevent the spread of SARS-CoV2 and induces the proliferation of macrophages and the release of cathelicidin and defensins, which are antimicrobial peptides active against a spectrum of microbes including viruses. Mg is a cofactor that is necessary for the synthesis, transport, and activation of vitamin D. ACE2: angiotensin-converting enzyme 2 receptor; DPP-4/CD26: dipeptidyl peptidase-4 receptor.

It is proposed that vitamin D may affect the response to COVID-19 infection by (i) supporting the production of antimicrobial peptides in the respiratory epithelium, thus making virus infection and development of COVID-19 symptoms less likely and (ii) helping to reduce the inflammatory response to SARS-CoV-2 infection. Deregulation of this response is characteristic of COVID-19 and the degree of overactivation is associated with poorer prognosis.

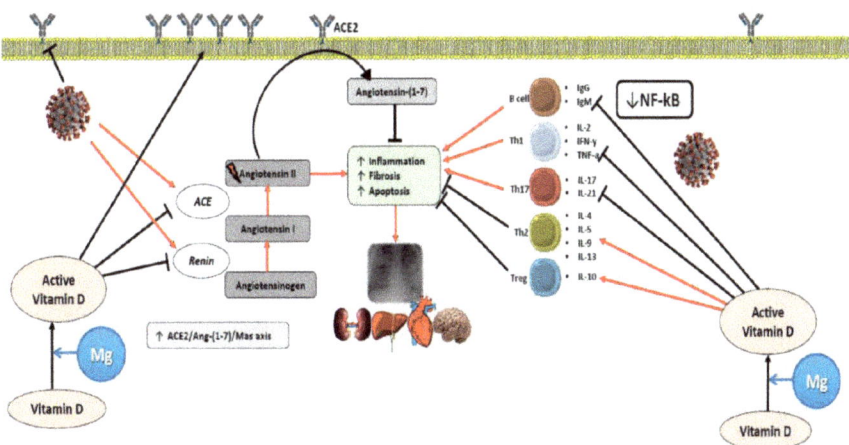

Figure 4. Proposed mechanisms by which vitamin D and Mg can exert actions against COVID-19. ACE, angiotensin-converting enzyme; ACE2: angiotensin-converting enzyme 2; Ang-(1-7), angiotensin (1-7); Ig, immunoglobulin; IFN-γ, interferon gamma; IL, interleukin; NF-κB, nuclear factor kappa-light-chain-enhancer of activated B cells; TNF-a, tumor necrosis factor alpha; Th, T helper cell; Treg, regulatory T cells.

The medical literature on the possible actions of vitamin D in COVID-19 has exploded in recent months. Small observational studies and trials have shown encouraging results. For example, a retrospective study in a single center showed that the deficit of vitamin D was associated with increased COVID-19 risk [159], and a meta-analysis of 27 studies found that severe cases of COVID-19 more frequently had vitamin D deficiency compared with mild cases, while vitamin D insufficiency was associated with an increased possibility of hospitalization and mortality [184]. Another retrospective observational trial in 186 cases of severe COVID-19 found that low 25(OH)D levels on admission were associated with COVID-19 disease stage and mortality [185]. A study including 91 asymptomatic participants and 63 severely ill patients with COVID-19 reported a vitamin D deficiency of 33% and 97%, respectively. Serum inflammatory markers and fatality rate were higher in those with vitamin D deficiency [186]. All these results are encouraging, but it is essential to keep in mind that Mg is an indispensable cofactor for the synthesis, transport, and activation of vitamin D (Figure 1). As mentioned above, the combination of oral supplementation with Mg, vitamin D, and vitamin B12 in a sample of patients with COVID-19 showed a reduction in the need for oxygen support, intensive care hospitalization, or both [156]. Therefore, it would be advisable to correct not only vitamin D deficiency, but also Mg deficiency.

7. Conclusions

In this review, we reported the potential role of Mg in infectious diseases, particularly those affecting older people, a population frequently affected by deficiency of this fundamental cation. The evidence regarding the importance of Mg in these kinds of diseases is derived from animal models reporting that low-Mg diets were associated with an unfavorable profile in the immune response, oxidative stress, and inflammatory markers. These findings have been confirmed in humans by epidemiological observational studies. The discovery of XMEN, an immunodeficiency characterized by chronic Epstein–Barr virus infection, opened a particularly interesting field of research demonstrating for the first time that a cation can be a second messenger in cellular signaling and revealed the potential key role of Mg in viral infections. Mg is a cofactor for the synthesis, transport, and activation of vitamin D, which has evidence of being an important immunomodulator in several infectious diseases, including SARS-Cov2 infection responsible for the current

COVID-19 pandemic. Other mechanisms described in COVID-19, such as the immune hyperresponsiveness with excessive release of inflammatory mediators leading to the cytokine storm, endothelial dysfunction, thrombotic complications, and preexisting predisposing conditions that worsen the prognosis of the COVID-19 clinical course, such as old age, diabetes, and hypertension, have all been associated with Mg deficit. Although direct data are not yet available, these concepts introduce the importance of Mg in COVID-19, a recent pandemic that is particularly harmful in older people also at higher risk for Mg deficiency and for which a definitive therapy or vaccination is still not available. It is foreseeable that an optimal Mg status might also provide healthy persons and patients that will be vaccinated against SARS-Cov2/COVID-19 with better tolerance due to the same mechanisms proposed above for possible therapeutic and disease-modulating actions.

Figure 5 summarizes the mechanisms by which maintaining an optimal Mg status may be of benefit in COVID-19.

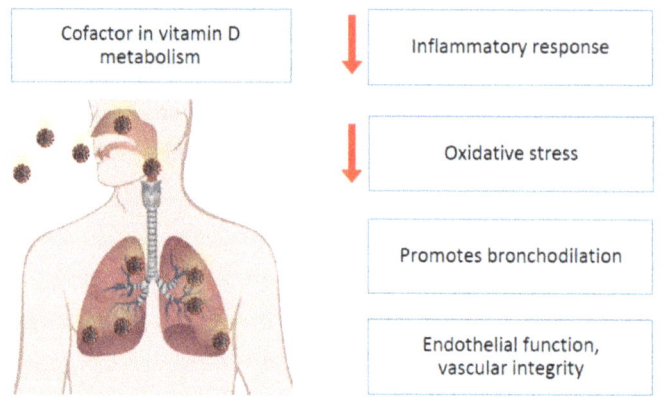

Figure 5. Summary of Mg's possible effects in COVID-19.

We all are struggling to decode a new and unknown hazard which has alarmed everyone, from health providers to scientists, economists, sociologists, and rulers since December 2019. Even if Mg is not curative, it is important to ensure the correction of its deficit in order to eventually help reduce the severity of the clinical course of COVID-19. Nevertheless, further research showing the potential association between poor Mg status and COVID-19 prevalence and outcomes is consequently necessary.

Author Contributions: Writing—original draft preparation, L.J.D., N.V.; writing—review and editing, L.J.D., N.V., M.B., F.G.-R. All authors have read and agreed to the published version of the manuscript.

Funding: This research received no external funding.

Institutional Review Board Statement: Not applicable.

Informed Consent Statement: Not applicable.

Data Availability Statement: No new data were created or analyzed in this study. Data sharing is not applicable to this article.

Conflicts of Interest: Authors declare no conflict of interest.

References

1. Wolfe, N.D.; Dunavan, C.P.; Diamond, J. Origins of major human infectious diseases. *Nat. Cell Biol.* **2007**, *447*, 279–283. [CrossRef]
2. Global burden of 369 diseases and injuries in 204 countries and territories, 1990–2019: A systematic analysis for the Global Burden of Disease Study 2019. *Lancet* **2020**, *396*, 1204–1222.

3. WHO. *World Report on Ageing and Health*; World Health Organisation: Geneva, Switzerland, 2015; Available online: https://www.who.int/ageing/events/world-report-2015-launch/en/ (accessed on 1 December 2020).
4. Caspi, R.; Altman, T.; Dreher, K.; Fulcher, C.A.; Subhraveti, P.; Keseler, I.M.; Kothari, A.; Krummenacker, M.; Latendresse, M.; Mueller, L.A.; et al. The MetaCyc database of metabolic pathways and enzymes and the BioCyc collection of pathway/genome databases. *Nucleic Acids Res.* 2011, 40, D742–D753. [CrossRef]
5. Saris, N.-E.L.; Mervaala, E.; Karppanen, H.; Khawaja, J.A.; Lewenstam, A. Magnesium: An update on physiological, clinical and analytical aspects. *Clin. Chim. Acta* 2000, 294, 1–26.
6. Barbagallo, M.; Gupta, R.K.; Dominguez, L.J.; Resnick, L.M. Cellular Ionic Alterations with Age: Relation to Hypertension and Diabetes. *J. Am. Geriatr. Soc.* 2000, 48, 1111–1116. [CrossRef]
7. Barbagallo, M.; Dominguez, L.J. Magnesium Metabolism in Type 2 Diabetes Mellitus. *Encycl. Metalloproteins* 2013, 458, 1277–1281. [CrossRef]
8. Tam, M.; Gómez, S.; GonzalezGross, M.; Marcos, A. Possible roles of magnesium on the immune system. *Eur. J. Clin. Nutr.* 2003, 57, 1193–1197. [CrossRef]
9. Mazur, A.; Maier, J.A.; Rock, E.; Gueux, E.; Nowacki, W.; Rayssiguier, Y. Magnesium and the inflammatory response: Potential physiopathological implications. *Arch. Biochem. Biophys.* 2007, 458, 48–56. [CrossRef]
10. Wolf, F.I.; Trapani, V.; Simonacci, M.; Ferrè, S.; Maier, J.A.M. Magnesium deficiency and endothelial dysfunction: Is oxidative stress involved? *Magnes. Res.* 2008, 21, 58–64.
11. Barbagallo, M.; Belvedere, M.; Dominguez, L.J. Magnesium homeostasis and aging. *Magnes. Res.* 2009, 22, 235–246.
12. Li, F.-Y.; Chaigne-Delalande, B.; Kanellopoulou, C.; Davis, J.C.; Matthews, H.F.; Douek, D.C.; Cohen, J.I.; Uzel, G.; Su, H.C.; Lenardo, M.J. Second messenger role for Mg2+ revealed by human T-cell immunodeficiency. *Nat. Cell Biol.* 2011, 475, 471–476. [CrossRef]
13. Chaigne-Delalande, B.; Li, F.-Y.; O'Connor, G.M.; Lukacs, M.J.; Jiang, P.; Zheng, L.; Shatzer, A.; Biancalana, M.; Pittaluga, S.; Matthews, H.F.; et al. Mg2+ Regulates Cytotoxic Functions of NK and CD8 T Cells in Chronic EBV Infection Through NKG2D. *Science* 2013, 341, 186–191. [CrossRef]
14. Li, F.-Y.; Chaigne-Delalande, B.; Su, H.; Uzel, G.; Matthews, H.; Lenardo, M.J. XMEN disease: A new primary immunodeficiency affecting Mg2+ regulation of immunity against Epstein-Barr virus. *Blood* 2014, 123, 2148–2152. [CrossRef]
15. Barbagallo, M.; Dominguez, L. Magnesium and Aging. *Curr. Pharm. Des.* 2010, 16, 832–839. [CrossRef]
16. Galland, L. Magnesium and immune function: An overview. *Magnesium* 1988, 7, 290–299.
17. Sugimoto, J.; Romani, A.M.; Valentin-Torres, A.M.; Luciano, A.A.; Kitchen, C.M.R.; Funderburg, N.; Mesiano, S.; Bernstein, H.B. Magnesium Decreases Inflammatory Cytokine Production: A Novel Innate Immunomodulatory Mechanism. *J. Immunol.* 2012, 188, 6338–6346. [CrossRef]
18. Feske, S.; Skolnik, E.Y.; Prakriya, M. Ion channels and transporters in lymphocyte function and immunity. *Nat. Rev. Immunol.* 2012, 12, 532–547. [CrossRef]
19. Bussière, F.; Tridon, A.; Zimowska, W.; Mazur, A.; Rayssiguier, Y. Increase in complement component C3 is an early response to experimental magnesium deficiency in rats. *Life Sci.* 2003, 73, 499–507. [CrossRef]
20. Kraeuter, S.L.; Schwartz, R. Blood and Mast Cell Histamine Levels in Magnesium-Deficient Rats. *J. Nutr.* 1980, 110, 851–858. [CrossRef]
21. Takemoto, S.; Yamamoto, A.; Tomonaga, S.; Funaba, M.; Matsui, T. Magnesium Deficiency Induces the Emergence of Mast Cells in the Liver of Rats. *J. Nutr. Sci. Vitaminol.* 2013, 59, 560–563. [CrossRef]
22. Chien, M.M.; Zahradka, K.E.; Newell, M.K.; Freed, J.H. Fas-induced B cell apoptosis requires an increase in free cytosolic magnesium as an early event. *J. Biol. Chem.* 1999, 274, 7059–7066. [CrossRef]
23. Bussière, F.I.; Gueux, E.; Rock, E.; Mazur, A.; Rayssiguier, Y. Protective effect of calcium deficiency on the inflammatory response in magnesium-deficient rats. *Eur. J. Nutr.* 2002, 41, 197–202. [CrossRef]
24. Malpuech-Brugère, C.; Nowacki, W.; Daveau, M.; Gueux, E.; Linard, C.; Rock, E.; Lebreton, J.-P.; Mazur, A.; Rayssiguier, Y. Inflammatory response following acute magnesium deficiency in the rat. *Biochim. Biophys. Acta Mol. Basis Dis.* 2000, 1501, 91–98. [CrossRef]
25. Petrault, I.; Zimowska, W.; Mathieu, J.; Bayle, D.; Rock, E.; Favier, A.; Rayssiguier, Y.; Mazur, A. Changes in gene expression in rat thymocytes identified by cDNA array support the occurrence of oxidative stress in early magnesium deficiency1Presented in part at the 9th International Magnesium Symposium, 10–15 September 2000, Vichy, France.1. *Biochim. Biophys. Acta Mol. Basis Dis.* 2002, 1586, 92–98. [CrossRef]
26. Zimowska, W.; Girardeau, J.P.; Kuryszko, J.; Bayle, D.; Rayssiguier, Y.; Mazur, A. Morphological and immune response alterations in the intestinal mucosa of the mouse after short periods on a low-magnesium diet. *Br. J. Nutr.* 2002, 88, 515–522. [CrossRef]
27. Malpuech-Brugère, C.; Nowacki, W.; Gueux, E.; Kuryszko, J.; Rock, E.; Rayssiguier, Y.; Mazur, A. Accelerated thymus involution in magnesium-deficient rats is related to enhanced apoptosis and sensitivity to oxidative stress. *Br. J. Nutr.* 1999, 81, 405–411. [CrossRef]
28. Romani, A. Magnesium Homeostasis in Mammalian Cells. *Metal Ions Life Sci.* 2012, 12, 69–118. [CrossRef]
29. Quamme, G.A. Molecular identification of ancient and modern mammalian magnesium transporters. *Am. J. Physiol. Physiol.* 2010, 298, C407–C429. [CrossRef]

30. Ryazanova, L.V.; Rondon, L.J.; Zierler, S.; Hu, Z.; Galli, J.; Yamaguchi, T.P.; Mazur, A.; Fleig, A.; Ryazanov, A.G. TRPM7 is essential for Mg2+ homeostasis in mammals. *Nat. Commun.* **2010**, *1*, 109. [CrossRef]
31. Brandao, K.; Deason-Towne, F.; Perraud, A.-L.; Schmitz, C. The role of Mg2+ in immune cells. *Immunol. Res.* **2012**, *55*, 261–269 [CrossRef]
32. Van Der Wijst, J.; Hoenderop, J.G.; Bindels, R.J. Epithelial Mg2+ channel TRPM6: Insight into the molecular regulation. *Magnes. Res.* **2009**, *22*, 127–132. [CrossRef]
33. Schmitz, C.; Perraud, A.-L.; O Johnson, C.; Inabe, K.; Smith, M.K.; Penner, R.; Kurosaki, T.; Fleig, A.; Scharenberg, A.M. Regulation of Vertebrate Cellular Mg2+ Homeostasis by TRPM7. *Cell* **2003**, *114*, 191–200. [CrossRef]
34. Jin, J.; Desai, B.N.; Navarro, B.; Donovan, A.; Andrews, N.C.; Clapham, D.E. Deletion of Trpm7 Disrupts Embryonic Development and Thymopoiesis Without Altering Mg2+ Homeostasis. *Science* **2008**, *322*, 756–760. [CrossRef]
35. Desai, B.N.; Krapivinsky, G.; Navarro, B.; Krapivinsky, L.; Carter, B.C.; Febvay, S.; Delling, M.; Penumaka, A.; Ramsey, I.S.; Manasian, Y.; et al. Cleavage of TRPM7 Releases the Kinase Domain from the Ion Channel and Regulates Its Participation in Fas-Induced Apoptosis. *Dev. Cell* **2012**, *22*, 1149–1162. [CrossRef]
36. Mandt, T.; Song, Y.; Scharenberg, A.M.; Sahni, J. SLC41A1 Mg2+ transport is regulated via Mg2+-dependent endosomal recycling through its N-terminal cytoplasmic domain. *Biochem. J.* **2011**, *439*, 129–139. [CrossRef]
37. Sahni, J.; Nelson, B.; Scharenberg, A.M. SLC41A2 encodes a plasma-membrane Mg2+ transporter. *Biochem. J.* **2006**, *401*, 505–513. [CrossRef]
38. Rink, T.J.; Tsien, R.Y.; Pozzan, T. Cytoplasmic pH and free Mg2+ in lymphocytes. *J. Cell Biol.* **1982**, *95*, 189–196. [CrossRef]
39. Rijkers, G.T.; Griffioen, A.W. Changes in free cytoplasmic magnesium following activation of human lymphocytes. *Biochem. J.* **1993**, *289*, 373–377. [CrossRef]
40. Goytain, A.; Quamme, G.A. Identification and characterization of a novel mammalian Mg2+ transporter with channel-like properties. *BMC Genom.* **2005**, *6*, 48. [CrossRef]
41. Zhou, H.; Clapham, D.E. Mammalian MagT1 and TUSC3 are required for cellular magnesium uptake and vertebrate embryonic development. *Proc. Natl. Acad. Sci. USA* **2009**, *106*, 15750–15755. [CrossRef]
42. Klinken, E.M.; Gray, P.E.; Pillay, B.; Worley, L.; Edwards, E.S.J.; Payne, K.; Bennetts, B.; Hung, D.; Wood, B.A.; Chan, J.J.; et al. Diversity of XMEN Disease: Description of 2 Novel Variants and Analysis of the Lymphocyte Phenotype. *J. Clin. Immunol.* **2019**, *40*, 299–309. [CrossRef]
43. Matsuda-Lennikov, M.; Biancalana, M.; Zou, J.; Ravell, J.C.; Zheng, L.; Kanellopoulou, C.; Jiang, P.; Notarangelo, G.; Jing, H.; Masutani, E.; et al. Magnesium transporter 1 (MAGT1) deficiency causes selective defects in N-linked glycosylation and expression of immune-response genes. *J. Biol. Chem.* **2019**, *294*, 13638–13656. [CrossRef]
44. Ravell, J.C.; Chauvin, S.D.; He, T.; Lenardo, M.J. An Update on XMEN Disease. *J. Clin. Immunol.* **2020**, *40*, 671–681. [CrossRef]
45. Dominguez, L.J.; Barbagallo, M.; Di Lorenzo, G.; Drago, A.; Scola, S.; Morici, G.; Caruso, C. Bronchial reactivity and intracellular magnesium: A possible mechanism for the bronchodilating effects of magnesium in asthma. *Clin. Sci.* **1998**, *95*, 137–142.
46. A Jones, L.; Goodacre, S. Magnesium sulphate in the treatment of acute asthma: Evaluation of current practice in adult emergency departments. *Emerg. Med. J.* **2009**, *26*, 783–785. [CrossRef]
47. Britton, J.; Pavord, I.; Richards, K.; Wisniewski, A.; Knox, A.; Lewis, S.; Tattersfield, A.; Weiss, S. Dietary magnesium, lung function, wheezing, and airway hyperreactivity in a random adult population sample. *Lancet* **1994**, *344*, 357–362.
48. Liang, R.-Y.; Wu, W.; Huang, J.; Jiang, S.-P.; Lin, Y. Magnesium Affects the Cytokine Secretion of CD4+T Lymphocytes in Acute Asthma. *J. Asthma* **2012**, *49*, 1012–1015. [CrossRef]
49. Franceschi, C.; Campisi, J. Chronic Inflammation (Inflammaging) and Its Potential Contribution to Age-Associated Diseases. *J. Gerontol. Ser. A Biomed. Sci. Med. Sci.* **2014**, *69*, S4–S9. [CrossRef]
50. Kramer, J.H.; Mak, I.T.; Phillips, T.M.; Weglicki, W.B. Dietary Magnesium Intake Influences Circulating Pro-Inflammatory Neuropeptide Levels and Loss of Myocardial Tolerance to Postischemic Stress. *Exp. Biol. Med.* **2003**, *228*, 665–673. [CrossRef]
51. Stankovic, M.; Janjetovic, K.; Velimirović, M.; Milenković, M.; Stojković, T.; Puskas, N.; Zaletel, I.; De Luka, S.R.; Jankovic, S.; Stefanovic, S.; et al. Effects of IL-33/ST2 pathway in acute inflammation on tissue damage, antioxidative parameters, magnesium concentration and cytokines profile. *Exp. Mol. Pathol.* **2016**, *101*, 31–37. [CrossRef]
52. Maier, J.A.; Malpuech-Brugere, C.; Zimowska, W.; Rayssiguier, Y.; Mazur, A. Low magnesium promotes endothelial cell dysfunction: Implications for atherosclerosis, inflammation and thrombosis. *Biochim. Biophys. Acta* **2004**, *1689*, 13–21.
53. Su, N.-Y.; Peng, T.-C.; Tsai, P.-S.; Huang, C.-J. Phosphoinositide 3-kinase/Akt pathway is involved in mediating the anti-inflammation effects of magnesium sulfate. *J. Surg. Res.* **2013**, *185*, 726–732. [CrossRef]
54. Lin, C.Y.; Tsai, P.-S.; Hung, Y.C.; Huang, C.-J. L-type calcium channels are involved in mediating the anti-inflammatory effects of magnesium sulphate. *Br. J. Anaesth.* **2010**, *104*, 44–51. [CrossRef]
55. King, D.E.; Mainous, I.I.I.A.G.; Geesey, M.E.; Woolson, R.F. Dietary magnesium and C-reactive protein levels. *J. Am. Coll. Nutr.* **2005**, *24*, 166–171.
56. Guerrero-Romero, F.; Bermudez-Peña, C.; Rodríguez-Morán, M. Severe hypomagnesemia and low-grade inflammation in metabolic syndrome. *Magnes. Res.* **2011**, *24*, 45–53. [CrossRef]
57. Song, Y.; Li, T.Y.; Van Dam, R.M.; E Manson, J.; Hu, F.B. Magnesium intake and plasma concentrations of markers of systemic inflammation and endothelial dysfunction in women. *Am. J. Clin. Nutr.* **2007**, *85*, 1068–1074. [CrossRef]

58. Song, Y.; Ridker, P.M.; Manson, J.E.; Cook, N.R.; Buring, J.E.; Liu, S.-M. Magnesium Intake, C-Reactive Protein, and the Prevalence of Metabolic Syndrome in Middle-Aged and Older U.S. Women. *Diabetes Care* **2005**, *28*, 1438–1444. [CrossRef]
59. Mazidi, M.; Kengne, A.P.; Mikhailidis, D.P.; Cicero, A.F.; Banach, M. Effects of selected dietary constituents on high-sensitivity C-reactive protein levels in U.S. adults. *Ann. Med.* **2017**, *50*, 1–6. [CrossRef]
60. Konstari, S.; Sares-Jäske, L.; Heliövaara, M.; Rissanen, H.; Knekt, P.; Arokoski, J.; Sundvall, J.; Karppinen, J. Dietary magnesium intake, serum high sensitivity C-reactive protein and the risk of incident knee osteoarthritis leading to hospitalization—A cohort study of 4,953 Finns. *PLoS ONE* **2019**, *14*, e0214064. [CrossRef]
61. Mazidi, M.; Rezaie, P.; Banach, M. Effect of magnesium supplements on serum C-reactive protein: A systematic review and meta-analysis. *Arch. Med. Sci.* **2018**, *14*, 707–716. [CrossRef]
62. Bussière, F.I.; Mazur, A.; Fauquert, J.L.; Labbé, A.; Rayssiguier, Y.; Tridon, A. High magnesium concentration in vitro decreases human leukocyte activation. *Magnes. Res.* **2002**, *15*, 43–48.
63. Kuzniar, A.; Mitura, P.; Kurys, P.; Szymonik-Lesiuk, S.; Florianczyk, B.; Stryjecka-Zimmer, M. The influence of hypomagnesemia on erythrocyte antioxidant enzyme defence system in mice. *BioMetals* **2003**, *16*, 349–357. [CrossRef]
64. Weglicki, W.B.; Mak, I.T.; Kramer, J.H.; Dickens, B.F.; Cassidy, M.M.; Stafford, R.E.; Phillips, T.M. Role of free radicals and substance P in magnesium deficiency. *Cardiovasc. Res.* **1996**, *31*, 677–682.
65. Calviello, G.; Ricci, P.; Lauro, L.; Palozza, P.; Cittadini, A. Mg deficiency induces mineral content changes and oxidative stress in rats. *Biochem. Mol. Boil. Int.* **1994**, *32*, 903–911.
66. Kolisek, M.; Launay, P.; Beck, A.; Sponder, G.; Serafini, N.; Brenkus, M.; Froschauer-Neuhauser, E.; Martens, H.; Fleig, A.; Schweigel, M. SLC41A1 Is a Novel Mammalian Mg2+Carrier. *J. Biol. Chem.* **2008**, *283*, 16235–16247. [CrossRef]
67. Yamanaka, R.; Tabata, S.; Shindo, Y.; Hotta, K.; Suzuki, K.; Soga, T.; Oka, K. Mitochondrial Mg2+ homeostasis decides cellular energy metabolism and vulnerability to stress. *Sci. Rep.* **2016**, *6*. [CrossRef]
68. Mastrototaro, L.; Smorodchenko, A.; Aschenbach, J.R.; Kolisek, M.; Sponder, G. Solute carrier 41A3 encodes for a mitochondrial Mg(2+) efflux system. *Sci. Rep.* **2016**, *6*, 27999.
69. Liu, M.; Jeong, E.-M.; Liu, H.; Xie, A.; So, E.Y.; Shi, G.; Jeong, G.E.; Zhou, A.; Dudley, S.C. Magnesium supplementation improves diabetic mitochondrial and cardiac diastolic function. *JCI Insight* **2019**, *4*. [CrossRef]
70. Liu, M.; Liu, H.; Xie, A.; Kang, G.J.; Feng, F.; Zhou, X.; Zhao, Y.; Dudley, S.C. Magnesium deficiency causes reversible diastolic and systolic cardiomyopathy. *Biophys. J.* **2020**, *118*, 245a.
71. Gout, E.; Rébeillé, F.; Douce, R.; Bligny, R. Interplay of Mg2+, ADP, and ATP in the cytosol and mitochondria: Unravelling the role of Mg2+ in cell respiration. *Proc. Natl. Acad. Sci. USA* **2014**, *111*, E4560–E4567. [CrossRef]
72. Panov, A.; Scarpa, A. Mg2+Control of Respiration in Isolated Rat Liver Mitochondria†. *Biochemistry* **1996**, *35*, 12849–12856. [CrossRef]
73. Rodríguez-Zavala, J.; Moreno-Sánchez, R.; Rodriguez-Zavala, J.S. Modulation of Oxidative Phosphorylation by Mg2+in Rat Heart Mitochondria. *J. Biol. Chem.* **1998**, *273*, 7850–7855. [CrossRef]
74. Kramer, J.H.; Mišík, V.; Weglicki, W.B. Magnesium-deficiency potentiates free radical production associated with postischemic injury to rat hearts: Vitamin E affords protection. *Free Radic. Biol. Med.* **1994**, *16*, 713–723. [CrossRef]
75. Morais, J.B.; Severo, J.S.; Santos, L.R.; de Sousa Melo, S.R.; de Oliveira Santos, R.; de Oliveira, A.R.S.; Cruz, K.J.C.; do Nascimento Marreiro, D. Role of Magnesium in Oxidative Stress in Individuals with Obesity. *Biol. Trace Elem. Res.* **2017**, *176*, 20–26.
76. Shah, N.C.; Liu, J.-P.; Iqbal, J.; Hussain, M.; Jiang, X.-C.; Li, Z.; Li, Y.; Zheng, T.; Li, W.; Sica, A.C.; et al. Mg deficiency results in modulation of serum lipids, glutathione, and NO synthase isozyme activation in cardiovascular tissues: Relevance to de novo synthesis of ceramide, serum Mg2+ and atherogenesis. *Int. J. Clin. Exp. Med.* **2011**, *4*, 103–118.
77. Kumar, B.P.; Shivakumar, K. Depressed antioxidant defense in rat heart in experimental magnesium deficiency implications for the pathogenesis of myocardial lesions. *Biol. Trace Element Res.* **1997**, *60*, 139–144. [CrossRef]
78. Racay, P. Effect of magnesium on calcium-induced depolarisation of mitochondrial transmembrane potential. *Cell Biol. Int.* **2008**, *32*, 136–145. [CrossRef]
79. Blomeyer, C.A.; Bazil, J.N.; Stowe, D.F.; Dash, R.K.; Camara, A.K. Mg2+ differentially regulates two modes of mitochondrial Ca2+ uptake in isolated cardiac mitochondria: Implications for mitochondrial Ca2+ sequestration. *J. Bioenerg. Biomembr.* **2016**, *48*, 175–188. [CrossRef]
80. Chen, Y.; Wei, X.; Yan, P.; Han, Y.; Sun, S.; Wu, K.-C.; Fan, D. Human mitochondrial Mrs2 protein promotes multidrug resistance in gastric cancer cells by regulating p27, cyclin D1 expression and cytochrome C release. *Cancer Biol. Ther.* **2009**, *8*, 607–614. [CrossRef]
81. Salvi, M.; Bozac, A.; Toninello, A. Gliotoxin induces Mg2+ efflux from intact brain mitochondria. *Neurochem. Int.* **2004**, *45*, 759–764.
82. Sponder, G.; Abdulhanan, N.; Fröhlich, N.; Mastrototaro, L.; Aschenbach, J.R.; Röntgen, M.; Pilchova, I.; Cibulka, M.; Racay, P.; Kolisek, M. Overexpression of Na+/Mg2+ exchanger SLC41A1 attenuates pro-survival signaling. *Oncotarget* **2017**, *9*, 5084–5104. [CrossRef]
83. Bednarczyk, P.; Dołowy, K.; Szewczyk, A. Matrix Mg2+regulates mitochondrial ATP-dependent potassium channel from heart. *FEBS Lett.* **2005**, *579*, 1625–1632. [CrossRef]
84. Beavis, A.D.; Powers, M.F. On the regulation of the mitochondrial inner membrane anion channel by magnesium and protons. *J. Biol. Chem.* **1989**, *264*, 17148–17155.

85. Zoratti, M.; Szabò, I. The mitochondrial permeability transition. *Biochim. Biophys. Acta Rev. Biomembr.* **1995**, *1241*, 139–176. [CrossRef]
86. Gorgoglione, V.; Laraspata, D.; La Piana, G.; Marzulli, D.; Lofrumento, N.E. Protective effect of magnesium and potassium ions on the permeability of the external mitochondrial membrane. *Arch. Biochem. Biophys.* **2007**, *461*, 13–23. [CrossRef]
87. La Piana, G.; Gorgoglione, V.; Laraspata, D.; Marzulli, D.; Lofrumento, N.E. Effect of magnesium ions on the activity of the cytosolic NADH/cytochrome c electron transport system. *FEBS J.* **2008**, *275*, 6168–6179.
88. Seo, Y.-W.; Na Shin, J.; Ko, K.H.; Cha, J.H.; Park, J.Y.; Lee, B.R.; Yun, C.-W.; Kim, Y.M.; Seol, D.-W.; Kim, D.-W.; et al. The Molecular Mechanism of Noxa-induced Mitochondrial Dysfunction in p53-Mediated Cell Death. *J. Biol. Chem.* **2003**, *278*, 48292–48299. [CrossRef]
89. Sharikabad, M.N.; Ostbye, K.M.; Brors, O. Increased [Mg2+]o reduces Ca2+ influx and disruption of mitochondrial membrane potential during reoxygenation. *Am. J. Physiol. Heart Circ. Physiol.* **2001**, *281*, H2113–H2123.
90. Huang, C.-Y.; Hsieh, Y.-L.; Ju, D.-T.; Lin, C.-C.; Kuo, C.-H.; Liou, Y.-F.; Ho, T.-J.; Tsai, C.-H.; Tsai, F.-J.; Lin, J.-Y. Attenuation of Magnesium Sulfate on CoCl(2)-Induced Cell Death by Activating ERK1/2/MAPK and Inhibiting HIF-1alpha via Mitochondrial Apoptotic Signaling Suppression in a Neuronal Cell Line. *Chin. J. Physiol.* **2015**, *58*, 244–253.
91. Ferrari, R.; Albertini, A.; Curello, S.; Ceconi, C.; Di Lisa, F.; Raddino, R.; Visioli, O. Myocardial recovery during post-ischaemic reperfusion: Effects of nifedipine, calcium and magnesium. *J. Mol. Cell. Cardiol.* **1986**, *18*, 487–498. [CrossRef]
92. Boelens, A.D.; Pradhan, R.K.; Blomeyer, C.A.; Camara, A.K.S.; Dash, R.K.; Stowe, D.F. Extra-matrix Mg2+ limits Ca2+ uptake and modulates Ca2+ uptake–independent respiration and redox state in cardiac isolated mitochondria. *J. Bioenerg. Biomembr.* **2013**, *45*, 203–218. [CrossRef]
93. Li, Y.; Wang, J.; Yue, J.; Wang, Y.; Yang, C.; Cui, Q. High magnesium prevents matrix vesicle-mediated mineralization in human bone marrow-derived mesenchymal stem cells via mitochondrial pathway and autophagy. *Cell Biol. Int.* **2018**, *42*, 205–215. [CrossRef]
94. Franceschi, C.; Garagnani, P.; Vitale, G.; Capri, M.; Salvioli, S. Inflammaging and 'Garb-aging'. *Trends Endocrinol. Metab.* **2017**, *28*, 199–212.
95. Pike, J.W.; Christakos, S. Biology and Mechanisms of Action of the Vitamin D Hormone. *Endocrinol. Metab. Clin. N. Am.* **2017**, *46*, 815–843. [CrossRef]
96. Holick, M. Vitamin D Deficiency. *New Engl. J. Med.* **2007**, *357*, 266–281. [CrossRef]
97. Charoenngam, N.; Holick, M. Immunologic Effects of Vitamin D on Human Health and Disease. *Nutrients* **2020**, *12*, 2097. [CrossRef]
98. Rude, R.K.; Adams, J.S.; Ryzen, E.; Endres, D.B.; Niimi, H.; Horst, R.L.; Haddad, J.G.; Singer, F.R. Low Serum Concentrations of 1,25-Dihydroxyvitamin D in Human Magnesium Deficiency. *J. Clin. Endocrinol. Metab.* **1985**, *61*, 933–940. [CrossRef]
99. Reddy, V.; Sivakumar, B. MAGNESIUM-DEPENDENT VITAMIN-D-RESISTANT RICKETS. *Lancet* **1974**, *303*, 963–965. [CrossRef]
100. Uwitonze, A.M.; Razzaque, M.S. Role of Magnesium in Vitamin D Activation and Function. *J. Am. Osteopat. Assoc.* **2018**, *118*, 181–189. [CrossRef]
101. Zittermann, A. Magnesium deficit—overlooked cause of low vitamin D status? *BMC Med.* **2013**, *11*. [CrossRef]
102. Risco, F.; Traba, M.L. Influence of magnesium on the in vitro synthesis of 24,25-dihydroxyvitamin D3 and 1 alpha, 25-dihydroxyvitamin D3. *Magnes. Res.* **1992**, *5*, 5–14.
103. Anast, C.S.; Mohs, J.M.; Kaplan, S.L.; Burns, T.W. Evidence for Parathyroid Failure in Magnesium Deficiency. *Science* **1972**, *177*, 606–608. [CrossRef]
104. Medalle, R.; Waterhouse, C.; Hahn, T.J. Vitamin D resistance in magnesium deficiency. *Am. J. Clin. Nutr.* **1976**, *29*, 854–858. [CrossRef]
105. Rude, R.K.; Oldham, S.B.; Sharp, C.F.; Singer, F.R. Parathyroid Hormone Secretion in Magnesium Deficiency*. *J. Clin. Endocrinol. Metab.* **1978**, *47*, 800–806. [CrossRef]
106. Mutnuri, S.; Fernández, I.; Kochar, T. Suppression of Parathyroid Hormone in a Patient with Severe Magnesium Depletion. *Case Rep. Nephrol.* **2016**, *2016*, 1–3. [CrossRef]
107. Rude, R.K.; Oldham, S.B.; Singer, F.R. FUNCTIONAL HYPOPARATHYROIDISM AND PARATHYROID HORMONE END-ORGAN RESISTANCE IN HUMAN MAGNESIUM DEFICIENCY. *Clin. Endocrinol.* **1976**, *5*, 209–224. [CrossRef]
108. Rösler, A.; Rabinowitz, D. Magnesium-induced reversal of vitamin-D resistance in hypoparathyroidism. *Lancet* **1973**, *1*, 803–804.
109. Fuss, M.; Bergmann, P.; Bergans, A.; Bagon, J.; Cogan, E.; Pepersack, T.; Van Gossum, M.; Corvilain, J. CORRECTION OF LOW CIRCULATING LEVELS OF 1,25-DIHYDROXYVITAMIN D BY 25-HYDROXYVITAMIN D DURING REVERSAL OF HYPOMAGNESAEMIA. *Clin. Endocrinol.* **1989**, *31*, 31–38. [CrossRef]
110. Hardwick, L.L.; Jones, M.R.; Brautbar, N.; Lee, D.B.N. Magnesium Absorption: Mechanisms and the Influence of Vitamin D, Calcium and Phosphate. *J. Nutr.* **1991**, *121*, 13–23. [CrossRef]
111. Veronese, N.; Stubbs, B.; Solmi, M.; Noale, M.; Vaona, A.; Demurtas, J.; Maggi, S. Dietary magnesium intake and fracture risk: Data from a large prospective study. *Br. J. Nutr.* **2017**, *117*, 1570–1576. [CrossRef]
112. Deng, X.; Song, Y.; Manson, J.E.; Signorello, L.B.; Zhang, S.M.; Shrubsole, M.J.; Ness, R.M.; Seidner, D.L.; Dai, Q. Magnesium, vitamin D status and mortality: Results from US National Health and Nutrition Examination Survey (NHANES) 2001 to 2006 and NHANES III. *BMC Med.* **2013**, *11*. [CrossRef]

13. Dai, Q.; Zhu, X.; E Manson, J.; Song, Y.; Li, X.; A Franke, A.; Costello, R.B.; Rosanoff, A.; Nian, H.; Fan, L.; et al. Magnesium status and supplementation influence vitamin D status and metabolism: Results from a randomized trial. *Am. J. Clin. Nutr.* **2018**, *108*, 1249–1258. [CrossRef]
14. Chocano-Bedoya, P.; Ronnenberg, A.G. Vitamin D and tuberculosis. *Nutr. Rev.* **2009**, *67*, 289–293. [CrossRef]
15. Beard, J.A.; Bearden, A.; Striker, R. Vitamin D and the anti-viral state. *J. Clin. Virol.* **2011**, *50*, 194–200. [CrossRef]
16. Brighenti, S.; Bergman, P.; Martineau, A.R. Vitamin D and tuberculosis: Where next? *J. Intern. Med.* **2018**. [CrossRef]
17. Dini, C.; Bianchi, A. The potential role of vitamin D for prevention and treatment of tuberculosis and infectious diseases. *Annali dell'Istituto Superiore Sanità* **2012**, *48*, 319–327. [CrossRef]
18. Reid, D.; Toole, B.J.; Knox, S.; Talwar, D.; Harten, J.; O'Reilly, D.S.J.; Blackwell, S.; Kinsella, J.; McMillan, D.C.; Wallace, A.M.; et al. The relation between acute changes in the systemic inflammatory response and plasma 25-hydroxyvitamin D concentrations after elective knee arthroplasty. *Am. J. Clin. Nutr.* **2011**, *93*, 1006–1011. [CrossRef]
19. Borella, E.; Nesher, G.; Israeli, E.; Shoenfeld, Y. Vitamin D: A new anti-infective agent? *Ann. N. Y. Acad. Sci.* **2014**, *1317*, 76–83. [CrossRef]
20. Arboleda, J.F.; Urcuqui-Inchima, S. Vitamin D Supplementation: A Potential Approach for Coronavirus/COVID-19 Therapeutics? *Front. Immunol.* **2020**, *11*. [CrossRef]
21. Grant, W.B.; Lahore, H.; McDonnell, S.L.; Baggerly, C.A.; French, C.B.; Aliano, J.L.; Bhattoa, H.P. Evidence that Vitamin D Supplementation Could Reduce Risk of Influenza and COVID-19 Infections and Deaths. *Nutrients* **2020**, *12*, 988. [CrossRef]
22. Rejnmark, L.; Bislev, L.S.; Cashman, K.D.; Eiríksdottir, G.; Gaksch, M.; Gruebler, M.; Grimnes, G.; Gudnason, V.; Lips, P.; Pilz, S.; et al. Non-skeletal health effects of vitamin D supplementation: A systematic review on findings from meta-analyses summarizing trial data. *PLoS ONE* **2017**, *12*, e0180512. [CrossRef]
23. Martineau, A.R.; A Jolliffe, D.; Hooper, R.L.; Greenberg, L.; Aloia, J.F.; Bergman, P.; Dubnov-Raz, G.; Esposito, S.; Ganmaa, D.; Ginde, A.A.; et al. Vitamin D supplementation to prevent acute respiratory tract infections: Systematic review and meta-analysis of individual participant data. *BMJ* **2017**, *356*, i6583. [CrossRef]
24. Liu, M.; Yang, H.; Mao, Y. Magnesium and liver disease: An overview. *Ann. Transl. Med.* **2019**, *7*, 578. [CrossRef]
25. Liu, Y.; Xu, Y.; Ma, H.; Wang, B.; Xu, L.; Zhang, H.; Song, X.; Gao, L.; Liang, X.; Ma, C. Hepatitis B virus X protein amplifies TGF-beta promotion on HCC motility through down-regulating PPM1a. *Oncotarget* **2016**, *7*, 33125–33135.
26. Nasser, R.; Naffaa, M.E.; Mashiach, T.; Azzam, Z.S.; Braun, E. The association between serum magnesium levels and community-acquired pneumonia 30-day mortality. *BMC Infect. Dis.* **2018**, *18*, 698.
27. Bhatt, S.P.; Khandelwal, P.; Nanda, S.; Stoltzfus, J.C.; Fioravanti, G.T. Serum magnesium is an independent predictor of frequent readmissions due to acute exacerbation of chronic obstructive pulmonary disease. *Respir. Med.* **2008**, *102*, 999–1003. [CrossRef]
28. Tannou, T.; Koeberle, S.; Manckoundia, P.; Aubry, R. Multifactorial immunodeficiency in frail elderly patients: Contributing factors and management. *Méd. Mal. Infect.* **2019**, *49*, 167–172. [CrossRef]
29. Sadighi Akha, A.A. Aging and the immune system: An overview. *J. Immunol. Methods* **2018**, *463*, 21–26.
30. Herzig, C.T.A.; Dick, A.W.; Sorbero, M.; Pogorzelska-Maziarz, M.; Cohen, C.C.; Larson, E.L.; Stone, P.W. Infection Trends in US Nursing Homes, 2006-2013. *J. Am. Med. Dir. Assoc.* **2017**, *18*, 635.e9–635.e20. [CrossRef]
31. Yorita, K.L.; Holman, R.C.; Steiner, C.A.; Sejvar, J.J.; Stoll, B.J.; Schonberger, L.B. Infectious Disease Hospitalizations in the United States. *Clin. Infect. Dis.* **2009**, *49*, 1025–1035. [CrossRef]
32. WHO. *Global Health Estimates 2016: Estimated Deaths by Age, Sex and Cause*; WHO: Geneva, Switzerland, 2016; Available online: https://www.who.int/healthinfo/global_burden_disease/estimates/en/ (accessed on 1 December 2020).
33. Chiara, T.; Victoria, C.C.; Giulia, A.; Cristina, B.; Stefano, C.; Matilde, C.; Rita, D.M.; Viviana, G.; Beata, J.; Leopoldo, S.; et al. Health-Care-Associated Infections Management, sow the seed of good habits: A grounded theory study. *Acta Biomed.* **2019**, *90*, 26–33.
34. Freedman, V.A.; Martin, L.G. Contribution of chronic conditions to aggregate changes in old-age functioning. *Am. J. Public Health* **2000**, *90*, 1755–1760. [CrossRef]
35. Meurer, W.J.; Losman, E.D.; Smith, B.L.; Malani, P.N.; Younger, J.G. Short-term functional decline of older adults admitted for suspected sepsis. *Am. J. Emerg. Med.* **2011**, *29*, 936–942. [CrossRef]
36. Johnstone, J.; Eurich, D.T.; Majumdar, S.R.; Jin, Y.; Marrie, T.J. Long-term morbidity and mortality after hospitalization with community-acquired pneumonia: A population-based cohort study. *Medicine* **2008**, *87*, 329–334.
37. Curns, A.T.; Holman, R.C.; Sejvar, J.J.; Owings, M.F.; Schonberger, L.B. Infectious disease hospitalizations among older adults in the United States from 1990 through 2002. *Arch. Intern. Med.* **2005**, *165*, 2514–2520.
38. Elias, R.; Hartshorn, K.; Rahma, O.; Lin, N.; Snyder-Cappione, J.E. Aging, immune senescence, and immunotherapy: A comprehensive review. *Semin. Oncol.* **2018**, *45*, 187–200.
39. Agarwal, S.; Busse, P.J. Innate and adaptive immunosenescence. *Ann. Allergy Asthma Immunol.* **2010**, *104*, 183–190.
40. Castle, S.C.; Uyemura, K.; Fulop, T.; Makinodan, T. Host Resistance and Immune Responses in Advanced Age. *Clin. Geriatr. Med.* **2007**, *23*, 463–479. [CrossRef]
41. Shahid, Z.; Kalayanamitra, R.; McClafferty, B.; Kepko, D.; Ramgobin, D.; Nitasa Sahu, M.D.; Dhirisha Bhatt, M.D.; Kirk Jones, P.D.; Reshma Golamari, M.D.; Rohit Jain, M.D. COVID-19 and Older Adults: What We Know. *J. Am. Geriatr. Soc.* **2020**, *68*, 926–929.
42. Emami, A.; Javanmardi, F.; Pirbonyeh, N.; Akbari, A. Prevalence of Underlying Diseases in Hospitalized Patients with COVID-19: A Systematic Review and Meta-Analysis. *Arch. Acad. Emerg. Med.* **2020**, *8*, e35.

143. Zhou, P.; Yang, X.-L.; Wang, X.-G.; Hu, B.; Zhang, L.; Zhang, W.; Si, H.-R.; Zhu, Y.; Li, B.; Huang, C.-L.; et al. A pneumonia outbreak associated with a new coronavirus of probable bat origin. *Nat. Cell Biol.* **2020**, *579*, 270–273. [CrossRef]
144. WHO. Coronavirus Disease (COVID-19) Dashboard. Available online: https://covid19.who.int/?gclid=Cj0KCQjw0rr4BRCtARIsAB0_4 8NF8a417ap3xz5a6rC5bv4LHq4iaWP5iTQPyvEhFlQLpGa7fyo6R0aAhVTEALw_wcB (accessed on 14 December 2020).
145. Fajgenbaum, D.C.; June, C.H. Cytokine Storm. *N. Engl. J. Med.* **2020**, *383*, 2255–2273. [CrossRef]
146. Perrotta, F.; Corbi, G.; Mazzeo, G.; Boccia, M.; Aronne, L.; D'Agnano, V.; Komici, K.; Mazzarella, G.; Parrella, R.; Bianco, A. COVID-19 and the elderly: Insights into pathogenesis and clinical decision-making. *Aging Clin. Exp. Res.* **2020**, *32*, 1599–1608. [CrossRef]
147. Li, P.; Chen, L.; Liu, Z.; Pan, J.; Zhou, D.; Wang, H.; Gong, H.; Fu, Z.; Song, Q.; Min, Q.; et al. Clinical features and short-term outcomes of elderly patients with COVID-19. *Int. J. Infect. Dis.* **2020**, *97*, 245–250. [CrossRef]
148. Sepulveda, E.R.; Stall, N.M.; Sinha, S.K. A Comparison of COVID-19 Mortality Rates Among Long-Term Care Residents in 12 OECD Countries. *J. Am. Med Dir. Assoc.* **2020**, *21*, 1572–1574. [CrossRef]
149. Abebe, E.C.; Dejenie, T.A.; Shiferaw, M.Y.; Malik, T. The newly emerged COVID-19 disease: A systemic review. *Virol. J.* **2020**, *17*, 1–8. [CrossRef]
150. Nielsen, F.H. Magnesium, inflammation, and obesity in chronic disease. *Nutr. Rev.* **2010**, *68*, 333–340. [CrossRef]
151. Dominguez, L.; Barbagallo, M. The biology of the metabolic syndrome and aging. *Curr. Opin. Clin. Nutr. Metab. Care* **2016**, *19*, 5–11. [CrossRef]
152. Dietz, W.; Santos Burgoa, C. Obesity and its Implications for COVID-19 Mortality. *Obesity* **2020**, *28*, 1005.
153. Wadman, M. Why obesity worsens COVID-19. *Science* **2020**, *369*, 1280–1281. [CrossRef]
154. Iotti, S.; Wolf, F.; Mazur, A.; A Maier, J. The COVID-19 pandemic: Is there a role for magnesium? Hypotheses and perspectives. *Magnes. Res.* **2020**, *1*. [CrossRef]
155. Wallace, T. Combating COVID-19 and Building Immune Resilience: A Potential Role for Magnesium Nutrition? *J. Am. Coll. Nutr.* **2020**, *39*, 685–693. [CrossRef]
156. Tan, C.W.; Ho, L.P.; Kalimuddin, S.; Cherng, B.P.Z.; Teh, Y.E.; Thien, S.Y.; Wong, H.M.; Tern, P.J.W.; Chandran, M.; Chay, J.W.M.; et al. Cohort study to evaluate the effect of vitamin D, magnesium, and vitamin B12 in combination on progression to severe outcomes in older patients with coronavirus (COVID-19). *Nutrient* **2020**, *79*. [CrossRef]
157. Tang, C.-F.; Ding, H.; Jiao, R.-Q.; Wu, X.-X.; Kong, L.-D. Possibility of magnesium supplementation for supportive treatment in patients with COVID-19. *Eur. J. Pharmacol.* **2020**, *886*. [CrossRef]
158. Ilie, P.C.; Stefanescu, S.; Smith, L. The role of vitamin D in the prevention of coronavirus disease 2019 infection and mortality. *Aging Clin. Exp. Res.* **2020**, *32*, 1195–1198. [CrossRef]
159. Meltzer, D.O.; Best, T.J.; Zhang, H.; Vokes, T.; Arora, V.; Solway, J. Association of Vitamin D Status and Other Clinical Characteristics with COVID-19 Test Results. *JAMA Netw. Open* **2020**, *3*, e2019722. [CrossRef]
160. Bernheim, A.; Mei, X.; Huang, M.; Yang, Y.; Fayad, Z.A.; Zhang, N.; Diao, K.; Lin, B.; Zhu, X.; Li, K.; et al. Chest CT Findings in Coronavirus Disease-19 (COVID-19): Relationship to Duration of Infection. *Radiology* **2020**, *295*. [CrossRef]
161. Zheng, Y.-Y.; Ma, Y.-T.; Zhang, J.; Xie, X. COVID-19 and the cardiovascular system. *Nat. Rev. Cardiol.* **2020**, *17*, 259–260. [CrossRef]
162. Zimmer, H.G. Effects of magnesium orotate on rat heart function. *Cardioscience* **1994**, *5*, 55–61.
163. Gao, C.; Cai, Y.; Zhang, K.; Zhou, L.; Zhang, Y.; Zhang, X.; Li, Q.; Li, W.; Yang, S.; Zhao, X.; et al. Association of hypertension and antihypertensive treatment with COVID-19 mortality: A retrospective observational study. *Eur. Heart J.* **2020**, *41*, 2058–2066. [CrossRef]
164. Katulanda, P.; Dissanayake, H.A.; Ranathunga, I.; Vithiya, R.; Wijewickrama, P.S.A.; Yogendranathan, N.; Gamage, K.K.K.; De Silva, N.L.; Sumanatilleke, M.; Somasundaram, N.; et al. Prevention and management of COVID-19 among patients with diabetes: An appraisal of the literature. *Diabetologia* **2020**, *63*, 1440–1452. [CrossRef]
165. O'Driscoll, M.; Ribeiro Dos Santos, G.; Wang, L.; Cummings, D.A.T.; Azman, A.S.; Paireau, J.; Fontanet, A.; Cauchemez, S.; Salje, H. Age-specific mortality and immunity patterns of SARS-CoV-2. *Nature* **2020**. [CrossRef]
166. Barbagallo, M.; Dominguez, L.J.; Galioto, A.; Ferlisi, A.; Cani, C.; Malfa, L.; Pineo, A.; Paolisso, G. Role of magnesium in insulin action, diabetes and cardio-metabolic syndrome X. *Mol. Aspects Med.* **2003**, *24*, 39–52.
167. Chernow, B.; Bamberger, S.; Stoiko, M.; Vadnais, M.; Mills, S.; Hoellerich, V.; Warshaw, A.L. Hypomagnesemia in Patients in Postoperative Intensive Care. *Chest* **1989**, *95*, 391–397. [CrossRef]
168. Escuela, M.P.; Guerra, M.; Celaya, S.; Añón, J.M.; Martínez-Vizcaíno, V.; Zapatero, M.D.; García-Jalón, A. Total and ionized serum magnesium in critically ill patients. *Intensiv. Care Med.* **2005**, *31*, 151–156. [CrossRef]
169. Hansen, B.-A.; Bruserud, Ø. Hypomagnesemia in critically ill patients. *J. Intensiv. Care* **2018**, *6*, 1–11. [CrossRef]
170. Ackermann, M.; Verleden, S.E.; Kuehnel, M.; Haverich, A.; Welte, T.; Laenger, F.; Vanstapel, A.; Werlein, C.; Stark, H.; Tzankov, A.; et al. Pulmonary Vascular Endothelialitis, Thrombosis, and Angiogenesis in Covid-19. *N. Engl. J. Med.* **2020**, *383*, 120–128. [CrossRef]
171. Libby, P.; Luscher, T. COVID-19 is, in the end, an endothelial disease. *Eur. Heart J.* **2020**, *41*, 3038–3044.
172. Barbagallo, M.; Dominguez, L.; Galioto, A.; Pineo, A.; Belvedere, M. Oral magnesium supplementation improves vascular function in elderly diabetic patients. *Magnes. Res.* **2010**, *23*, 131–137.
173. Shechter, M.; Sharir, M.; Labrador, M.J.P.; Forrester, J.; Silver, B.; Merz, C.N.B. Oral Magnesium Therapy Improves Endothelial Function in Patients With Coronary Artery Disease. *Circulation* **2000**, *102*, 2353–2358. [CrossRef]

174. Marques, B.C.A.A.; Klein, M.R.S.T.; Da Cunha, M.R.; Mattos, S.D.S.; Nogueira, L.D.P.; De Paula, T.; Corrêa, F.M.; Oigman, W.; Neves, M.F. Effects of Oral Magnesium Supplementation on Vascular Function: A Systematic Review and Meta-analysis of Randomized Controlled Trials. *High Blood Press. Cardiovasc. Prev.* **2019**, *27*, 19–28. [CrossRef]
175. Coperchini, F.; Chiovato, L.; Croce, L.; Magri, F.; Rotondi, M. The cytokine storm in COVID-19: An overview of the involvement of the chemokine/chemokine-receptor system. *Cytokine Growth Factor Rev.* **2020**, *53*, 25–32. [CrossRef]
176. Altura, B.M.; Gebrewold, A.; Ising, H.; Gunther, T. Magnesium deficiency and hypertension: Correlation between magnesium-deficient diets and microcirculatory changes in situ. *Science* **1984**, *223*, 1315–1317. [CrossRef]
177. Iseri, L.T.; French, J.H. Magnesium: Nature's physiologic calcium blocker. *Am. Hear. J.* **1984**, *108*, 188–193. [CrossRef]
178. Louvet, L.; Büchel, J.; Steppan, S.; Passlick-Deetjen, J.; Massy, Z. Magnesium prevents phosphate-induced calcification in human aortic vascular smooth muscle cells. *Nephrol. Dial. Transplant.* **2012**, *28*, 869–878. [CrossRef]
179. Evans, P.C.; Rainger, G.E.; Mason, J.C.; Guzik, T.J.; Osto, E.; Stamataki, Z.; Neil, D.; E Hoefer, I.; Fragiadaki, M.; Waltenberger, J.; et al. Endothelial dysfunction in COVID-19: A position paper of the ESC Working Group for Atherosclerosis and Vascular Biology, and the ESC Council of Basic Cardiovascular Science. *Cardiovasc. Res.* **2020**, *116*, 2177–2184. [CrossRef]
180. Varga, Z.; Flammer, A.J.; Steiger, P.; Haberecker, M.; Andermatt, R.; Zinkernagel, A.S.; Mehra, M.R.; A Schuepbach, R.; Ruschitzka, F.; Moch, H. Endothelial cell infection and endotheliitis in COVID-19. *Lancet* **2020**, *395*, 1417–1418. [CrossRef]
181. Wiersinga, W.J.; Rhodes, A.; Cheng, A.C.; Peacock, S.J.; Prescott, H.C. Pathophysiology, Transmission, Diagnosis, and Treatment of Coronavirus Disease 2019 (COVID-19): A Review. *JAMA* **2020**, *324*, 782–793.
182. Maier, J. Endothelial cells and magnesium: Implications in atherosclerosis. *Clin. Sci.* **2011**, *122*, 397–407. [CrossRef]
183. Sheu, J.-R.; Hsiao, G.; Shen, M.-Y.; Fong, T.-H.; Chen, Y.-W.; Lin, C.-H.; Chou, D.-S. Mechanisms involved in the antiplatelet activity of magnesium in human platelets. *Br. J. Haematol.* **2002**, *119*, 1033–1041.
184. Pereira, M.; Damascena, A.D.; Azevedo, L.M.G.; Oliveira, T.D.A.; Santana, J.D.M. Vitamin D deficiency aggravates COVID-19: Systematic review and meta-analysis. *Crit. Rev. Food Sci. Nutr.* **2020**, 1–9. [CrossRef]
185. De Smet, D.; De Smet, K.; Herroelen, P.; Gryspeerdt, S.; Martens, G.A. Serum 25(OH)D Level on Hospital Admission Associated With COVID-19 Stage and Mortality. *Am. J. Clin. Pathol.* **2020**. [CrossRef]
186. Jain, A.; Chaurasia, R.; Sengar, N.S.; Singh, M.; Mahor, S.; Narain, S. Analysis of vitamin D level among asymptomatic and critically ill COVID-19 patients and its correlation with inflammatory markers. *Sci. Rep.* **2020**, *10*, 20191. [CrossRef]

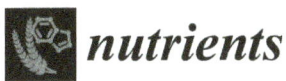

Article

Low Serum Magnesium is Associated with Incident Dementia in the ARIC-NCS Cohort

Aniqa B. Alam [1,*], Pamela L. Lutsey [2], Rebecca F. Gottesman [3], Adrienne Tin [4] and Alvaro Alonso [1]

1. Department of Epidemiology, Emory University School of Public Health, Atlanta, GA 30322, USA; alvaro.alonso@emory.edu
2. Division of Epidemiology and Community Health, University of Minnesota School of Public Health, Minneapolis, MN 55454, USA; lutsey@umn.edu
3. Department of Neurology, Johns Hopkins University School of Medicine, Baltimore, MD 21205, USA; rgottesm@jhmi.edu
4. Department of Medicine, University of Mississippi Medical Center, Jackson, MS 39216, USA; atin@umc.edu
* Correspondence: abalam@emory.edu; Tel.: +1-470-331-5188

Received: 24 September 2020; Accepted: 1 October 2020; Published: 9 October 2020

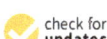

Abstract: Higher serum magnesium is associated with lower risk of multiple morbidities, including diabetes, stroke, and atrial fibrillation, but its potential neuroprotective properties have also been gaining traction in cognitive function and decline research. We studied 12,040 participants presumed free of dementia in the Atherosclerosis Risk in Communities (ARIC) study. Serum magnesium was measured in fasting blood samples collected in 1990–1992. Dementia status was ascertained through cognitive examinations in 2011–2013, 2016–2017, and 2018–2019, along with informant interviews and indicators of dementia-related hospitalization events and death. Participants' cognitive functioning capabilities were assessed up to five times between 1990–1992 and 2018–2019. The cognitive function of participants who did not attend follow-up study visits was imputed to account for attrition. We identified 2519 cases of dementia over a median follow-up period of 24.2 years. The lowest quintile of serum magnesium was associated with a 24% higher rate of incident dementia compared to those in the highest quintile of magnesium (HR, 1.24; 95% CI, 1.07, 1.44). No relationship was found between serum magnesium and cognitive decline in any cognitive domain. Low midlife serum magnesium is associated with increased risk of incident dementia, but does not appear to impact rates of cognitive decline.

Keywords: dementia; cognitive decline; magnesium

1. Introduction

Minerals and their role in cognition have been attracting attention in dementia and cognitive decline research. Magnesium, in particular, has a potential beneficial effect on multiple morbidities, including diabetes, stroke, atrial fibrillation, and other cardiovascular diseases [1–4]. Given the role of these conditions as risk factors for cognitive decline, interest in the role of magnesium as a preventive or therapeutic approach in cognitive decline and dementia is growing. Magnesium's potentially protective effect against cognitive decline has been demonstrated in several animal models [5–7], but human studies are limited with conflicting results, and mainly focus on dietary intake of magnesium [8,9]. The only study to date to examine the relation between serum magnesium and cognition within a cohort found a U-shaped—rather than linear—association of baseline serum magnesium with cognitive decline over a 10-year period (i.e.: high and low baseline serum magnesium were associated with increased risk of dementia) [10].

With the goal of growing our understanding on the role that magnesium can play in cognitive decline and dementia, we studied the association of mid-life circulating magnesium with incident dementia and cognitive decline over a 27-year period within a large community cohort.

2. Materials and Methods

2.1. Study Population

The Atherosclerosis Risk in Communities (ARIC) study is an ongoing, community-based cohort study based in four communities across the US: Jackson, Mississippi; Washington County, Maryland; Forsyth County, North Carolina; and select suburbs in Minneapolis, Minnesota [11]. To date, participants have been examined in 7 visits spanning a 30-year time period, with the first visits taking place in 1987–1989. Participants have also taken part in regular phone calls (annual until 2012, twice-yearly thereafter). The recruited sample was exclusively black in Jackson, and representative of the underlying population in the other three sites (white and black in Forsyth County, and predominately white in Washington County and Minneapolis). For the purposes of this study, visit 2 (1990-1992) was considered the baseline, since it was the first time that cognitive function was assessed. This study has been approved by each study center's institutional review board, with all ARIC participants having provided written informed consent at each visit.

Exclusion criteria for this analysis were based on the following: refusing consent for genetic testing for *APOE* genotyping ($n = 45$), prevalent dementia at visit 2 ($n = 9$), and missing magnesium measurements ($n = 58$). Additionally, because ARIC participants are predominately black and white, Asian and Native American participants were excluded ($n = 40$). Furthermore, black participants from Minneapolis and Washington County were excluded due to low counts ($n = 50$). Finally, those with missing covariates at visit 2 were also excluded ($n = 2106$). Selection into a secondary analysis looking at visit 5 as baseline can be found in Supplementary Figure S1.

2.2. Incident Dementia

ARIC utilized several approaches to ascertain dementia status. Briefly, starting from visit 5 (2011–2013), all participants who attended in-person evaluations underwent cognitive exams, with results of these assessments, along with earlier cognitive assessments (see below), evaluated and adjudicated by an expert committee. Of those that were unable or refused to attend visits, or to detect earlier cases of incident dementia (prior to visit 5), dementia status was based on over-the-phone dementia screeners and/or informant interviews. Additionally, hospitalization for, or death due to, dementia—as determined by ICD-9/10-CM discharge codes and/or death certificates—was classified as having dementia, with discharge codes reviewed from over the entire study follow-up. The methodology for diagnosing dementia in the ARIC study has been described in detail elsewhere [11].

2.3. Cognitive Function

We evaluated cognitive functioning at ARIC visits 2 (1990–1992), 4 (1996–1998), 5 (2011–2013), 6 (2016–2017), and 7 (2018–2019), using three cognitive tests designed to evaluate functioning in three cognitive domains. The delayed word recall test (DWRT) assesses verbal learning and short-term memory, by asking participants to memorize 10 words, use them in a sentence, and then recall the words again after a 5-min break. The digit symbol substitution test (DSST) evaluates executive functioning by giving the participant 90 s to draw symbols that correspond to a set of numbers based on a key. The word fluency test (WFT) measures expressive language by having the participant list as many words as they can in 60 s that start with the letters F, A, and S. The testing procedures have been described in detail elsewhere [11].

We calculated z-scores for each test at all study visits, and then scaled the results to the visit 2 mean and standard deviation. We also generated z-scores for overall cognition by averaging the z-scores and standardizing to the visit 2 mean and standard deviation.

2.4. Serum Magnesium

Blood was drawn at visit 2 into vacuum tubes designated for either lipids or chemistries, and then centrifuged for 10 min at 3000× g at 4 °C. The blood samples were stored at −70 °C and then shipped to the ARIC central laboratories for analysis. Serum magnesium was measured using the metallochromic dye calmagite [1-(1-hydroxy-4-methyl-2-phenylazo)-2-napthol-4sulfonic acid] under the Gindler and Heth method [12]. Repeated measurements in 40 participants were sent to the same lab, with at least one week in between samples, to assess between-person variability (magnesium reliability coefficient = 0.69) and in-person variability (coefficient of variation = 3.6%).

2.5. Covariates

Along with assessing the impact of magnesium categorized into quintiles, we also examined associations of magnesium as a continuous variable, expressed as per standard deviation decrease of serum magnesium. Except for education status and diet scores which were measured at visit 1 and visit 3, respectively, analyses using visit 2 as baseline used covariates measured at visit 2, whereas analyses using visit 5 as baseline used covariates measured at visit 5. Educational attainment was categorized into 3 levels: did not complete high school; completed high school or general education development (GED) or 1-3 years of vocational school; or at least some college. The following blood analytes were measured from fasting blood samples taken at respective visits: estimated glomerular filtration rate, C-reactive protein, potassium, sodium, calcium, total and HDL cholesterol. Smoking and drinking status were self-reported. Blood pressure estimates were the average of the 2nd and 3rd measurements taken over the course of 15 min. Participant diets were assessed through principal component analysis using food frequency questionnaires to analyze the consumption of 32 food groups, generating scores characterizing how much of their dietary patterns were considered "Western" (characterized by consumption of meats, processed foods, sweetened drinks, etc.) and "prudent" (characterized by consumption of whole grains, fresh fruits and vegetables, etc.) [13]. The prevalence of coronary heart disease was based on the presence of myocardial infarction (MI) from adjudicated visit 1 electrocardiogram data, history of MI, or previous coronary bypass. Stroke history was based on prevalent stroke at visit 1 or stroke hospitalization before or at visit 2. Diabetes status was based on serum glucose (fasting cutoff ≥126 mg/dL; non-fasting cutoff ≥200 mg/dL), self-reported physician diagnosis of diabetes, or use of diabetes medication.

2.6. Statistical Analysis

The association between serum magnesium (in quintiles) measured at baseline and incident dementia was measured using Cox proportional hazard models. Model 1 was adjusted for age, the combination of race and center (Jackson black people, Forsyth black people, Forsyth white people, Minneapolis white people, Washington white people), sex, and education (did not complete high school; high school graduate or vocational school; or at least some college). Model 2 adjusted for model 1 covariates, along with smoking history (ever smoked/never smoked), drinking status (current drinker/not current drinker), waist-to-hip ratio, diet scores, estimated glomerular filtration rate (mL/min/1.73m^2), C-reactive protein (mg/L), potassium (mmol/L), sodium (mmol/L), calcium (mmol/L), coronary heart disease (prevalent/not prevalent), history of stroke (yes/no), systolic blood pressure (mmHg), diastolic blood pressure (mmHg), antihypertensive medication use (antihypertensive diuretic, non-diuretic antihypertensive, no antihypertensive use), total cholesterol-to-HDL cholesterol ratio, diabetes status (diabetes/no diabetes), and *APOE* ε4 carrier status (allele/no allele). The proportional hazards assumption was checked by testing interactions with log-time.

In a secondary analysis, to determine if more proximal measurements of magnesium (i.e.: magnesium in late life) influenced rates of incident dementia, we estimated the association between visit 5 serum magnesium and incident dementia, using Cox proportional hazard models.

We used linear models to assess cognitive decline from visit 2 through visit 7, based on visit 2 serum magnesium quintiles and fit them with generalized estimating equations (GEE), with an unstructured correlation matrix to account for repeated testing. Time was modeled using two linear spline terms with knots at 6 years (corresponding to visit 4) and 21 years (corresponding to visit 5) to account for the pronounced decline that is typically expected in later life. Models also incorporated interaction terms with the time splines and covariates. We also assessed differences in baseline cognitive function at visit 2 across magnesium quintiles to better understand baseline cognition. Additionally, in order to evaluate potential floor effects, we conducted a sensitivity analysis, excluding the bottom 5% of test scores within each race at baseline.

Significant attrition was expected over the course of 27 years [14], so we utilized multiple imputation with chained equations (MICE) in order to impute missing values [15]. Twenty datasets with imputed values were calculated based on dementia diagnosis, surveillance information based on telephone screeners and informant interviews, and visit 2 covariates. All cognitive decline results presented have been imputed.

All analyses were conducted using SAS 9.4 (Cary, NC; SAS Institute Inc).

3. Results

Figure 1 presents a flowchart for selection into the study, using visit 2 as baseline. There were 14,348 participants at visit 2, and after applying the exclusion criteria, the final analytic cohort included 12,040 participants free of dementia and with available magnesium at visit 2 (mean age: 56.9 years (SD: 5.7), 56.3% female, 24.6% black). The median follow-up time was 24.2 years (25th, 75th percentiles: 17.3, 27.1 years).

Participants with lower baseline serum magnesium were more likely to be female, black, and have less education than those with higher magnesium (Table 1). Those with lower serum magnesium were also more likely to be diabetic and on antihypertensive medication.

Table 1. Cohort characteristics by baseline magnesium quintile, ARIC 1990–1992.

Characteristics	Magnesium Quintiles				
	1st (≤1.4 mg/dL)	2nd (1.5 mg/dL)	3rd (1.6 mg/dL)	4th (1.7 mg/dL)	5th (≥1.8 mg/dL)
	N = 1650	N = 2370	N = 3255	N = 2599	N = 2166
Age, years	57.1 (5.8)	56.7 (5.8)	56.8 (5.6)	57.0 (5.7)	57.2 (5.7)
Female, %	63.0	56.6	56.7	54.0	53.0
African American, %	43.8	29.2	22.0	18.5	16.3
Education, %					
Did not complete high school	29.8	22.4	20.0	18.5	18.5
High school graduate and/or vocational school	39.1	41.1	42.3	42.2	42.6
At least some college	31.1	36.5	37.7	39.4	39.0
Sodium, mmol/L	140.3 (2.6)	140.6 (2.3)	140.8 (2.3)	141.0 (2.2)	141.2 (2.2)
Potassium, mmol/L	4.06 (0.42)	4.15 (0.38)	4.18 (0.38)	4.22 (0.40)	4.24 (0.40)
Calcium, mmol/L	0.521 (0.027)	0.518 (0.023)	0.518 (0.023)	0.519 (0.023)	0.520 (0.023)
Waist-to-Hip Ratio	0.93 (0.08)	0.93 (0.08)	0.92 (0.08)	0.92 (0.08)	0.93 (0.08)
Ever smoked, %	59.0	60.5	59.1	59.2	61.6
Current drinker, %	48.1	54.8	57.8	59.0	60.5
Prevalent coronary heart disease, %	6.8	6.4	5.9	5.2	5.2
Previous stroke, %	2.9	1.9	1.5	1.6	1.6
Diabetes, %	33.4	19.4	13.1	11.0	9.0
Systolic BP, mmHg	125.4 (20.4)	121.7 (19.0)	121.0 (18.2)	119.5 (17.9)	120.6 (17.8)
Diastolic BP, mmHg	73.1 (10.6)	72.2 (10.2)	72.1 (10.3)	71.6 (10.1)	71.9 (10.0)
Total Cholesterol-to-HDL cholesterol ratio	4.76 (2.06)	4.73 (2.00)	4.62 (1.81)	4.65 (1.74)	4.76 (1.93)

Table 1. Cont.

Characteristics	Magnesium Quintiles				
	1st (≤1.4 mg/dL)	2nd (1.5 mg/dL)	3rd (1.6 mg/dL)	4th (1.7 mg/dL)	5th (≥1.8 mg/dL)
	N = 1650	N = 2370	N = 3255	N = 2599	N = 2166
Antihypertensive medication, %					
Diuretic	25.5	15.7	12.3	10.7	9.4
Non-diuretic, antihypertensive	5.0	3.0	3.1	3.3	2.6
No antihypertensive medication	69.6	81.3	84.7	86.0	88.0
eGFR, mL/min/1.73m^2	97.2 (20.1)	96.1 (17.2)	96.1 (16.1)	94.5 (15.7)	92.3 (16.3)
APOE ε4 allele, %	31.4	31.2	30.8	29.6	30.9
C-reactive Protein, mg/L	5.9 (8.8)	4.6 (6.9)	4.2 (7.1)	3.9 (7.1)	3.8 (6.3)
Western Diet Score	−0.018 (0.981)	−0.012 (1.000)	−0.031 (0.979)	−0.046 (0.967)	−0.009 (0.996)
Prudent Diet Score	−0.025 (0.988)	0.021 (1.027)	0.011 (0.950)	0.032 (0.987)	0.019 (1.00)

Values correspond to mean (standard deviation) or percentage.

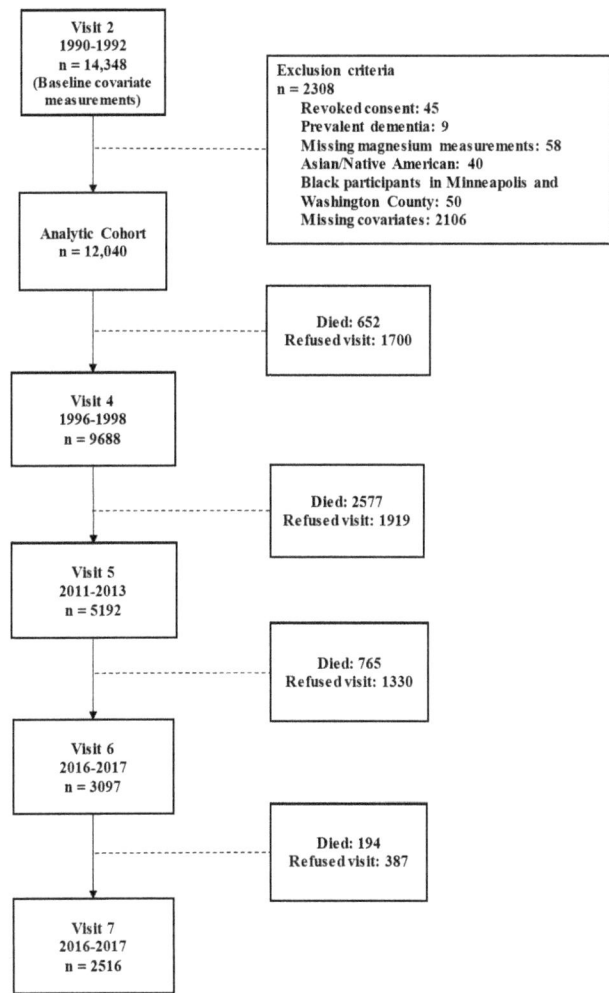

Figure 1. Diagram of the analytic cohort selection from visits 2 through 7 within Atherosclerosis Risk in Communities (ARIC) cohort.

3.1. Incident Dementia

A preliminary analysis found no evidence of a U-shaped association when using the 3rd quintile as the referent group. Therefore, subsequent analyses use the 5th quintile as the referent group. When minimally adjusting for sex, race and center, age, and education, participants in the lowest quintile had a 34% higher rate of dementia [HR: 1.34; 95%CI: 1.17, 1.54] (Table 2). Additional adjustment for diet, cardiovascular disease correlates, APOE4 carrier status, and other micronutrients resulted in a slight attenuation, but remained significant, with a 24% higher rate of incident dementia [HR: 1.24; 95%CI: 1.07, 1.44]. A one SD lower serum magnesium concentration [SD: ~0.009 mmol/L] was associated with a 7% higher rate of dementia when adjusted for model 2 covariates [95%CI: 2%–11%]. When using visit 5 as baseline, no significant associations or trends were found between magnesium and incident dementia (Supplementary Table S1).

Table 2. Association of baseline magnesium with incident dementia, ARIC 1990-2019.

Quintile of Magnesium	Person Years of Follow-Up	Dementia Cases	IR ‡	Model 1 * HR (95%CI)	Model 2 ** HR (95%CI)
Quintile 1	32,306	367	11.36	1.34 (1.17, 1.54)	1.24 (1.07, 1.44)
Quintile 2	49,507	475	9.59	1.11 (0.97, 1.26)	1.08 (0.95, 1.24)
Quintile 3	70,753	681	9.63	1.03 (0.91, 1.16)	1.03 (0.91, 1.16)
Quintile 4	56,470	559	9.90	1.07 (0.95, 1.21)	1.08 (0.95, 1.22)
Quintile 5	47,188	437	9.26	1 (Ref)	1 (Ref)
Per 1 standard deviation (~0.009 mmol/L) decrease in Mg				1.09 (1.05, 1.14)	1.07 (1.02, 1.11)

HR, hazard ratio; 95%CI, 95% confidence interval. ‡ Crude incidence rate, per 1000 person-years. * Model 1 adjusted for sex, race and center, education, and age. ** Adjusted for Model 1 variables, along with history of smoking, drinking status, western and prudent diet scores, waist-to-hip ratio, estimated glomerular filtration rate, c-reactive protein, sodium, potassium, calcium, prevalent coronary heart disease, previous stroke, antihypertensive medication use, systolic and diastolic blood pressure, total-cholesterol-to-HDL cholesterol ratio, apolipoprotein E4 carrier status, diabetes status.

Race- and sex-stratified models revealed similar patterns of association, with no real differences found between black people and white people [race interaction, $p = 0.51$] nor between men and women [sex interaction, $p = 0.46$] (Supplementary Tables S2 and S3).

3.2. Cognitive Decline

Low magnesium was associated with poorer performance at baseline in the DSST, WFT, and the global composite score (Supplementary Table S4). Table 3 presents rates of cognitive decline during the 27-year follow-up period by serum magnesium at visit 2. There was no clear association between serum magnesium and cognitive decline, with magnesium modeled in quintiles for the composite cognitive score or any of the individual cognitive tests, even after excluding the bottom 5% of test scores at baseline (Supplementary Table S5).

Table 3. Cognitive change over 27 years by baseline magnesium quintile, ARIC 1990-2019.

Test	Quintiles	Model 1 *	Model 2 **
Global			
	1	−0.031 (−0.092, 0.029)	0.003 (−0.060, 0.067)
	2	0.052 (−0.0004, 0.104)	0.063 (0.011, 0.115)
	3	0.027 (−0.022, 0.075)	0.030 (−0.017, 0.077)
	4	−0.021 (−0.074, 0.031)	−0.022 (−0.073, 0.028)
	5	0 (Referent)	0 (Referent)
Per 1-SD *** decrease in Mg		0.004 (−0.013, 0.020)	−0.003 (−0.022, 0.016)
DWR			
	1	−0.023 (−0.126, 0.080)	0.001 (−0.106, 0.107)
	2	0.058 (−0.033, 0.149)	0.066 (−0.027, 0.158)
	3	0.052 (−0.035, 0.139)	0.053 (−0.034, 0.141)
	4	−0.051 (−0.145, 0.043)	−0.054 (−0.146, 0.038)
	5	0 (Referent)	0 (Referent)
Per 1-SD decrease in Mg		0.011 (−0.017, 0.039)	0.007 (−0.028, 0.042)
DSS			
	1	−0.039 (−0.096, 0.017)	−0.0004 (−0.056, 0.055)
	2	0.048 (0.006, 0.090)	0.063 (0.021, 0.105)
	3	0.020 (−0.018, 0.059)	0.027 (−0.011, 0.065)
	4	−0.023 (−0.069, 0.022)	−0.023 (−0.068, 0.022)
	5	0 (Referent)	0 (Referent)
Per 1-SD decrease in Mg		0.002 (−0.014, 0.017)	−0.010 (−0.027, 0.008)
WF			
	1	−0.017 (−0.082, 0.047)	0.018 (−0.052, 0.089)
	2	0.034 (−0.017, 0.085)	0.047 (−0.003, 0.097)
	3	0.009 (−0.041, 0.059)	0.011 (−0.038, 0.061)
	4	0.013 (−0.039, 0.064)	0.012 (−0.039, 0.063)
	5	0 (Referent)	0 (Referent)
Per 1-SD decrease in Mg		−0.001 (−0.018, 0.017)	−0.007 (−0.030, 0.015)

SD, standard deviation; DWR, delayed word recall; DSS, digit symbol substitution; WF, word fluency. * Model 1 adjusted for sex, race and center, education, and age, and interactions of all covariates with time. Time modeled as spline term with knots at 6 years and 21 years. ** Adjusted for model 1 variables, along with history of smoking, drinking status, western and prudent diet scores, waist-to-hip ratio, estimated glomerular filtration rate, c-reactive protein, sodium, potassium, calcium, prevalent coronary heart disease, previous stroke, antihypertensive medication use, systolic and diastolic blood pressure, total-cholesterol-to-HDL cholesterol ratio, apolipoprotein E4 carrier status, and diabetes status, and interactions of all covariates with time. Time modeled as spline terms with knots at 6 years and 21 years. *** SD being equal to ~0.009 mmol/L.

4. Discussion

Within a large, community-based cohort, we found low levels of mid-life serum magnesium to be associated with an elevated risk of incident dementia, with a 24% increased risk of dementia for participants in the bottom compared to the top magnesium quintile, even when adjusting for demographics, lifestyle, cardiovascular risk factors, APOE4 carrier status, and other micronutrients. Mid-life magnesium, however, was not associated with decline over a 27-year period. No meaningful differences were found between race or sex.

The discrepancy between incident dementia and decline may in part be explained by differences in baseline cognition and education levels. Cognitive performance at visit 2 was poorer among participants with lower serum magnesium compared to those with higher magnesium. Low magnesium participants also on average had less formal education than their higher magnesium counterparts, which has been shown to primarily affect baseline cognition while remaining unrelated to cognitive change [16]. Even after excluding the lowest 5% of scores at baseline to account for possible floor effects, rates of decline did not appear to differ across magnesium levels. Based on our findings, though the rates of decline do not seem to differ across magnesium levels, it may not take much decline to reach the dementia "threshold" for low magnesium individuals.

Magnesium may target multiple pathways in dementia pathology. N-methyl-D-aspartate (NMDA) receptors play critical roles in learning processes and the formation of memories [17]. Through the glutamatergic excitation of NMDA receptors, calcium ions flow into cells and trigger other signaling pathways important in dementia and cognitive decline pathology [18]. Over-excitation of NDMA receptors, however, may impair synaptic activity and lead to neuronal necrosis [19]. Magnesium is able to block this NMDA-induced excitotoxicity by inhibiting NMDA receptors and subsequent cellular cascades [20,21]. Another pathway targets neuroinflammation triggered by beta-amyloid (Aβ) leakages through the blood brain barrier, which can lead to the release of proinflammatory cytokines, such as interleukins, tumor necrosis factor alpha (TNF-α), and nitric oxide [22,23], all resulting in a higher rate of neurodegeneration. Magnesium has shown to inhibit excessive Aβ production and prevent this inflammatory cascade [24]. Additionally, elevated magnesium may be able to induce amyloid precursor protein cleavage, which would also prevent the accumulation of Aβ [25].

Our results confirm much of the previous literature. Cross-sectional studies comparing those with diagnosed dementia against healthy controls found patients with dementia to have lower serum magnesium than their non-impaired peers [26]. In the Rotterdam study, serum magnesium at either extreme was associated with increased risk of dementia compared to the average serum levels (third quintile) [10]. Magnesium intake, whether through diet or supplements, seems to also be associated with better cognitive functioning in both mice and human models [7,27]. For instance, over a ten-year follow-up period, patients in Taiwan using magnesium oxide had a decreased risk of developing dementia compared to those not on magnesium oxide therapy [9]. Magnesium oxide is commonly prescribed as an antacid or laxative, and has been shown to increase serum magnesium [28]. Other studies have found benefits in having a more balanced intake of magnesium. In the Women's Health Initiative Memory Study, women in the third quintile of dietary magnesium intake (corresponding to about 216–263 mg/day) had a lower risk of mild cognitive impairment or dementia than those in the first quintile; no association was found comparing the fifth quintile against the first quintile [8].

Though the evidence is promising, determining the utility of serum measurements versus dietary intake of magnesium in dementia pathology requires a critical examination of each of their shortcomings. Magnesium homeostasis is dependent on its interaction with calcium and phosphorus within the small intestines, bones, and kidneys [29]. Consequently, it is difficult to separate the effects of dietary magnesium from the overall quality of one's diet. Conversely, though serum magnesium offers a more direct measurement of circulating magnesium than perhaps through supplement or dietary intake, serum magnesium has very little correlation with total body magnesium, most of which is present in either the bones and teeth or in the intracellular space [30]. When blood concentrations are low, magnesium may be pulled out of the cells to maintain normal levels in the blood [30], which could mask possible hypomagnesemia when determined through serum measurements alone. That said, though the association of blood magnesium with brain magnesium has been difficult to establish up to this point, previous research has found that both brain [31] and serum magnesium levels [32] are diminished in Alzheimer's patients, suggesting some level of positive correlation between the two measurements.

Strengths of this study include the ability to use data from a large, prospective cohort study, which grants us significant time to follow-up with participants. We were also able to adjust our models for a variety of cardiovascular risk factors, diet, and other micronutrients. On the other hand, the limitations of this study warrant a cautious interpretation of the results. First, even though we were able to assess the impact of both mid-life and late-life magnesium on dementia and cognitive function, two measurements may not be enough to account for the impact of micronutrient fluctuations over a life course. Second, the cognitive change analyses may be influenced by possible "floor effects", though we attempted to account for this in a sensitivity analysis by excluding the bottom 5% of scores within each race. Furthermore, though the MICE method for imputing missing data has been previously validated in the ARIC cohort [33], estimation errors may occur for data over 50% missing [34], and with over 80% of the cohort missing by visit 7, results should be interpreted with caution. Additionally, though we were able to follow-up with the cohort for over two and a half decades, because the baseline for this analysis corresponds to mid-life for our participants, we are unlikely to fully capture cognitive trajectories over a life course. Finally, though we adjusted for many biological and lifestyle factors and undertook the rigorous adjudication of dementia status, there may be some level of confounding by socioeconomic factors or possible malnutrition, biasing our results and potentially inflating the effect of serum magnesium in dementia pathology.

5. Conclusions

In conclusion, consistent with some prior studies, we found that low circulating magnesium in midlife was associated with increased risk of dementia. Confirming this association across multiple forms of magnesium intake and measurements (i.e.: blood magnesium, brain magnesium) and elucidating the underlying pathways may offer new avenues for the prevention of dementia in the community.

Supplementary Materials: The following are available online at http://www.mdpi.com/2072-6643/12/10/3074/s1, Figure S1: Diagram of analytic cohort selection for visits 5 through 7, using visit 5 as baseline. Table S1: Association of visit 5 magnesium quintiles with incident dementia, ARIC 2011–2019; Table S2: Association of baseline magnesium quintiles with incident dementia, stratified by race, ARIC 1990-2019; Table S3: Association of baseline magnesium quintiles with incident dementia, stratified by sex, ARIC 1990–2019; Table S4: Difference in cognitive functioning at visit 2 by baseline magnesium quintile, ARIC 1990–1992; Table S5: Cognitive change over 27 years by baseline magnesium quintile, excluding the bottom 5% of test scores at baseline, ARIC 1990–2019.

Author Contributions: Conceptualization: A.B.A. and A.A. Methodology: A.B.A., A.A., P.L.L., R.F.G., and A.T. Formal analysis: A.B.A. Writing—original draft preparation: A.B.A. and A.A. Writing—review and editing: A.B.A., A.A., P.L.L., R.F.G., and A.T. All authors have read and agreed to the published version of the manuscript.

Funding: The Atherosclerosis Risk in Communities Study was carried out as a collaborative study, supported by National Heart, Lung, and Blood Institute contracts (HHSN268201700004I, HHSN268201700003I, HHSN268201700002I, HHSN268201700005I, HHSN268201700001I). Neurocognitive data were collected by U01 2U01HL096917, 2U01HL096899, 2U01HL096814, 2U01HL096902, 2U01HL096812 from the NIH (NHLBI, NINDS, NIA and NIDCD), and with previous brain MRI examinations funded by R01-HL70825 from the NHLBI. Additional support was provided by the National Heart, Lung, And Blood Institute of the National Institutes of Health under Award Number K24HL148521. The content is solely the responsibility of the authors and does not necessarily represent the official views of the National Institutes of Health.

Acknowledgments: The authors thank the staff and participants of the ARIC study for their important contributions.

Conflicts of Interest: The authors declare no conflict of interest.

References

1. Zhao, B.; Hu, L.; Dong, Y.; Xu, J.; Wei, Y.; Yu, D.; Xu, J.; Zhang, W. The Effect of Magnesium Intake on Stroke Incidence: A Systematic Review and Meta-Analysis With Trial Sequential Analysis. *Front. Neurol.* **2019**, *10*, 852. [CrossRef] [PubMed]
2. Barbagallo, M.; Dominguez, L.J. Magnesium and type 2 diabetes. *World J. Diabetes* **2015**, *6*, 1152–1157. [CrossRef] [PubMed]
3. Misialek, J.R.; Lopez, F.L.; Lutsey, P.L.; Huxley, R.R.; Peacock, J.M.; Chen, L.Y.; Soliman, E.Z.; Agarwal, S.K.; Alonso, A. Serum and dietary magnesium and incidence of atrial fibrillation in whites and in African Americans–Atherosclerosis Risk in Communities (ARIC) study. *Circ. J.* **2013**, *77*, 323–329. [CrossRef] [PubMed]
4. Zhao, L.; Hu, M.; Yang, L.; Xu, H.; Song, W.; Qian, Y.; Zhao, M. Quantitative Association Between Serum/Dietary Magnesium and Cardiovascular Disease/Coronary Heart Disease Risk: A Dose-Response Meta-analysis of Prospective Cohort Studies. *J. Cardiovasc. Pharm.* **2019**, *74*, 516–527. [CrossRef] [PubMed]
5. Huang, Y.; Huang, X.; Zhang, L.; Han, F.; Pang, K.L.; Li, X.; Shen, J.Y. Magnesium boosts the memory restorative effect of environmental enrichment in Alzheimer's disease mice. *CNS Neurosci.* **2018**, *24*, 70–79. [CrossRef] [PubMed]

6. Wang, P.; Yu, X.; Guan, P.P.; Guo, J.W.; Wang, Y.; Zhang, Y.; Zhao, H.; Wang, Z.Y. Magnesium ion influx reduces neuroinflammation in Abeta precursor protein/Presenilin 1 transgenic mice by suppressing the expression of interleukin-1beta. *Cell Mol. Immunol.* **2017**, *14*, 451–464. [CrossRef]
7. Li, W.; Yu, J.; Liu, Y.; Huang, X.; Abumaria, N.; Zhu, Y.; Huang, X.; Xiong, W.; Ren, C.; Liu, X.G.; et al. Elevation of brain magnesium prevents synaptic loss and reverses cognitive deficits in Alzheimer's disease mouse model. *Mol. Brain* **2014**, *7*, 65. [CrossRef]
8. Lo, K.; Liu, Q.; Madsen, T.; Rapp, S.; Chen, J.C.; Neuhouser, M.; Shadyab, A.; Pal, L.; Lin, X.; Shumaker, S.; et al. Relations of magnesium intake to cognitive impairment and dementia among participants in the Women's Health Initiative Memory Study: A prospective cohort study. *BMJ Open* **2019**, *9*, e030052. [CrossRef]
9. Tzeng, N.S.; Chung, C.H.; Lin, F.H.; Huang, C.F.; Yeh, C.B.; Huang, S.Y.; Lu, R.B.; Chang, H.A.; Kao, Y.C.; Yeh, H.W.; et al. Magnesium oxide use and reduced risk of dementia: A retrospective, nationwide cohort study in Taiwan. *Curr. Med. Res. Opin.* **2018**, *34*, 163–169. [CrossRef]
10. Kieboom, B.C.T.; Licher, S.; Wolters, F.J.; Ikram, M.K.; Hoorn, E.J.; Zietse, R.; Stricker, B.H.; Ikram, M.A. Serum magnesium is associated with the risk of dementia. *Neurology* **2017**, *89*, 1716–1722. [CrossRef]
11. The ARIC Investigators. The Atherosclerosis Risk in Communities (ARIC) Study: Design and objectives. *Am. J. Epidemiol.* **1989**, *129*, 687–702.
12. Gindler, E.; Heth, D. Colorimetric determination with bound calmagite of magnesium in human blood serum. In *Clinical Chemistry*; American Association Clinical Chemistry: Washington, DC, USA, 1971; p. 20037-1526.
13. Lutsey, P.L.; Steffen, L.M.; Stevens, J. Dietary intake and the development of the metabolic syndrome: The Atherosclerosis Risk in Communities study. *Circulation* **2008**, *117*, 754–761. [CrossRef] [PubMed]
14. Siegler, I.C.; Botwinick, J. A long-term longitudinal study of intellectual ability of older adults: The matter of selective subject attrition. *J. Gerontol.* **1979**, *34*, 242–245. [CrossRef] [PubMed]
15. White, I.R.; Royston, P.; Wood, A.M. Multiple imputation using chained equations: Issues and guidance for practice. *Stat. Med.* **2011**, *30*, 377–399. [CrossRef] [PubMed]
16. Gottesman, R.F.; Rawlings, A.M.; Sharrett, A.R.; Albert, M.; Alonso, A.; Bandeen-Roche, K.; Coker, L.H.; Coresh, J.; Couper, D.J.; Griswold, M.E.; et al. Impact of differential attrition on the association of education with cognitive change over 20 years of follow-up: The ARIC neurocognitive study. *Am. J. Epidemiol.* **2014**, *179*, 956–966. [CrossRef]
17. Olivares, D.; Deshpande, V.K.; Shi, Y.; Lahiri, D.K.; Greig, N.H.; Rogers, J.T.; Huang, X. N-methyl D-aspartate (NMDA) receptor antagonists and memantine treatment for Alzheimer's disease, vascular dementia and Parkinson's disease. *Curr. Alzheimer Res.* **2012**, *9*, 746–758. [CrossRef] [PubMed]
18. Lynch, M.A. Long-term potentiation and memory. *Physiol. Rev.* **2004**, *84*, 87–136. [CrossRef]
19. Zipfel, G.J.; Babcock, D.J.; Lee, J.M.; Choi, D.W. Neuronal apoptosis after CNS injury: The roles of glutamate and calcium. *J. Neurotrauma* **2000**, *17*, 857–869. [CrossRef]
20. Hynd, M.R.; Scott, H.L.; Dodd, P.R. Glutamate-mediated excitotoxicity and neurodegeneration in Alzheimer's disease. *Neurochem. Int.* **2004**, *45*, 583–595. [CrossRef]
21. Greene, J.G.; Greenamyre, J.T. Bioenergetics and glutamate excitotoxicity. *Prog. Neurobiol.* **1996**, *48*, 613–634. [CrossRef]
22. Wenzel, T.J.; Klegeris, A. Novel multi-target directed ligand-based strategies for reducing neuroinflammation in Alzheimer's disease. *Life Sci.* **2018**, *207*, 314–322. [CrossRef] [PubMed]
23. Rakic, S.; Hung, Y.M.A.; Smith, M.; So, D.; Tayler, H.M.; Varney, W.; Wild, J.; Harris, S.; Holmes, C.; Love, S.; et al. Systemic infection modifies the neuroinflammatory response in late stage Alzheimer's disease. *Acta Neuropathol. Commun.* **2018**, *6*, 88. [CrossRef] [PubMed]
24. Yu, X.; Guan, P.P.; Zhu, D.; Liang, Y.Y.; Wang, T.; Wang, Z.Y.; Wang, P. Magnesium Ions Inhibit the Expression of Tumor Necrosis Factor alpha and the Activity of gamma-Secretase in a beta-Amyloid Protein-Dependent Mechanism in APP/PS1 Transgenic Mice. *Front. Mol. Neurosci.* **2018**, *11*, 172. [CrossRef] [PubMed]
25. Yu, J.; Sun, M.; Chen, Z.; Lu, J.; Liu, Y.; Zhou, L.; Xu, X.; Fan, D.; Chui, D. Magnesium modulates amyloid-beta protein precursor trafficking and processing. *J. Alzheimers Dis.* **2010**, *20*, 1091–1106. [CrossRef]
26. Veronese, N.; Zurlo, A.; Solmi, M.; Luchini, C.; Trevisan, C.; Bano, G.; Manzato, E.; Sergi, G.; Rylander, R. Magnesium Status in Alzheimer's Disease: A Systematic Review. *Am. J. Alzheimers Dis. Other Demen* **2016**, *31*, 208–213. [CrossRef]

27. Ozawa, M.; Ninomiya, T.; Ohara, T.; Hirakawa, Y.; Doi, Y.; Hata, J.; Uchida, K.; Shirota, T.; Kitazono, T.; Kiyohara, Y. Self-reported dietary intake of potassium, calcium, and magnesium and risk of dementia in the Japanese: The Hisayama Study. *J. Am. Geriatr. Soc.* **2012**, *60*, 1515–1520. [CrossRef]
28. Horibata, K.; Tanoue, A.; Ito, M.; Takemura, Y. Relationship between renal function and serum magnesium concentration in elderly outpatients treated with magnesium oxide. *Geriatr. Gerontol. Int.* **2016**, *16*, 600–605. [CrossRef]
29. Blaine, J.; Chonchol, M.; Levi, M. Renal control of calcium, phosphate, and magnesium homeostasis. *Clin. J. Am. Soc. Nephrol.* **2015**, *10*, 1257–1272. [CrossRef]
30. Razzaque, M.S. Magnesium: Are We Consuming Enough? *Nutrients* **2018**, *10*, 1863. [CrossRef]
31. Andrasi, E.; Pali, N.; Molnar, Z.; Kosel, S. Brain aluminum, magnesium and phosphorus contents of control and Alzheimer-diseased patients. *J. Alzheimers Dis.* **2005**, *7*, 273–284. [CrossRef]
32. Balmus, I.M.; Strungaru, S.A.; Ciobica, A.; Nicoara, M.N.; Dobrin, R.; Plavan, G.; Stefanescu, C. Preliminary Data on the Interaction between Some Biometals and Oxidative Stress Status in Mild Cognitive Impairment and Alzheimer's Disease Patients. *Oxid. Med. Cell Longev.* **2017**, *2017*, 7156928. [CrossRef] [PubMed]
33. Rawlings, A.M.; Sang, Y.; Sharrett, A.R.; Coresh, J.; Griswold, M.; Kucharska-Newton, A.M.; Palta, P.; Wruck, L.M.; Gross, A.L.; Deal, J.A.; et al. Multiple imputation of cognitive performance as a repeatedly measured outcome. *Eur. J. Epidemiol.* **2017**, *32*, 55–66. [CrossRef] [PubMed]
34. Johnson, D.R.; Young, R. Toward best practices in analyzing datasets with missing data: Comparisons and recommendations. *J. Marriage Fam.* **2011**, *73*, 926–945. [CrossRef]

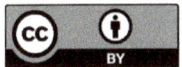

© 2020 by the authors. Licensee MDPI, Basel, Switzerland. This article is an open access article distributed under the terms and conditions of the Creative Commons Attribution (CC BY) license (http://creativecommons.org/licenses/by/4.0/).

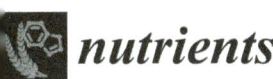

Review

Magnesium and Hypertension in Old Age

Ligia J. Dominguez, Nicola Veronese and Mario Barbagallo *

Geriatric Unit, Department of Medicine, University of Palermo, 90100 Palermo, Italy; ligia.dominguez@unipa.it (L.J.D.); nicola.veronese@unipa.it (N.V.)
* Correspondence: mario.barbagallo@unipa.it; Tel.: +39-091-655-4828; Fax: +39-091-655-2952

Abstract: Hypertension is a complex condition in which various actors and mechanisms combine, resulting in cardiovascular and cerebrovascular complications that today represent the most frequent causes of mortality, morbidity, disability, and health expenses worldwide. In the last decades, there has been an exceptional amount of experimental, epidemiological, and clinical studies confirming a close relationship between magnesium deficit and high blood pressure. Multiple mechanisms may help to explain the bulk of evidence supporting a protective effect of magnesium against hypertension and its complications. Hypertension increases sharply with advancing age, hence older persons are those most affected by its negative consequences. They are also more frequently at risk of magnesium deficiency by multiple mechanisms, which may, at least in part, explain the higher frequency of hypertension and its long-term complications. The evidence for a favorable effect of magnesium on hypertension risk emphasizes the importance of broadly encouraging the intake of foods such as vegetables, nuts, whole cereals and legumes, optimal dietary sources of magnesium, avoiding processed food, which are very poor in magnesium and other fundamental nutrients, in order to prevent hypertension. In some cases, when diet is not enough to maintain an adequate magnesium status, magnesium supplementation may be of benefit and has been shown to be well tolerated.

Keywords: magnesium; hypertension; aging; ions; insulin resistance; cardiovascular disease; diet; supplement

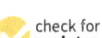

Citation: Dominguez, L.J.; Veronese, N.; Barbagallo, M. Magnesium and Hypertension in Old Age. *Nutrients* **2021**, *13*, 139. https://doi.org/10.3390/nu13010139

Received: 12 November 2020
Accepted: 29 December 2020
Published: 31 December 2020

Publisher's Note: MDPI stays neutral with regard to jurisdictional claims in published maps and institutional affiliations.

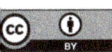

Copyright: © 2020 by the authors. Licensee MDPI, Basel, Switzerland. This article is an open access article distributed under the terms and conditions of the Creative Commons Attribution (CC BY) license (https://creativecommons.org/licenses/by/4.0/).

1. Introduction

Magnesium is the most present divalent intracellular cation in the human body, and the second intracellular ion after potassium. This primary cation has been traditionally considered as cofactor of about 300 regulatory enzymes [1], but current databases list over 600 enzymes for which magnesium is cofactor [2]. Magnesium is involved in fundamental cellular reactions comprising ATP-dependent biochemical processes as part of the activated MgATP complex, DNA synthesis, RNA expression, muscular and neural cell signaling, glucose metabolism, and blood pressure control [3,4].

Although magnesium was first recommended as treatment for malignant hypertension as early as 1925 [5], subsequent studies failed to demonstrate reliable results. In 1983, a study by Resnick et al. [6], showed a close inverse relationship of serum ionized magnesium and plasma renin activity. The following year (1984) Resnick and Gupta, using novel ^{31}P-NMR technique that allowed precise assessment of intracellular cytosolic magnesium concentrations, published a seminal paper showing that persons with essential hypertension had consistently lower levels of intracellular magnesium with an inverse relationship between these concentrations and blood pressure values, the lower intracellular magnesium, the higher blood pressure [7]. This close quantitative relationship confirmed the presence of a powerful link between magnesium deficiency and human essential hypertension. Afterwards, a number of experimental, clinical and epidemiological studies exploring the relationship of this key cation with hypertension have been undertaken. Magnesium is involved in blood pressure regulation by diverse mechanisms including modulation of vascular tone and reactivity acting as a calcium antagonist [8,9], the renin–angiotensin–aldosterone system (RAAS) [6], endothelial function [10–12], vascular remodeling and stiffness [13], and catecholamine release [14]. Magnesium deficiency has been also related to low-grade inflammation, oxidative stress [12,15,16], insulin resistance, and metabolic syndrome [3].

High blood pressure is the strongest independent and modifiable risk factor for heart failure, ischemic heart disease, cerebrovascular events, chronic kidney disease, and cognitive decline worldwide [17]. Hypertension was associated with 4.9, 2.0, and 1.5 million deaths due to ischemic heart disease, hemorrhagic stroke, and ischemic stroke, respectively, in 2015 [18]. According to the World Health Organization, 1.13 billion adults have hypertension currently [19]. The prevalence of hypertension rises remarkably with advancing age and due to the continuous and global increase in aging populations, the prevalence of hypertension and its derived detrimental consequences are still increasing [20]. Hence, public health preventive actions are urgently needed, comprising nutrition, to combat the hypertension pandemic.

A number of investigations have assessed the association of dietary and supplemental magnesium with the development of high blood pressure and meta-analyses on cohort studies and RCTs have confirmed protective effects [21–24]. A recent summary of meta-analyses on the effects of electrolytes on hypertension revealed that the greatest beneficial effect on blood pressure lowering was ascribed to magnesium intake followed by potassium intake and by salt reduction [25]. Dietary magnesium intake is deficient in a large proportion of European and US populations where Western dietary patterns full of processed food are very frequent [26–29]. Indeed, magnesium is abundant in green leafy vegetables, nuts, legumes, and whole cereals, while it is practically absent in processed food and sugar sweetened beverages [30]. Chronic inadequate magnesium intake, particularly frequent in old age, has been associated with an increased risk of multiple clinical conditions including hypertension and stroke [3,8,31]. The Dietary Guidelines for Americans recommend a daily intake of 420 mg of magnesium for men and 320 mg for women [32], but estimates indicate that more than 60% of Americans are under the recommendation [28].

Most studies have shown inverse associations of dietary magnesium intake with hypertension [33–35] or risk of incident hypertension [36–40], while fewer studies have reported negative or inconclusive results [41–43]. A systematic review and meta-analysis of cohort studies reported that a 100 mg/day increment of magnesium dietary intake was significantly associated with 5% reduction in incident hypertension [21]. Three meta-analyses of 11, 34, and 28 RCTs found that supplementation with oral magnesium resulted in significant reductions in blood pressure vs. controls [22,23,44]. Earlier meta-analyses suggested benefit with less prominent effect, possibly due to heterogeneity and to the inclusion of persons with and without other chronic diseases in the analyses [24,45].

The present article aims to review the role of alterations of magnesium metabolism in the pathophysiology of high blood pressure, condition which is particularly frequent in old age. We discuss the possible mechanisms involved and the available evidence of the effects of dietary and supplemental magnesium on blood pressure lowering and risk of hypertension.

2. Magnesium Metabolism, Dietary Sources, and Requirements

Approximately 24 g (1 mole) of magnesium are present in the human body, of which almost 2/3 stored in the bone and 1/3 in the cellular compartment. Blood serum contains less than 1% of the total body magnesium with normal concentrations ranging between 0.75 and 0.95 mmol/L (1.7–2.5 mg/dL or 1.5–1.9 meq/L). Magnesium concentrations in the serum are extremely constant and are tightly controlled and kept within this narrow range by the kidney and small intestine increasing their fractional magnesium absorption during magnesium deprivation. If the lack of magnesium persists, bone stores help maintaining serum magnesium concentration through exchange with extracellular fluid [3].

Serum magnesium exists in three forms: 25% is bound to albumin and 8% bound to globulins (protein-bound fraction); 12% corresponds to the chelated fraction; while 55% represents the metabolically active ionized fraction. Hypomagnesemia is generally identified as a serum magnesium concentration below 0.75 mmol/L [3]. Magnesium is an intracellular regulator of the cell cycle physiology and apoptosis; its intracellular concentrations are as well highly regulated. Most intracellular magnesium exists in bound form. Circulating magnesium concentrations do not always correspond to intracellular or total magnesium.

Magnesium equilibrium depends on magnesium intake, its absorption through intestine (mainly small intestine), its renal excretion, and its requirements in all tissues [46]. Magnesium's requirement per day in healthy adults is estimated at 300–400 mg (5 to 6 mg/kg/day) but in several physiological conditions this requirement may be increased (i.e., exercise, aging, pregnancy, etc.), as well as in some pathological conditions (diabetes, infections, etc.). Because magnesium stored in bone tissue cannot be quickly exchanged with magnesium in the extracellular fluids, the rapid magnesium needs are provided by magnesium stored in the intracellular compartment. About 120 mg of magnesium are eliminated into the urine every day contributing substantially to magnesium homeostasis [47]. Renal magnesium exchanges are closely dependent on magnesium body status, because magnesium depletion increases magnesium reabsorption. Thus, urinary excretion is reduced in magnesium-depleted conditions [48]. Diuretic, drugs that are commonly used in hypertension and heart failure, may as well modify renal magnesium exchanges by reducing the reabsorption of magnesium [49]. No known hormonal factor is specifically involved as a main regulator of magnesium homeostasis. Nevertheless, several hormones have been shown to exert actions on magnesium balance and transport, including parathyroid hormone, calcitonin, catecholamines, and insulin [3,50].

Table 1 depicts some food sources of magnesium, which correspond to foods belonging to dietary patterns generally considered healthy. Contrariwise, the foods contained in the Western diet, most of them ultra-processed, are very poor in magnesium. Ultra-processed food, according to NOVA classification, the most widely used classification of processed food, is defined as the "formulations of food substances often modified by chemical processes and then assembled into ready-to-consume hyper-palatable food and drink products using flavors, colors, emulsifiers and other cosmetic additives" [51]. In the last decades, the global supply of food products derived from industrial processes has increased substantially. The percentage of energy intake derived from ultra-processed foods has been reported to be 29.1% in France [52], 42% in Australia [53] and 57.9% in the USA [54]. Parallel to this transition towards diets based on processed food, a remarkable increase of non-communicable diseases, including obesity and hypertension, has been reported worldwide [55]. There is growing evidence linking consumption of this type of foods with poor diet quality, increased cardiovascular risk factors (e.g., hypertension, dyslipidemia), and harmful health outcomes such as obesity, metabolic syndrome [51] and also with increased mortality risk [52,56,57]. Negative nutritional characteristics of ultra-processed foods include its high content of low-quality fat, added salt and sugar, as well as low vitamin, mineral and fiber content [51].

Regarding the actual dietary sources of magnesium, in the USA, where 57.9% of energy intake comes from ultra-processed food [54], a study analyzing data from the National Health and Nutrition Examination Survey (NHANES) 2003 to 2008 among 25,351 participants, found that minimally processed food contributed only 27.6% to total magnesium intake, whereas ready-to-eat foods and packaged ready-to-eat foods contributed 28.8% and 26.3% to dietary magnesium intake, respectively [58]. This corresponds with the low consumption of foods rich in magnesium reported by the Dietary Guidelines for Americans (estimated % of persons below recommendation across all ages and both sexes in the USA was near 100% for whole grains, near 90% for total vegetables, over 80% for beans and peas, and near 60% for nuts, according to data from NHANES 2007–2010), which also indicated that 49% of the USA population, considering all age-groups, had a magnesium intake below the estimated average requirement [32]. Other estimates indicated that over 60% of Americans are under the recommended daily intake [28].

Table 1. Some Food Sources of Magnesium.

Food	Serving	Magnesium (mg)
Cereal all bran	1/2 cup	112
Cereal oat bran	1/2 cup dry	96
Brown rice, medium-grain, cooked	1 cup	86
Fish, mackerel, cooked	3 ounces	82
Spinach, frozen, chopped, cooked	1/2 cup	78
Almonds	1 ounce (23 almonds)	77
Swiss chard, chopped, cooked	1/2 cup	75
Lima beans, large, cooked	1/2 cup	63
Cereal, shredded wheat	2 biscuits	61
Peanuts	1 ounce	48
Molasses, blackstrap	1 tablespoon	48
Hazelnuts	1 ounce (21 hazelnuts)	46
Walnuts	1 ounce (14 walnuts)	44
Okra, frozen, cooked	1/2 cup	37
Milk, 1% fat	8 fluid ounces	34
Banana	1 medium	32

Data from the European Prospective Investigation into Cancer and Nutrition (EPIC) study reported that in Nordic and central European countries (i.e., Germany, UK, the Netherlands, Denmark, Sweden, and Norway), a large proportion (76 to 79%) of magnesium intake comes from highly processed foods. In Southern European countries, (i.e., Italy, Spain, and Greece) a lower proportion of magnesium intake derives from highly processed foods (43 to 67%), which is lower than in Nordic and central European countries, but still high [59]. Because highly processed foods are in general poor in magnesium, this may mean that people, both from the USA and European countries, consume large amounts of this type of foods to obtain magnesium, which is in any case insufficient, as indicated by the finding of frequent dietary magnesium deficiency at the population level [26–29].

The main sources of dietary magnesium, some examples shown in Table 1, contain also other components known to have beneficial health effects, i.e., other minerals and micronutrients, vitamins, fiber, and phytochemicals with recognized antioxidant and anti-inflammatory actions. Therefore, magnesium intake may be a marker of adherence to a healthy diet at a population level. Analyses of data from the Seguimiento Universidad de Navarra (SUN) prospective project showed that a higher adherence to the Mediterranean dietary pattern was associated with a lower prevalence of inadequacy for the intake of vitamins and minerals, including magnesium. Conversely, participants with a higher adherence to the Western dietary pattern (with greater consumption of red and processed meat, eggs, sauces, precooked food, fast-food, energy soft drinks, sweets, whole dairy and potatoes) were less likely to achieve adequate intakes of vitamins and minerals, including magnesium. Participants in the fifth quintile of adherence to Western dietary pattern had a 2.5-fold increased risk for having more than ten nutrient intake recommendations unmet, comprising magnesium, when compared to the first quintile of adherence to Western dietary pattern [60].

3. Mechanistic Insights on the Relationship of Magnesium and Hypertension

Several mechanisms can help explain the connection between magnesium and high blood pressure, including its calcium antagonist actions and its effects on endothelial function, vascular tone, reactivity, vascular cells growth, vascular calcification, oxidative stress and chronic inflammation, and glucose metabolism, as will be discussed in the below subsections (Table 2).

Table 2. Main Mechanisms of Magnesium-related Blood Pressure Regulation.

- Regulation of vascular tone and contraction
    - Calcium antagonism
    - Endothelial function
    - RAAS
    - Catecholamine secretion
    - Vascular calcification
- Insulin resistance
- Oxidative stress and inflammation

RASS: Renin-Angiotensin-Aldosterone System.

3.1. Regulation of Vascular Tone and Contraction

Magnesium is a major physiological regulator of vascular tone, and modulates peripheral vascular resistance by enhancing relaxation responses and mitigating agonist-induced vasoconstriction. The effects of magnesium as a modulator of vascular tone are also connected to its competitive action with calcium, while other mechanisms may be also involved as discussed below.

3.1.1. Magnesium as a Calcium Antagonist

Calcium ion plays a crucial role in the control of vascular smooth muscle cells excitation, contraction and impulse propagation. All modifications of the endogenous magnesium status determine changes in vascular tone and, consequently, variations in blood pressure [4,8]. Although magnesium is not directly involved in the contraction process, it plays a role in blood pressure regulation through modulation of vascular smooth muscle tone and contractility by controlling calcium ion concentrations and availability [61,62]. Thus, a reduction of magnesium levels raises smooth muscle calcium content; while on the contrary, an increase of magnesium concentrations reciprocally lowers calcium content in the cells [63,64]. Extracellular magnesium levels and cellular-free magnesium concentrations modulate vascular smooth muscle cells tone by voltage-dependent L-type calcium channels [64]. Furthermore, magnesium can itself function as a natural physiologic calcium channel blocker [65], modulating the activity of the calcium-channels [66]. Thus, magnesium counteracts calcium and functions as physiological calcium blocker, similarly to synthetic calcium antagonists [67].

Magnesium binds hydration water more than calcium. Hence, the hydrated magnesium, with a radius of about four hundred times larger than its radius after dehydration, is more challenging to dehydrate. This dissimilarity clarifies many of magnesium biological properties, including its calcium antagonistic actions, in spite of similar chemical charge and reactivity of both ions. As such, it is almost impossible for magnesium to pass through narrow channels in biological membranes, opposite to calcium, because of its hydration cover [68].

Two mechanisms are proposed for the extracellular magnesium-inhibition of calcium current in vascular smooth muscle cells. On one hand, extracellular magnesium would stabilize the excitable membranes and raise the excitation threshold which diminishes the current via the voltage-gated calcium channels by neutralizing the negative charges on the external surface of the cell membrane. On the other hand, it has been suggested that extracellular magnesium may reduce calcium current by directly binding to the calcium channels. Magnesium may either cause an allosteric modulation of the channel gating, or mechanically block the channel pore, thus causing its closure [69].

In vascular smooth muscle cells, the concentration of intracellular magnesium modulates their tone by means of its effects on ion channels and calcium signal transduction pathways. As mentioned, decreased extracellular magnesium activates calcium influx, while raised extracellular magnesium levels inhibit calcium influx through calcium channels [64]. Variations in intracellular magnesium modulates channels activity by altering its amplitude, activation/inactivation kinetics, and by factors such as phosphorylation, thus reducing calcium entry. The magnesium-related activation of the calcium-ATPase pump in the sarcoplasmic/endoplasmic reticulum sequesters intracellular calcium into the sarcoplasmic reticulum. Elevated intracellular magnesium stimulates inositol-1,4,5-trisphosphate (IP3) breakdown, inhibits IP3-induced calcium release from the sarcoplasmic reticulum, and competes with intracellular calcium for cytoplasmic and reticular binding sites [69] Contrariwise, low concentrations of intracellular magnesium stimulate IP3-mediated mobilization of calcium from the sarcoplasmic reticulum and reduce calcium-ATPase activity, reducing calcium efflux and reuptake by the sarcoplasmic reticulum. This causes an accumulation of cytosolic calcium and a raised cellular calcium concentration, which is a crucial factor for vasoconstriction [64]. Magnesium can also block sarcoplasmic reticulum calcium release through the ryanodine receptor [70]. The action of magnesium to compete with calcium for binding sites on troponin C also modulates the activity of contractile proteins and their dynamics [71]. In addition, intracellular magnesium regulates vascular smooth muscle cells G-protein-coupled activity of various receptors, including those for angiotensin II (type 1), endothelin-1, vasopressin, and norepinephrine and epinephrine, as well as intracellular calcium signal transduction pathways, such as translocation of phospholipase C and activation of protein kinase C [69].

Considering all those previously described direct and indirect actions of magnesium on the vascular smooth muscle cells, it is plausible to propose a role of magnesium deficiency in the pathophysiology of alterations of blood pressure homeostasis, such as hypertension. Thus, elevation of blood pressure and vascular hyperreactivity can be induced in experimental models by diminishing magnesium both in the in vitro environment, or depleting magnesium in experimental animals [72].

3.1.2. Magnesium and Endothelial Function

Magnesium stimulates vascular endothelial functions by affecting the release of nitric oxide, endothelin-1, and prostacyclin [73]. Magnesium ions directly trigger the production of prostacyclin and nitric oxide [74,75] and its concentrations were found inversely related to endothelin-1 in hypertension experimental models [76], further supporting the ability of magnesium to modulate vasodilatation. Magnesium deficit have been shown to potentiate endothelial dysfunction by means of the activation of nuclear factor kappa-light-chain-enhancer of activated B cells (NF-kB), a well-known transcription mediator of proinflammatory pathways [77], Low concentrations of extracellular magnesium reduces endothelial cell proliferation, stimulates monocytes adhesion, and impairs vasoactive molecules, such as nitric oxide and prostacycline [78]. Another key mediator of magnesium's effects on the endothelium is interleukin (IL)-1alpha, regulated by NF-kB, which in turn may be an inducer of NF-kB. IL-1alpha increases sharply in a low magnesium content environment and induces the production of various chemokines and adhesion molecules in vascular endothelial cells by activating NF-kB, hence, provoking adhesion, aggregation, and diapedesis of monocytes. Reduced magnesium concentrations trigger the secretion of IL-8 and chemokines overexpressed in human atherosclerotic plaques, promoting monocyte adhesion and chemotaxis to endothelial cells. IL-8 also stimulates proliferation and migration of vascular smooth muscle cells. The secretion of IL-1alpha induced by low serum magnesium stimulates overexpression of vascular cell adhesion molecule (VCAM)-1 on the surface of endothelial cells, which contributes to leukocyte migration. Granulocyte-macrophage colony-stimulating factor is also significantly higher in endothelial cells with magnesium deficit [78].

Supporting the key role of magnesium on endothelial function, oral magnesium supplementation was significantly associated with improvement in exercise tolerance and brachial artery endothelial function, in patients with coronary artery disease [11]. Likewise, oral magnesium improved endothelial function in type 2 diabetic older adults evaluated by non-invasive flow-mediated dilatation of the brachial artery [10]. A recent systematic review and meta-analysis summarized the effects of oral magnesium supplementation on vascular function in RCTs. Even if available studies were scarce and heterogeneity was high among the studies included, in subgroup analyses oral magnesium significantly improved flow-mediated dilation in studies longer than 6 months, including unhealthy persons, older than 50 years, or with BMI higher than 25 kg/m^2 [79].

3.1.3. Magnesium and the Renin-Angiotensin-Aldosterone System (RAAS)

In 1983, a study by Resnick et al. evaluated the relationship between plasma renin activity and serum concentrations of ionized calcium and magnesium in normotensive and hypertensive patients clustered into low-renin, normal-renin, and high-renin groups. Overall, the range of plasma renin activity in hypertensive participants showed a continuous and close inverse relation with serum ionized magnesium concentrations and a positive relation with serum ionized calcium [6]. The authors concluded that plasma renin activity may reflect modifications in calcium and magnesium fluxes across cell membranes in hypertension.

In experimental models, it has been shown that magnesium has some direct effects on the synthesis of aldosterone and indirect effects through the RAAS [80]. Aldosterone secretion is a calcium-dependent process, which can be affected by magnesium due to its calcium antagonist properties mentioned above. Rats maintained in a magnesium-deficient diet exhibited a slight reduction of the thickness of the inner zones and an increment of the juxtaglomerular granulation index and width of the zona glomerulosa of the adrenal cortex. When magnesium was restored in the diet, the thickness of the zona glomerulosa returned to normal [81]. Infusion of magnesium in humans decreased the production of aldosterone induced by angiotensin II, and on the contrary, dietary-induced magnesium deficiency enhanced angiotensin-induced aldosterone synthesis [82]. Magnesium supplementation has been shown to improve the pressor effects of angiotensin II and stimulate the production of vasodilator prostacyclin [74,75].

3.1.4. Magnesium and Catecholamines

The release of catecholamines from the adrenal gland and from adrenergic nerve terminals in response to sympathetic stimulation is a calcium-mediated process. As discussed above, magnesium competes with calcium for membrane channels, blocking the calcium entrance, and consequently modifying these calcium-linked responses. The ability of magnesium to prevent the release of catecholamines from both the adrenal gland and peripheral adrenergic nerve terminals was shown in earlier laboratory experiments [83]. Based on these effects, magnesium sulfate was used with benefit in patients with phaeochromocytoma undergoing surgery in order to help control cardiovascular changes at induction and tracheal intubation during anesthesia [84]. Subsequent cases confirmed the beneficial effects of magnesium sulfate on life-threatening pheochromocytoma crisis with hypertensive encephalopathy and catecholamine-induced cardiomyopathy [85]. Also in patients undergoing anesthesia for other reasons, pretreatment with magnesium sulfate attenuated the systolic blood pressure upsurge and the rise in norepinephrine and epinephrine after tracheal intubation [86]. Magnesium is needed for the catalytic action of adenylate cyclase. As such, in the absence of magnesium the decreased activity of adenylate cyclase leads to an increased secretion of acetylcholine from preganglionic nerves, which in turn triggers further release of catecholamines from the adrenal glands [87].

Experimental animals fed with a magnesium-deficient diet showed a significant rise in catecholamines excretion [88]. Also in an experimental model of hypertension, it has been reported that magnesium has important sympatholytic effects by blocking N-type calcium channels at nerve endings, inhibiting norepinephrine release, and decreasing blood pressure independently of its direct vasodilating actions [89]. These effects are very relevant considering that sympathetic stimulation plays a pivotal role in the regulation of arterial blood pressure [83]. A recent systematic review and meta-analysis evaluating the effectiveness of intravenous magnesium sulfate on the hemodynamic fluctuations associated with the creation of pneumoperitoneum in adults undergoing laparoscopic surgery showed a consistent reduction in the magnesium treated groups compared to placebo in heart rate, systolic, diastolic and mean blood pressures, at 5 min, 10 to 15 min, and 30 min after pneumoperitoneum, confirming its ability to blunt the physiologic sympathetic response associated with exposure to injurious stimuli [90].

3.1.5. Magnesium and Vascular Calcification

Vascular calcification refers to the deposit of calcium in the arterial wall and is closely linked to high blood pressure. Hypertension is a risk factor for atherosclerosis and intimal calcification. Nevertheless, not all vascular calcifications take place with atherosclerosis, while calcification of the vessel media is associated with reduced elasticity and arterial stiffness, a major cause of isolated systolic hypertension particularly frequent in old age. Notably, vascular calcification, independent of its anatomical site, is itself a risk factor for cardiovascular mortality [91]. Some studies have indicated a protective effect of magnesium against vascular calcification, attributable to its calcium antagonistic effects including hydroxyapatite formation and calcium transport into the cells [92,93]. The possible mechanism to explain such protective effect has not been yet fully clarified. In experimental models, it has been reported that calcium deposition in the rat aortic wall dramatically increased when the magnesium concentration was increased considering also calcium concentration (ratio of magnesium:calcium = 1:1) compared to low magnesium concentration and high calcium concentration (ratio magnesium:calcium = 1:3), suggesting that the impact of magnesium on vascular calcification might be studied in association with calcium levels [9].

In primary human aortic vascular smooth muscle cells, increasing magnesium concentrations improved cell viability and normalized the release of proteins involved in vascular calcification [94]. In this in vitro experimental model, the formation of calcium–phosphate–apatite crystals assessed with a qualitative analysis suggested a potential beneficial effect of magnesium in reducing the number and intensities of crystal formation. The authors suggested that their results seem to exclude a physicochemical role of magnesium in altering crystal growth, composition or structure, but that this attenuating effect should be linked to an active cellular role [67]. Also in bovine vascular smooth muscle cells higher magnesium concentrations prevented calcification and inhibited the expression of osteogenic proteins, apoptosis and further progression of already established calcification [95]. One of the intracellular mechanisms identified as possible mediator of magnesium's anti-calcifying effect is the inhibition of the Wnt/beta-catenin signaling pathway [96].

In community-dwelling participants of the Framingham Heart Study without any cardiovascular disease at baseline, self-reported dietary and supplemental magnesium intake was inversely associated with coronary and abdominal artery calcification [97], supporting a protective role of magnesium on vascular calcification and derived complications, such as isolated systolic hypertension, stroke and coronary heart disease events.

3.2. Magnesium, Insulin Action, Diabetes, and Cardiometabolic Syndrome

Hypertension is common among patients with diabetes, and it is a strong risk factor for atherosclerotic cardio-vascular disease, heart failure, and microvascular complications in diabetic patients [98]. A recent analysis of the tendency of diabetics to develop hypertension and of hypertensives to develop diabetes concluded that the development of diabetes and hypertension track each other over time and that a reduced insulin sensitivity is a common feature of both pre-diabetes and pre-hypertension and an index of progression to the two conditions [99]. The constellation of risk factors known as metabolic syndrome including hypertension, obesity, and impaired glucose tolerance/insulin resistance has compelling evidence of its association with magnesium deficiency [3,39,50,100–104]. Cardiometabolic syndrome represents a strong risk factor for cardiovascular events and for the progression to type 2 diabetes. There is also convincing evidence of the link between magnesium deficit and diabetes. Type 2 diabetes has been associated with both intracellular and extracellular magnesium depletion, mostly in patients with poorly controlled glycemic profiles, longer duration of the disease, and in those with macro- and microvascular chronic complications [50,105–107]. Reduction in intracellular and/or ionized plasma magnesium has been reported in diabetic patients with normal values of total magnesium [108–110].

One of the key mechanisms that may induce magnesium depletion in diabetes is a low dietary magnesium intake and an increase in magnesium urinary loss, while absorption and retention of dietary magnesium appears to be unmodified in these patients [111]. A diet deficient in magnesium, very common in western dietary patterns full of ultra-processed food, has been associated with an impaired cellular insulin-mediated glucose uptake and with a remarkably high risk of developing glucose intolerance and type 2 diabetes [50]. On the other hand, magnesium depletion in diabetic patients has been related to renal calcium and magnesium wasting. It has been suggested that both, hyperglycemia and hyperinsulinemia, may play a role in the increased urinary magnesium excretion contributing to magnesium reduction. Urinary magnesium excretion rates were more than doubled in diabetic patients during hyperglycemia, in parallel with a reduction in plasma magnesium [112]. An effective metabolic control is associated with a reduced urinary magnesium wasting [107]. In addition, hyperinsulinemia, associated with insulin resistant conditions, may contribute per se to the urinary magnesium depletion, while reduced insulin sensitivity may itself affect magnesium transport [113]. In this way, lower magnesium levels may not only be a consequence, but may also predispose to the development of diabetes. Insulin resistance reduces renal magnesium reabsorption leading to urinary magnesium wasting. Thus, persons with type 2 diabetes may end up in a vicious circle in which hypomagnesemia causes insulin resistance and insulin resistance reinforces magnesium depletion [50,105].

After the introduction of insulin-containing extracts from animal pancreas as a lifesaving therapy for diabetes in the early 1920s [114], a study published in 1933 reported increased blood magnesium and sodium concentrations during therapy with impure insulin extracts [115]. Only 30 years later in 1960 when synthetic insulin was available and methods of magnesium measurements improved, it became apparent that insulin regulates magnesium renal reabsorption [116]. Afterwards, microperfusion experiments in mouse thick ascending limb of Henle loop showed an increased magnesium permeability after addition of insulin [117]. Furthermore, insulin stimulated magnesium uptake in mouse distal convoluted tubule cells [118]. It seems then clear that magnesium transport is a key molecular target to help explain the actions of insulin in the kidney.

In the last decades there have been advances in the study of magnesium transport systems, but the results of the available studies are still inconsistent. For example, in 2012, transient receptor potential melastatin type 6 (TRPM6) was identified as the molecular target of insulin signaling and some mutations in TRPM6 were proposed as responsible for rendering the channel insensitive to insulin stimulation in patch clamp analyses [119]. This was not confirmed when higher amounts of magnesium intake were examined together with possible genetic variations. Analyses of fifteen studies from the CHARGE (Cohorts for Heart and Aging Research in Genomic Epidemiology) Consortium providing data from 52,684 participants showed that magnesium intake was significantly and inversely associated with fasting glucose and insulin, after adjustment for age, sex, energy intake, body mass index, and behavioral risk factors. No magnesium-related SNP (single nucleotide polymorphism) or interaction between any SNP and magnesium reached significance after correction for multiple testing [120]. Also in experimental models, the mRNA expression of TRPM6 in diabetic rats, are contradictory with some reports showing increased TRPM6 expression [121], and others showing downregulation of TRPM6 [122]. These inconsistencies, as in other animal studies, may depend on the different experimental model used. Moreover, because hypomagnesemia may per se stimulate TRPM6 expression [123], it is difficult to isolate the effects of hypomagnesemia from those of diabetes itself.

Another transport system involved in the renal actions of insulin is the thiazide-sensitive Na-Cl cotransporter in the distal convoluted tubule [124–127]. Insulin stimulation of this system has been shown to increase sodium reabsorption by activating an intracellular signaling cascade that includes mTOR complex 2 and stress-activated protein kinase/oxidative stress responsive kinase to increase Na-Cl cotransporter phosphorylation and activity [124,126,127]. It is noteworthy that, as mentioned above, all phosphorylation reactions are magnesium dependent. It has been suggested that hyperinsulinemia in patients with diabetes may cause an increased activation of Na-Cl cotransporter, hence, of renal sodium reabsorption, contributing to hypertension that is so common in type 2 diabetic patients [98]. This assumption is backed by studies in Zucker obese rats and db/db mice showing hypertension, hyperinsulinemia, and increased Na-Cl cotransporter activity [125,126].

In epidemiological studies magnesium deficit has been linked to an increased risk of glucose intolerance, type 2 diabetes and cardio-metabolic syndrome [39,100,128] Depletion of intracellular magnesium inducing an altered activity of the tyrosine kinase insulin receptor, as well as all other magnesium-dependent kinases of the insulin signaling, impairs insulin sensitivity and may contribute to the development of clinical conditions associated with a reduced insulin sensitivity, such as glucose intolerance, type 2 diabetes and hypertension. Additional mechanisms proposed to explain the link of magnesium with insulin resistance/metabolic syndrome are inflammation and oxidative stress. In general, conditions commonly associated with magnesium deficiency, such as diabetes and aging, are also associated with increased free radical formation and derived damage to cellular processes [50,129]. The view that a dietary magnesium deficit may cause and/or exacerbate insulin resistance is confirmed by data, both in experimental animals [130] and in humans [82], showing that a diet poor in magnesium is associated with insulin resistance. A magnesium-deficient diet caused a significant impairment of insulin-mediated glucose uptake in sheep [131], while magnesium supplementation delayed the development of diabetes in a rat model of diabetes [132]. A higher intake of magnesium was related to lower fasting insulin concentrations among non-diabetic women [133], and a significant inverse association was present between total dietary magnesium intake and the insulin responses to an oral glucose tolerance test [134]. Because of this reported increased risk for developing glucose intolerance and type 2 diabetes in persons with dietary magnesium deficits, it has been proposed a potential benefit of dietary magnesium supplementation, as a preventive tool in persons with diabetes or at risk for developing type 2 diabetes. However, the number of studies concerning magnesium supplementation in people with or at risk of diabetes is still limited [135]. Benefits of Mg supplementation on glucose control improvements have been suggested in most, but not all, studies. A systematic review and meta-analysis from our group including eighteen double-blind randomized controlled trials (RCTs), twelve in people with diabetes and six in people at high risk of diabetes, showed that magnesium supplementation appears to have a beneficial effect improving glucose parameters in persons with diabetes and also improving insulin-sensitivity parameters in those at high risk of diabetes [136].

3.3. Magnesium, Oxidative Stress and Chronic Inflammation

The etiology of hypertension involves the complex interaction among various elements, including genetic, environmental, anatomic, adaptive, neural, endocrine, humoral, and hemodynamic factors, first described by Irvine Page in his mosaic theory [137]. Since then, with the enormous progress in hypertension research it has become apparent that common molecular and cellular events in various organs lie beneath many features of the original mosaic theory. In 2013, David Harrison highlighted oxidative stress and inflammation as major drivers harmonizing diverse cellular events and organ systems involvement in hypertension, revisiting Page's theory. Harrison proposed that oxidative stress and inflammation increase neuronal firing in specific brain centers, increase sympathetic outflow, alter vascular tone and morphology, and cause sodium retention in the kidney together with other cellular signals, including calcium signaling and endoplasmic reticulum stress [138]. The crucial role of inflammation in cardiovascular and metabolic disease was first proposed by Ross in the 1990s, showing that excessive inflammatory-fibroproliferative responses to various forms of injury to arterial endothelium and smooth muscle are soundly involved in atherogenesis [139]. Nowadays, there is compelling experimental and clinical evidence indicating that hypertension is associated with inflammation, fibrosis, and activation of immune cells, processes that are driven in large part by oxidative stress [140]. Expression of vascular cell adhesion molecules (VCAMs), production of inflammatory mediators (e.g., tumor necrosis factor [TNF], IL-1, IL-6, 1L-17), stimulation of proinflammatory signaling pathways (e.g., mitogen-activated protein kinase [MAPK], signal transducer and activator of transcription [STAT]), activation of transcription factors (e.g., NF-kB, STAT activator protein 1, hypoxia-inducible factor 1), and circulating levels of inflammatory biomarkers (e.g., C-reactive protein [CRP], plasminogen activator inhibitor [PAI]-1, ILs) are all increased in hypertension [141–143]. Although it still remains unclear whether inflammation is a cause or an effect of hypertension, it is clear that the immune system and oxidative stress are important players.

Along with all the above-mentioned actions on key mediators of hypertension, it has been convincingly shown that low blood concentrations of magnesium are associated with an increased production of oxygen free radicals also known as reactive oxygen species (ROS). Also diets with poor magnesium content have been linked to a low-grade chronic inflammatory state, mainly by two mechanisms: first, by initiating an excessive production and release of IL-1beta and TNF-alfa, and second, by triggering the synthesis of nitric oxide and of some inflammatory markers [144,145]. Magnesium deficiency increases platelet aggregation and adhesiveness, and inhibits growth and migration of endothelial cell, potentially altering microvascular functions [145].

Several studies in experimental models have shown that magnesium deficiency causes: (i) elevation of proinflammatory molecules TNF-alfa, IL-1-beta, IL-6, VCAM-1, and PAI-1 [145,146]; (ii) increased circulating inflammatory cells [147]; and (iii) increased hepatic production and release of acute phase proteins (i.e., complement, alfa2-macroglobulin, fibrinogen) [145,148]. As mentioned above, endothelial dysfunction associated with low magnesium exposure has been linked to the release of inflammatory mediators [149].

In humans, clinical data have demonstrated that reduced serum magnesium levels as well as low dietary magnesium intakes are strongly associated with low-grade systemic inflammation [12,28,150]. Other studies have shown an inverse relationship of dietary magnesium intake and serum magnesium with inflammation markers. The Women's Health Study has shown that magnesium dietary intake was inversely related to systemic inflammation, measured by serum CRP concentrations, as well as with the prevalence of the metabolic syndrome in adult women [103]. Magnesium intake was inversely longitudinally related to incident diabetes in a large population of American adults, at least in part explained by the inverse association of magnesium intake with systemic inflammation and insulin resistance [151]. In addition, using the 1999–2002 NHANES databases, it was found that magnesium intake was inversely associated with CRP levels. Among 70% of the population studied, not taking magnesium supplements, dietary magnesium intake below the RDA was significantly related to an increased risk of having elevated CRP [28]. A recent investigation confirmed the significantly inverse relationship of low dietary magnesium intake with serum hs-CRP concentrations in a large Finish population [152].

Magnesium deficits have also been associated with decreased antioxidant defense competence and increased oxidative stress. There is evidence showing that magnesium depletion may cause an increased production of oxygen-derived free radicals in different tissues, decreased antioxidant enzyme expression and activity, decreased cellular and tissue antioxidant levels, increased production of superoxide anion by inflammatory cells and increased oxygen peroxide production and increased oxidative tissue damage [145,153].

Low serum magnesium (i.e., extracellular) can trigger magnesium transporters such as TRPM7 and solute carrier family 41 A1 (SLC41A1), a mammalian magnesium carrier [154], inducing magnesium efflux from cells to increase serum magnesium concentrations. This may decrease intracellular magnesium altering magnesium- and ATP-dependent cellular signaling functions. A decreased intracellular magnesium may trigger magnesium stores in the mitochondria to release magnesium [155] through SLC41A3 [156]. Reduced mitochondrial magnesium content may further compromise magnesium- and ATP-associated mitochondrial signaling and functions. This may explain the mitochondrial overproduction of ROS and decreased ATP observed in magnesium deficient mice [157,158]. Recently, it has been shown that magnesium deficiency in diabetic mice increased mitochondrial oxidative stress and contributed to cardiac diastolic dysfunction, which was reversed by magnesium supplementation [157]. Thus, magnesium can act as a mitochondrial antioxidant. Magnesium deficiency has been shown to alter mitochondrial function by several mechanisms, including alterations in coupled respiration [159–161], increasing mitochondrial ROS production [157,158,162], suppressing the antioxidant defense system (e.g., superoxide dismutase, glutathione, catalase, vitamin E) [163–166], inducing calcium overload via the mitochondrial calcium uniporter [157,167,168], attenuating pro-survival signaling [169–171], and promoting opening of mitochondrial ATP-sensitive potassium channel [172], inner membrane anion channel [173], and mitochondrial permeability transition pore [174]. These effects result in depolarization of the mitochondrial membrane potential [167]. Conversely, magnesium repletion has been shown to improve mitochondrial function by suppression of mitochondrial ROS overproduction [157,158], inhibition of mitochondrial permeability transition pore opening and cytochrome C release [175–177], preservation of mitochondrial membrane potential [178,179], reduction of mitochondrial calcium accumulation [180–182], increase of protein expression of the anti-apoptotic B-cell lymphoma 2 (Bcl-2) family and concurrently decreasing pro-apoptotic protein expression such as Bcl-2-associated X protein [169,179], decrease of apoptosis by suppressing activation of hypoxia-inducible factor 1alpha and p38 mitogenactivated protein kinase/c-Jun N-terminal kinase (p38/JNK) signaling [179], and by downregulation of autophagy [182].

We have previously proposed a link between the action of magnesium to alter the antioxidant capacity and to increase oxidative stress, inflammation, and lipid oxidation with the possible development of insulin resistance, type 2 diabetes, hypertension and cardio-metabolic syndrome [50]. Aging, very frequently associated with cardiovascular disease including hypertension, as well as with other chronic diseases, is characterized by a chronic, low-grade inflammatory state that involves several tissues and organs, and that has been named "inflammaging" [183]. Our group has suggested a link between the magnesium deficit through its role in causing a pro-oxidant –pro-inflammatory state to several age-related diseases and the low-grade inflammation associated with aging [15,129]. Magnesium itself has antioxidant properties scavenging oxygen radicals possibly by affecting the rate of spontaneous dismutation of the superoxide ion [184] and all the other mechanisms described above.

4. Hypertension in Old Age and Magnesium Deficit—Two Frequent Coexisting Conditions

Aging is accompanied by significant hemodynamic changes, leading to an ever-growing pandemic of hypertension. Modifications in central arterial structures are characterized initially by a decline in aortic distensibility with an increased diastolic blood pressure, followed by a sharp increase in pulse wave velocity (PWV), pulse pressure (PP) and systolic blood pressure, beyond the sixth decade. These trajectories of PWV and PP differ with advancing age. In addition, there is an increased prevalence of salt-sensitive hypertension in old age [185]. Epidemiological data from the Framingham Study suggest that the lifetime risk of incident hypertension is over 90% for a person aged 55 to 65 years [186]. Arterial stiffness is the major cause of elevated systolic blood pressure and PP (systolic minus diastolic blood pressure) as well as lower diastolic blood pressure in older adults. These age-related vascular alterations are powerful determinants of major cardiovascular disease events and all-cause mortality [187–191]. Vascular aging entails modifications in the properties of all the elements of the vascular wall, including endothelium, vascular smooth muscle, and extracellular matrix, leading to vascular stiffness and possible elevation of systolic blood pressure. These age-related arterial changes and those associated with hypertension (and with diabetes and atherosclerosis) are strictly connected at the cellular and molecular levels [192]. In the young adult, arterial vessels adapt blood flow and pressure during cardiac systole to facilitate perfusion to tissues during diastole. This is largely determined by elasticity, distensibility, and compliance of the arterial wall. Increased stiffness and loss of elasticity need greater force to accommodate blood flow, leading to increased systolic blood pressure and consequent increased cardiac work load. Various interrelating factors at the systemic (blood pressure, hemodynamics), vascular (vascular contraction/dilatation, extracellular matrix remodeling), cellular (cytoskeletal organization and inflammatory responses in endothelial cells and vascular smooth muscle), and molecular (oxidative stress, intracellular signaling, and mechanotransduction) levels contribute to arterial stiffness in hypertension [187–189]. Modifications in magnesium status and cellular content play a key role in many of these processes as discussed in previous subsections. Hence, interventions focused on correcting magnesium deficiency and maintaining an optimal magnesium balance may prove to be an appropriate strategy against arterial aging due to its positive effects on various mediators of the vascular aging process.

In experimental models, the effects of magnesium deficit and supplementation on the mechanical properties of common carotid artery were assessed continuously with an echo-tracking device. Histological examination showed a larger cross-sectional area, increased intima-media thickness and a greater media:lumen value in carotid artery of magnesium-deficient rats, suggesting growth and/or proliferation of arterial wall components in this condition. A negative linear relationship between intima-media thickness and plasma magnesium concentration was reported [193]. Another experimental study compared young and old rats with long-term magnesium-deficient diet vs. magnesium-supplemented diet. Old rats fed a normal diet (not deficient or supplemented) showed increased PP, increased aortic wall thickness, loss of endothelium-dependent relaxation, and a decrease of the aortic wall elastin/collagen ratio. Long-term magnesium deficiency progressively increased systolic blood pressure and intra-arterial PP. Histological examination showed that magnesium deficiency increased the age-induced deleterious effects on composition and structure of aorta (media thickness, increased collagen content and reduction in the elastin/collagen ratio), which led to large artery rigidity [194]. In humans, aortic distensibility measured with MRI imaging in the descending thoracic and abdominal aorta in relation to ^{31}P-MR spectroscopic measurement of in situ intracellular free magnesium levels in brain and skeletal muscle showed that aortic distensibility in hypertensive patients was consistently and significantly reduced as was brain and muscle intracellular magnesium, while systolic blood pressure was inversely related to aortic distensibility [13]. Another frequent characteristic of hypertension associated with aging is sodium sensitivity [195]. It has been shown that the ability of a high salt diet to elevate blood pressure is related to intracellular free magnesium in humans [196].

Along with the higher prevalence of hypertension, especially systolic due to arterial stiffness, aging is frequently associated with magnesium deficiency [129]. The total body and intracellular magnesium content tend to decrease with age. Aging is often associated with magnesium deficiency due to reduce intake and/or absorption, increased renal wasting and/or reduced tubular reabsorption, as well as age-related diseases and their treatment with certain pharmacological therapies [129]. In general, total plasma magnesium concentrations do not change with age [197]. Variability in magnesium circulating concentrations is generally associated with the presence of age-related diseases and modifications in renal function. An increased magnesium retention rate has been shown in old age, suggesting a significant subclinical magnesium deficit, not detected by the usual measurements of total serum magnesium [198]. We observed a decline in intracellular free magnesium with age; specifically, we studied the trend of intracellular magnesium content with age, using the gold standard method (^{31}P-NMR spectroscopy) in healthy young and older persons and observed a continuous age-dependent fall of intracellular magnesium levels in red blood cells of healthy older adults [199], while total serum magnesium was not modified in the different age groups. Many older adults are susceptible to chronic latent magnesium deficiency and epidemiological data from the US and Europe have confirmed that low magnesium intake is very common [26–29,200], in societies in which it is usual that processed and ultra-processed foods are the basis of the diet [51,53,54]. This type of dietary pattern is very poor in components of high nutritional value, that is, essential macro and micronutrients including magnesium [30].

Malnutrition is a common geriatric syndrome, frequently connected to frailty [201,202], particularly in very old persons. A multicenter study from Ireland showed that 63% of persons aged over 70 years were malnourished or at risk for malnutrition [203]. Another multicenter study including 4500 older adults from twelve European countries in diverse geriatric settings reported that two-thirds of participants were at risk of malnutrition or malnourished [204]. Numerous factors contribute to malnutrition in old age including decreased appetite due to reduced sense of smell and taste, poor oral health, loss of vision and hearing, and depression-associated anorexia; decreased ability to purchase and prepare food, altered energy need, decreased physical activity and sarcopenia, loss of self-sufficiency, isolation, and financial limited access to food [201]. All these factors may certainly result in poor diets lacking essential nutrients including magnesium. A former study showed that magnesium intake in older persons was near half of recommended dietary allowance (RDA) [205]. Other studies confirmed the fact that older populations have low dietary intake of magnesium [206–208]. Perhaps older adults are more likely to experience low magnesium intake for the reasons described above, but indeed, this is a problem in the whole population regardless of age [209]. The RDA of magnesium in the US is 420 mg/day for men and 320 mg/day for women, requirement that do not seem to change with age [210], but the mean intake of magnesium in the US older population is far below this recommendation (225 and 166 mg/day for men and women, respectively) [26]. Sixty-eight per cent of US adult population has been shown to consume less than the RDA of magnesium, 45% consume less than 75% of the RDA, and 19% consume less than 50% of the RDA [28]. The "Suppléments en Vitamines et Minéraux AntioXydants" (SU.VI.MAX) French study showed that 77% of women and 72% of men had dietary magnesium intakes lower than RDA; and 23% of women and 18% of men consumed less than two thirds of the RDA [200]. The problem of dietary magnesium deficiency is even worse in nursing home residents [211–217].

Data from the NHANES III showed that magnesium intake tend to decrease with age [26]. Additionally, older people who suffer from chronic diseases and who use multiple medications have a higher risk of magnesium deficiency [15]. Decreased intestinal magnesium absorption may further contribute to its deficiency in old age [218]. Magnesium absorption occurs mainly in the duodenum and ileum by both passive and active transport. Alterations of magnesium intestinal absorption in old age may be worsen by the common age-related impaired vitamin D homeostasis [29]. Latent primary renal disorders frequent in older adults may also be associated with an increased magnesium loss linked to a reduced renal tubular reabsorption.

Secondary magnesium deficiencies may be associated with the use of multiple medicaments, known as polypharmacotherapy (i.e., loop diuretics, thiazides, proton pump inhibitors, cytotoxic drugs, digoxin, aminoglycosides, steroids), or with some pathological conditions (e.g., type 2 diabetes, insulin resistance, alcoholism, hyperadrenoglucocorticism, HIV/AIDS, acute myocardial infarction, stroke, etc.). One of the most frequently used drugs in the cure of hypertension are diuretics, which by increasing magnesium urinary loss can be a frequent cause of hypomagnesemia [219]. It has been reported the finding of hypomagnesemia in 38% to 42% of hypokalemic patients. The correction of potassium and/or calcium deficits may be difficult to achieve unless the magnesium deficit is also corrected, hence in patients with hypokalemia and/or hypocalcemia, a magnesium deficiency should be considered [220]. Unfortunately, there are no readily and easy methods to accurately assess magnesium status. The serum magnesium (only 1% of total body magnesium) is easily available but may not adequately reflect body magnesium stores which are mostly intracellular. Normal circulating concentrations may be found even if intracellular magnesium is depleted because intracellular stores are recruited to keep serum concentrations within normal range [3,110]. Therefore, as no fully accurate and robust method to measure magnesium status is available, the biochemical measurements should always be supported by a clinical assessment of patients at risk for magnesium deficiency in order to timely star a proper therapy.

Many other medications may reduce magnesium absorption and/or diminish magnesium circulating concentrations (e.g., proton pump inhibitors, antacids, H2 blockers, antibiotics, antivirals, antiepileptic drugs, and antihistamines, among others) [220]. Hypomagnesemia can become severe when different factors are combined, such as those described in a case report of posterior reversible encephalopathy syndrome (PRES) with associated hypertension, and reversal of symptoms after normalization of magnesium blood levels by magnesium administration and suspension of a proton pump inhibitor [221].

Western diets are generally very low in green vegetables and whole grains (as those examples in Table 1), and rich in refined foods, and are often severely deficient in magnesium. Most of the magnesium present in processed food is lost in refining procedures, and thus, diets that provide a high proportion of daily calorie requirements from refined or processed foods are likely to be low in magnesium [222]. Magnesium deficiency in plants is becoming an increasingly severe problem linked to the development of industrial agriculture [223]. Moreover, some pesticide agents, commonly used in the crops, such as glyphosate, may chelate minerals including magnesium [224] further decreasing the content of magnesium in soil and in some crops. Organic food, from pesticide-free soils, has been reported to have significantly more magnesium than non-organic control food [225]. Table 3 summarizes the mechanisms of magnesium deficiency in old age.

Table 3. Main Mechanisms of Magnesium Deficit with Aging.

- Primary magnesium deficit:
    - Inadequate magnesium dietary intake
    - Reduced efficiency of magnesium absorption (associated with reduced vitamin D levels)?
    - Increased urinary excretion of magnesium (associated with age-dependent reduction of kidney function and of magnesium tubular reabsorption)
- Secondary magnesium deficiency:
    - Associated with age-related diseases and comorbidities
    - Increased urinary magnesium loss secondary to drugs (i.e., diuretics) frequently used in hypertensive older adults

5. Methods

We searched, from database inception to 16 December 2020, in Pubmed the topics of magnesium and hypertension using the following search for including all the studies (observational or interventional) eligible: "hypertension" [tiab] AND "magnesium" [tiab] Filters: Meta-Analysis, Observational Study, Randomized Controlled Trial, Systematic Review. A similar search was made in Scopus. Altogether, 200 title/abstracts were eligible from Pubmed and 627 from Scopus. After removing the duplicates, 758 title/abstracts were retrieved for a total of 40 works potentially eligible. Finally, a total of 18 eligible studies were considered for this narrative review (Figure 1 and Table 4).

Papers were considered eligible if: a. they included magnesium as treatment in placebo-controlled RCTs or if they assessed circulating or dietary magnesium in cohort studies, including meta-analyses of these works; b. they investigated hypertension as main condition in RCTs or as outcome in cohort studies. Concomitant supplementations (e.g., vitamin D), not clear definition of age or hypertension or cross-sectional/case–control design/no randomized controlled trials, studies made in children/adolescents/pregnant women were reasons of exclusion.

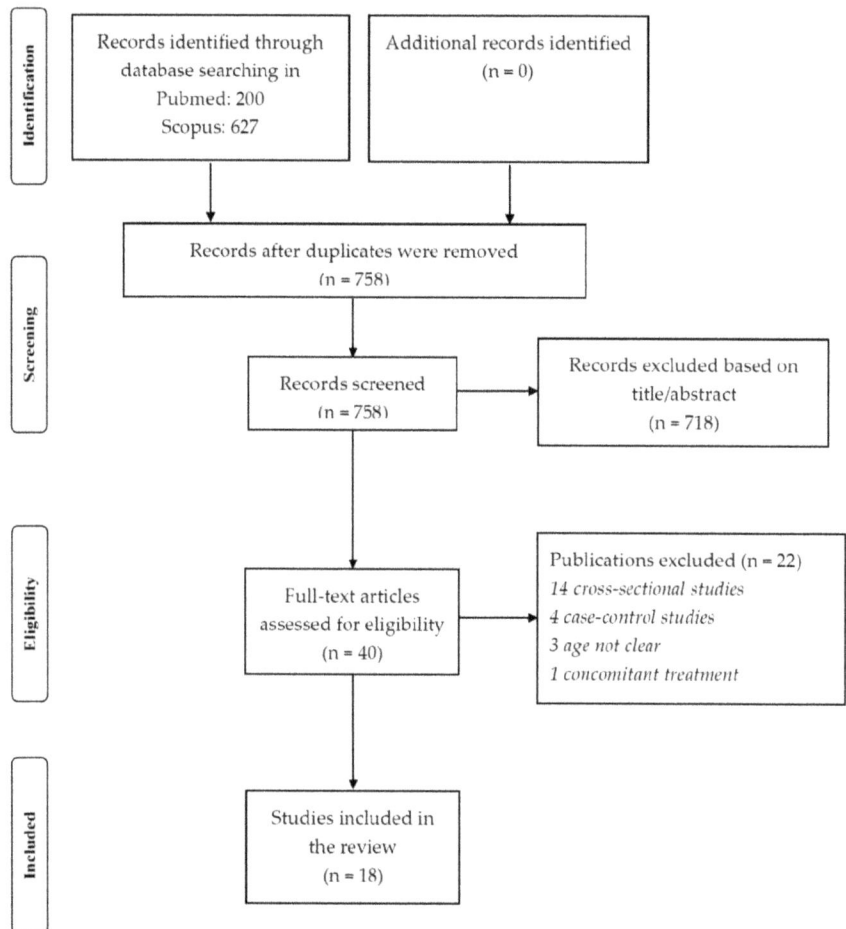

Figure 1. PRISMA flow-chart for the search and study selection.

Table 4. Summary of results from prospective studies and meta-analyses of trials and cohort studies on the association of magnesium and hypertension included in the review.

Authors/Country	Year	N. of Trials or Prospective Cohort Studies	N. of Participants/Cases	Study Characteristics	Magnesium Dose	Duration of Follow-up or Trials	Summary of Results
Witteman et al. USA [36]	1989	-	58,218/3275	Prospective cohort	-	4 years	For women with high intakes of magnesium vs. low intakes, the RR of hypertension was 0.65 (95% CI, 0.53–0.80).
Ascherio et al. USA [38]	1992	-	30,681/1248	Prospective cohort	-	4 years	Among male health professionals, dietary magnesium was significantly associated with lower risk of hypertension after adjustment for age, relative weight, alcohol consumption, and energy intake.
Ascherio et al. USA [37]	1996	-	41,541/2526	Prospective cohort	-	4 years	Among women who did not report hypertension during follow-up, magnesium was significantly inversely associated with self-reported systolic and diastolic BP, after adjusting for age, BMI, alcohol consumption, and energy intake. Dietary magnesium was not significantly associated with risk of hypertension, after adjusting for age, BMI, alcohol, and energy intake.
Peacock et al. USA [41]	1999	-	7731/1577	Prospective cohort	-	6 years	Significant trend for the association of serum magnesium and incident hypertension in women, after adjustment for age, race, and other risk factors (p trend = 0.01) but not in men (p trend = 0.16). No association between dietary magnesium intake and incident hypertension.
Townsend et al. USA [43]	2005	-	10,033/1045 in NHANES III 2311/299 in NHANES IV	Two waves national survey	-	-	Similar intakes of magnesium and other minerals in hypertensive and non-hypertensive participants in both surveys. The pattern of significantly lower mineral intake (potassium + calcium + magnesium) emerged as unique to persons with isolated systolic hypertension in both waves.
He et al. USA [39]	2006	-	4637/608 MS	Prospective cohort	-	15 years	Magnesium intake was inversely associated with incidence of metabolic syndrome after adjustment for major lifestyle and dietary variables and baseline status of each component of the metabolic syndrome. The inverse associations were not modified by gender and race. Magnesium intake was also inversely related with individual component of the metabolic syndrome.

Table 4. Cont.

Authors/Country	Year	N. of Trials or Prospective Cohort Studies	N. of Participants/Cases	Study Characteristics	Magnesium Dose	Duration of Follow-up or Trials	Summary of Results
Song et al. USA [40]	2006	-	28,349/8544	Prospective cohort	-	9.8 years	Among women, magnesium intake was inversely associated with the risk of hypertension (p for trend < 0.0001 of magnesium quintiles). This inverse association was attenuated but remained significant after further adjustment for known risk factors (p for trend = 0.03). Similar associations were observed for women who never smoked and reported no history of high cholesterol or diabetes at baseline.
Jee et al. Korea, USA [45]	2002	20 (14 in hypertensives)	1220	Meta-analysis of interventional studies	10–40 mmol/d	3–24 wks	Apparent dose-dependent effect of magnesium on BP, with reductions of 4.3 mm Hg in systolic BP and of 2.3 mm Hg in diastolic BP for each 10 mmol/d increase in magnesium dose. Limiting the analysis to the 14 trials in hypertensives, for each 10 mmol/d of magnesium SBP was reduced by 3.3 mm Hg and DBP by 2.3 mm Hg.
Dickinson et al. UK [226]	2006	12	545	Cochrane review-Meta-analysis of RCTs	10–40 mmol/d	8–26 wks	On average, people receiving magnesium achieved slightly but significantly lower DBP (mean difference: −2.2 mmHg). Poor quality and heterogeneity of the trials. None of the studies reported any serious side effects.
Kass et al. UK [24]	2012	22	1173	Meta-analysis of interventional studies	120–973 mg/d	3–24 wks	Small but significant reduction in SBP of 3–4 mm Hg and DBP of 2–3 mm Hg, with greater increased in trials with crossover design and magnesium dose >370 mg/d.
Rosanoff et al. USA [227]	2013	7	135	Meta-analysis of interventional studies	10.5–18.5 mmol/d	6–17 wks	Significant mean reduction in SBP (mean −18.7 mmHg) and DBP (mean −10.9 mmHg) in hypertensives on continuous anti-hypertensive medication for at least six months, with no more than a two-week washout, and mean starting SPB > 155 mmHg.
Zhang et al. USA, China, Canada, Japan [23]	2016	34	2028	Meta-analysis of RCTs	238–960 mg/d	3 wks to 6 months	Significant reduction in SBP (mean −2.0 mmHg) and DBP (mean −1.78 mmHg) accompanied by 0.05 mmol/L rise in serum magnesium vs. placebo. Greater BP reduction found in trials with high quality or low dropout rate.
Dibaba et al. USA, Israel [22]	2017	11	543	Meta-analysis of RCTs	365–450 mg/d	1–6 months	Significant decrease in BP: mean reduction of 4.18 mm Hg in SBP and 2.27 mm Hg in DBP in participants with insulin resistance, prediabetes, or other noncommunicable chronic diseases.

Table 4. Cont.

Authors/Country	Year	N. of Trials or Prospective Cohort Studies	N. of Participants/Cases	Study Characteristics	Magnesium Dose	Duration of Follow-up or Trials	Summary of Results
Verma et al. India [44]	2017	28 (19 trials included for HTN analyses, 4 in hypertensives)	1694	Meta-analysis of RCTs	300–1006 mg/d	4–24 wks	Significant reduction in SBP (weighted mean difference = −3.056 mmHg) with greater beneficial effect in diabetic patients with hypomagnesaemia. High heterogeneity of the trials. In meta-regression, elemental magnesium dose was inversely DBP ($p < 0.001$).
Han et al. China, Sweden, USA, Norway [21]	2017	9	180,566/4437	Meta-analysis of prospective cohort studies	-	4–15 years	Inverse association between dietary magnesium intake and the risk of hypertension. A 100 mg/d increment in magnesium intake was associated with a 5% reduction in the risk of hypertension. The association of serum magnesium concentration with the risk of hypertension was marginally significant.
Wu et al. China, USA [228]	2017	11 (3 on HTN)	Total: 38,808/4437 HTN: 14,876/3149	Meta-analysis of prospective cohort studies	-	6–8 years	Comparing highest vs. lowest category of circulating magnesium concentration, the pooled RR was 0.91 (95% CI 0.80, 1.02) for incident hypertension. Every 0.1 mmol/L increment in circulating magnesium levels was associated with 4% (RR 0.96; 95% CI: 0.94, 0.99) reduction in hypertension incidence.
Ikbal et al. Austria [25]	2019	8 (5 of RCTs, 3 of observational studies)	RCTs: 135–1694	Summary of meta-analyses	120–1006 mg/d	RCTs: 3–24 wks; observational studies: 4–15 years	The summary showed SBP reductions in the range of −0.2 and −18.7 mmHg, and DBP reductions between −0.3 and −10.9 mmHg. The meta-analysis [227] showing the largest effect, included a small sample of treated hypertensive patients, which probably responded highly to magnesium. When omitting this meta-analysis, the BP lowering effects of magnesium were attenuated to a low to moderate level. Observational studies showed a lower risk for hypertension with increasing magnesium intake or higher circulating magnesium levels.
Veronese et al. Italy, UK, Australia, Spain [31]	2020	16 meta-analyses	RCTs: 2262 participants in 34 RCTs; Observational studies: 180,566/20119	Umbrella review of systematic reviews and meta-analyses	120–1006 mg/d	RCTs: 3–24 wks; observational studies: 4–15 years	High class evidence for the association of diastolic blood pressure and magnesium in intervention studies with magnesium supplementation vs. placebo and moderate class evidence for systolic blood pressure. Large heterogeneity found for this outcome. The evidence was suggestive for the association of a higher dietary magnesium intake with a lower risk of stroke in observational studies.

BMI: body mass index; BP: blood pressure; CI: confidence interval; d: day; DBP: diastolic blood pressure; HTN: hypertension; MS: metabolic syndrome; RR: relative risk; SBP: systolic blood pressure; wks: weeks.

6. Available Evidence of the Effects of Dietary and Supplemental Magnesium on Hypertension

The role of magnesium as a therapy for hypertension in young and older adults, although first reported over 90 years ago for malignant hypertension and pre-eclamptic pregnancies [5], remains not completely defined. It is noteworthy that the use of intravenous magnesium sulfate in pregnancy-associated hypertension and especially in the prevention and treatment of seizures and PRES in eclampsia is well-established. This is based on evidence of beneficial effects in RCTs like the Magpie trial [229] and recommended in current guidelines [230–232], which prospects its validity in the third millennium after practically one hundred years of use. It should be noted that very high doses are used in pre-eclampsia and eclampsia and that the collateral effects are minimal considering that pregnant women are patients in whom particular caution is warranted due to the eventual consequences for both the mother and the newborn. Older hypertensive adults are frequently frail persons with multiple comorbidities who could potentially benefit from magnesium treatment.

Following the first use in 1925, magnesium continued to be utilized in hypertension associated with eclampsia, acute nephritis, and various vascular disorders, as testified by an article from 1942 including 40 cases with variable results [233], which discouraged further studies and recommendations of a regular use at that time. Results from different small trials remained non-homogeneous later on. Subsequent epidemiologic cross-sectional studies in the 1980's and 1990's suggested an inverse relationship between magnesium dietary intake and hypertension [33–35,234]. Straightforward recommendations were not possible upon cross-sectional studies, but the results suggested that foods rich in magnesium, such as vegetables, nuts, legumes, and whole grains may be protective against hypertension. The heterogeneous results of magnesium supplementation on the risk of hypertension, with some positive and some negative results, gave rise to a 2006 Cochrane review and meta-analysis suggesting that there was not yet enough information to recommend a wide use of magnesium in hypertension despite a small statistical reduction in diastolic blood pressure [226].

Currently, in addition to the former cross-sectional studies mentioned above [33–35,234], there is convincing evidence from prospective studies of an inverse relationship of dietary magnesium intake and of magnesium supplementation with the risk of incident hypertension [36–40], confirming a protective effect of the ion. There are few studies with non-optimal designs, two cross-sectional and one longitudinal, reporting negative or inconclusive results: one cross-sectional study from South Africa including a multi-ethnic heterogeneous population of 325 participants was inconclusive for a relationship between magnesium intake and blood pressure [42]; a longitudinal analysis of data from the Atherosclerosis Risk in Communities Study showed a significant inverse association of serum magnesium concentrations with incident hypertension in women that did not reach statistical significance in men (although the trend confirmed an inverse relationship), and no association between dietary magnesium intake and incident hypertension [41]; a cross-sectional analysis in two waves of data from the NHANES III and NHANES IV reported similar intakes of magnesium and other minerals in hypertensive and non-hypertensive participants in both surveys. However, the pattern of significantly lower mineral intake (potassium + calcium + magnesium) emerged as unique to persons with isolated systolic hypertension in both NHANES III and NHANES IV [43].

Three meta-analyses of RCTs found that participants receiving magnesium supplementation had a significant reduction in blood pressure values vs. controls [22,23,44]. The meta-analysis by Dibaba et al. included 11 RCTs and 543 participants followed up for periods ranging from one to six months. The daily dose of elemental magnesium used in the trials ranged from 365 to 450 mg. The pooled results indicated that magnesium supplementation had a significantly greater reduction in systolic and diastolic blood pressure when compared to controls without supplementation in patients with insulin resistance, prediabetes, or other non-communicable chronic diseases [22]. A second meta-analysis by

Zhang et al. included 34 RCTs and 2028 participants with a median dose of magnesium supplementation of 368 mg/d for a median duration of 3 months. The authors reported a significant reduction in systolic and diastolic blood pressure, accompanied with an elevation of serum magnesium concentrations when compared to placebo. One month of therapy with 300 mg/d was sufficient to elevate serum magnesium and reduce blood pressure according to restricted cubic spline curve analyses. A greater reduction of blood pressure were found in trials with high quality or low dropout rate, but residual heterogeneity was also found when these factors were considered [23]. A third meta-analysis of RCTs by Verma et al. evaluating the effect of magnesium supplementation on cardiovascular risk factors (including hypertension) in diabetic and nondiabetic participants found a favorable effect of magnesium supplementation on systolic blood pressure, together with reductions in fasting plasma glucose, high-density lipoprotein and low-density lipoprotein cholesterol and triglycerides, effects that were stronger in diabetic participants with hypomagnesemia. The meta-analysis included 28 RCTs, but only four were conducted in hypertensive participants [44].

Former meta-analyses suggested benefit with less prominent but still positive effects, possibly due to heterogeneity of the studies included in the analyses [24,45]. A meta-analysis by Kass et al., included 22 RCTs and 1173 participants with a range of follow-up between 3 and 24 weeks, and a daily dose of elemental magnesium ranging from 120 to 973 (mean dose of 410 mg/d). Although not all trials showed a significant blood pressure reduction, combining them there was a significant decrease in systolic (minus 3–4 mm Hg) and diastolic (minus 2–3 mm Hg) blood pressure, which was stronger for trials with crossover designed and doses higher than 370 mg per day. Overall, the size of the effect increased in parallel with the dose increment. The authors concluded that magnesium supplementation had a small but significant reducing effect on blood pressure, which warranted the implementation of larger RCTs [24]. Another meta-analysis by Jee et al., including 20 RCTs, most of them very small, with a total 1220 participants and a daily dose of magnesium supplementation ranging from 241 to 964 mg (median dose 371.1 mg/d), resulted in a small but significant effect for systolic blood pressure; diastolic blood pressure was also reduced without reaching the statistical significance. Nevertheless, there was an apparent dose-dependent effect of magnesium on blood pressure with reductions of 4.3 mm Hg in systolic blood pressure and of 2.3 mm Hg in diastolic blood pressure for each 241 mg/day increment in magnesium dose. Because the trials included were heterogeneous, the authors suggested that adequately powered trials with sufficiently high doses of magnesium supplements were needed to confirm their results [45].

Another meta-analysis with a different design by Rosanoff et al., examining 44 studies that were sorted according to hypertension status, magnesium dose and anti-hypertensive medication usage, showed that some studies reported significant lowering of blood pressure with magnesium supplementation, while others did not. Therefore, they performed analyses of a uniform subset of seven studies from the original studies identified involving 135 hypertensive participants on anti-hypertensive medication continuously for at least six months, with no more than a two-week washout, and with a mean starting systolic blood pressure higher than 155 mm Hg. In this subset of studies, the authors showed significant blood pressure reductions with magnesium supplementation (mean reductions in mm Hg of 18.7 mm Hg for systolic blood pressure and 10.9 mm Hg for diastolic blood pressure). The rest of the original trials, not fulfilling the characteristics described above, showed heterogeneous results, probably including high- and low- or non-responder participants combined [227]. The authors argued that the modest results reporter in former meta-analyses by Kass et al. [24], Jee et al. [45], and the Cochrane review by Dickinson et al. [226], were probably due to the fact that they blended dissimilar studies, which contributed to underestimate the potential of magnesium in hypertension in some (but not all) participants. Un umbrella review of systematic reviews and meta-analyses of observational and interventions studies from our group found a high-class evidence for the association of diastolic blood pressure and magnesium in intervention studies with magnesium supplementation vs. placebo and moderate class evidence for systolic blood pressure. The evidence was suggestive for the association of a higher dietary magnesium intake with a lower risk of stroke in observational studies [31].

Regarding dietary magnesium intake, a systematic review and meta-analysis of cohort prospective studies assessed the association of dietary magnesium intake and serum magnesium with incident hypertension. The meta-analysis included nine studies (6 on dietary magnesium, 2 on serum magnesium, and 1 in both) of ten cohorts and 20,119 cases of hypertension in 180,566 participates. Results showed a significant inverse relationship between dietary magnesium intake and the risk of incident hypertension when comparing the highest intake group with the lowest. For each 100 mg/day increment in magnesium intake there was a 5% lower risk of incident hypertension. The relation between the serum magnesium levels and the risk of hypertension was only marginally significant [21]. Dietary patterns reported to significantly reduce blood pressure in hypertensive and prehypertensive patients include Dietary Approaches to Stop Hypertension (DASH) and Mediterranean diet [235], both rich in foods such as vegetables, nuts, whole cereals and legumes—optimal dietary sources of magnesium. Interestingly, DASH, ranked as the most effective dietary model in reducing blood pressure [235], emphasizes the high content of minerals, including magnesium.

Concerning blood magnesium levels, a meta-analysis of cohort studies evaluated the association of circulating magnesium concentrations with the incidence of coronary heart disease, hypertension, and type 2 diabetes, including 11 studies (3 with results on hypertension, 14,876 participants with 3149 cases and mean 6.7-year follow-up). The pooled relative risk of incident hypertension was 0.91 (95% confidence intervals 0.80, 1.02; NS) comparing the highest to the lowest category of circulating magnesium concentration. However, the trend was significant with every 0.1 mmol/L increment in circulating magnesium being associated with a 4% reduction in hypertension incidence [228]. A recent review examining meta-analyses on the effects of electrolytes on hypertension including 32 meta-analyses showed that magnesium had the greatest blood pressure lowering effect followed by potassium and by sodium/salt reduction [25]. Table 4 summarizes the results from prospective studies and meta-analyses of trials or cohort studies on the association of magnesium and hypertension included in the review.

In summary, almost all (five out of seven) prospective observational studies exploring the association of dietary magnesium intake with incident hypertension reported significant inverse associations, sometimes varying among men and women. Only one of these studies reported data on serum magnesium showing a significant inverse association of serum magnesium with incident hypertension in women but not in men. All seven meta-analyses on RCTs testing the effects of magnesium supplementation on blood pressure reported significant blood pressure lowering effects. A meta-analysis of observational studies evaluating the association of dietary magnesium with the risk of hypertension reported a significant inverse association with each 100 mg/d increment of magnesium intake being associated with a 5% reduction in hypertension risk. A meta-analysis of serum magnesium concentrations with the risk of hypertension reported marginally significant effects. A summary of meta-analyses and an umbrella review reported generally positive effects as well. Nevertheless, it should be taken into account that all meta-analyses indicated the presence of large heterogeneity among the hitherto available trials.

7. Conclusions

Over the past decades, there has been an outstanding amount of experimental, epidemiological, and clinical evidence showing a close relationship between magnesium deficit and high blood pressure. As shown in Figure 2, the multiple effects of magnesium on key mechanisms linked to the generation of arterial hypertension and its complications make this link strongly plausible and help to explain the bulk of evidence supporting a protective effect of magnesium against hypertension.

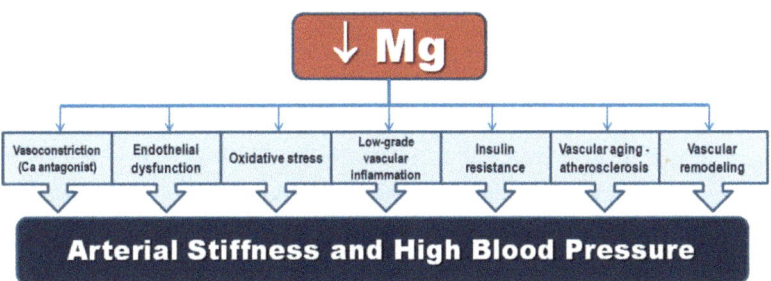

Figure 2. Combination of effects of magnesium by which magnesium deficit may lead to hypertension.

Magnesium has been used empirically for a century to treat severe hypertensive conditions, and in some cases, the most severe, such as pre-eclampsia, eclampsia-associated seizures and PRES, continues to be included in the guidelines of the third millennium, a century after having started its use. Hypertension is a complex condition in which various actors and mechanisms combine, resulting in cardiovascular and cerebrovascular complications that today represent the most frequent causes of mortality, morbidity, disability, and health expenses worldwide. This condition increases sharply with advancing age, hence older persons are those most affected by the negative consequences of hypertension. They are also more frequently at risk of magnesium deficiency by multiple mechanisms (Table 3), which may, at least in part, explain the higher frequency of hypertension and its long-term complications. Thus, older people have concurrently a higher risk for these two complex conditions. Moreover, the frequent use of diuretics as a therapy for hypertension and for one of its long-term complications, heart failure, can even worsen the magnesium deficiency.

Notwithstanding the convincing evidence that validates the possible key role of magnesium in hypertension, it is important to keep in mind that magnesium alone is not enough for hypertension prevention and/or treatment purposes. As mentioned, hypertension involves complex interactions among numerous endogenous and environmental factors; hence, the idea that it can be prevented or treated with a "magic bullet" is overstated and senseless. Furthermore, the main sources of dietary magnesium, i.e., vegetables, legumes, whole cereals, and nuts, contain also other components with health benefits, such as vitamins, other minerals and micronutrients, fiber, and phytochemicals with anti-inflammatory and antioxidant effects. At present, nutrition research emphasizes the impact of foods and nutrients combinations, as opposed to the reductionist approach based on single nutrients or foods, which was extensively considered in the past when diseases due to specific nutritional deficiencies were described and prevailing. Nevertheless, studies adjusted for multiple confounders have still reported independent associations of magnesium and hypertension. Moreover, at a population level, magnesium may be a marker of other significant risk factors for hypertension and of adherence to a healthy diet. Other non-dietary components of a healthy lifestyle are generally associated with a healthy diet [236]. Hence, dietary magnesium intake may be a marker of a healthy diet and lifestyle and may not only reflect the biological effect of an isolated healthy nutritional component.

The evidence for a beneficial effect of magnesium on hypertension risk emphasizes the importance of broadly encouraging the consumption of foods such as vegetables, nuts, whole cereals and legumes, optimal dietary sources of magnesium, avoiding processed foods, which are very poor in magnesium and lack other fundamental nutrients as well, in order to prevent hypertension. In some cases when diet is not enough to maintain an adequate magnesium status, magnesium supplementation may be of benefit and has been shown to be well tolerated.

Author Contributions: Writing—original draft preparation, L.J.D., M.B.; writing—review and editing, N.V. All authors have read and agreed to the published version of the manuscript.

Funding: This research received no external funding.

Data Availability Statement: No new data were created or analyzed in this study. Data sharing is not applicable to this article.

Conflicts of Interest: The authors declare no conflict of interest.

References

1. Ebel, H.; Günther, T.; Günther, H.E.T. Magnesium metabolism: A review. *Clin. Chem. Lab. Med.* **1980**, *18*, 257–270. [CrossRef] [PubMed]
2. Caspi, R.; Altman, T.; Dreher, K.; Fulcher, C.A.; Subhraveti, P.; Keseler, I.M.; Kothari, A.; Krummenacker, M.; Latendresse, M.; Mueller, L.A.; et al. The metacyc database of metabolic pathways and enzymes and the BioCyc collection of pathway/genome databases. *Nucleic Acids Res.* **2011**, *40*, D742–D753. [CrossRef] [PubMed]
3. Barbagallo, M.; Dominguez, L.J.; Galioto, A.; Ferlisi, A.; Cani, C.; Malfa, L.; Pineo, A.; Busardo', A.; Paolisso, G. Role of magnesium in insulin action, diabetes and cardio-metabolic syndrome X. *Mol. Asp. Med.* **2003**, *24*, 39–52. [CrossRef]
4. Gröber, U.; Schmidt, J.; Kisters, K. Magnesium in prevention and therapy. *Nutrients* **2015**, *7*, 8199–8226. [CrossRef] [PubMed]
5. Blackfan, K.; Hamilton, B. Uremia in acute glomerular nephritis: The cause and treatment in children. *Med. Surg. J.* **1925**, *193*, 617–628.
6. Resnick, L.M.; Laragh, J.H.; Sealey, J.E.; Alderman, M.H. Divalent cations in essential hypertension. relations between serum ionized calcium, magnesium, and plasma renin activity. *N. Engl. J. Med.* **1983**, *309*, 888–891. [CrossRef]
7. Resnick, L.M.; Gupta, R.K.; Laragh, J.H. Intracellular free magnesium in erythrocytes of essential hypertension: Relation to blood pressure and serum divalent cations. *Proc. Natl. Acad. Sci. USA* **1984**, *81*, 6511–6515. [CrossRef]
8. Barbagallo, M.; Dominguez, L.J.; Resnick, L.M. Magnesium metabolism in hypertension and type 2 diabetes mellitus. *Am. J. Ther.* **2007**, *14*, 375–385. [CrossRef]
9. Villa-Bellosta, R. Impact of magnesium: Calcium ratio on calcification of the aortic wall. *PLoS ONE* **2017**, *12*, e0178872. [CrossRef]
10. Barbagallo, M.; Dominguez, L.; Ligia, J.; Galioto, A.; Pineo, A.; Belvedere, M. Oral magnesium supplementation improves vascular function in elderly diabetic patients. *Magnes. Res.* **2010**, *23*, 131–137.
11. Shechter, M.; Sharir, M.; Labrador, M.J.P.; Forrester, J.; Silver, B.; Merz, C.N.B. Oral magnesium therapy improves endothelial function in patients with coronary artery disease. *Circulation* **2000**, *102*, 2353–2358. [CrossRef]
12. Song, Y.; Li, T.Y.; Van Dam, R.M.; Manson, J.E.; Hu, F.B. Magnesium intake and plasma concentrations of markers of systemic inflammation and endothelial dysfunction in women. *Am. J. Clin. Nutr.* **2007**, *85*, 1068–1074. [CrossRef] [PubMed]
13. Resnick, L.M.; Militianu, D.; Cunnings, A.J.; Pipe, J.G.; Evelhoch, J.L.; Soulen, R.L. Direct magnetic resonance determination of aortic distensibility in essential hypertension: Relation to age, abdominal visceral fat, and in situ intracellular free magnesium. *Hypertension* **1997**, *30*, 654–659. [CrossRef]
14. Soave, P.; Conti, G.; Costa, R.; Arcangeli, A. Magnesium and anaesthesia. *Curr. Drug Targets* **2009**, *10*, 734–743. [CrossRef] [PubMed]
15. Barbagallo, M.; Belvedere, M.; Dominguez, L.J. Magnesium homeostasis and aging. *Magnes Res.* **2009**, *22*, 235–246. [CrossRef] [PubMed]
16. King, D.E.; Mainous, A.G., 3rd; Geesey, M.E.; Ellis, T. Magnesium intake and serum C-reactive protein levels in children. *Magnes. Res.* **2007**, *20*, 32–36.
17. Benjamin, E.J.; Muntner, P.; Alonso, A.; Bittencourt, M.S.; Callaway, C.W.; Carson, A.P.; Chamberlain, A.M.; Chang, A.R.; Cheng, S.; Das, S.R.; et al. Heart disease and stroke statistics—2019 update: A report from the American heart association. *Circulation* **2019**, *139*, e56–e528. [CrossRef]
18. Forouzanfar, M.H.; Liu, P.; Roth, G.A.; Ng, M.; Biryukov, S.; Marczak, L.; Alexander, L.; Estep, K.; Abate, K.H.; Akinyemiju, T.F.; et al. Global burden of hypertension and systolic blood pressure of at Least 110 to 115 mm Hg, 1990–2015. *JAMA* **2017**, *317*, 165–182. [CrossRef]
19. World Health Organization. Global Health Observatory (GHO) Data. Blood Pressure. 2018. Available online: http://www.who.int/gho/ncd/risk_factors/blood_pressure_prevalence/en/ (accessed on 26 October 2020).
20. Olsen, M.H.; Angell, S.Y.; Asma, S.; Boutouyrie, P.; Burger, D.; Chirinos, J.A.; Damasceno, A.; Delles, C.; Gimenez-Roqueplo, A.-P.; Hering, D.; et al. A call to action and a lifecourse strategy to address the global burden of raised blood pressure on current and future generations: The Lancet Commission on hypertension. *Lancet* **2016**, *388*, 2665–2712. [CrossRef]
21. Han, H.; Fang, X.; Wei, X.; Liu, Y.; Jin, Z.; Chen, Q.; Fan, Z.; Aaseth, J.; Hiyoshi, A.; He, J.; et al. Dose-response relationship between dietary magnesium intake, serum magnesium concentration and risk of hypertension: A systematic review and meta-analysis of prospective cohort studies. *Nutr. J.* **2017**, *16*, 26. [CrossRef]
22. Dibaba, D.T.; Xun, P.; Song, Y.; Rosanoff, A.; Shechter, M.; He, K. The effect of magnesium supplementation on blood pressure in individuals with insulin resistance, prediabetes, or noncommunicable chronic diseases: A meta-analysis of randomized controlled trials. *Am. J. Clin. Nutr.* **2017**, *106*, 921–929. [CrossRef] [PubMed]
23. Zhang, X.; Li, Y.; Gobbo, D.; Liana, C.; Zhang, W.; Rosanoff, A.; Wang, J.; Song, Y. Effects of magnesium supplementation on blood pressure: A meta-analysis of randomized double-blind placebo-controlled trials. *Hypertension* **2016**, *68*, 324–333. [CrossRef] [PubMed]

24. Kass, L.S.; Weekes, J.; Carpenter, L.W. Effect of magnesium supplementation on blood pressure: A meta-analysis. *Eur. J. Clin. Nutr.* **2012**, *66*, 411–418. [CrossRef] [PubMed]
25. Iqbal, S.; Klammer, N.; Ekmekcioglu, C. The effect of electrolytes on blood pressure: A brief summary of meta-analyses. *Nutrients* **2019**, *11*, 1362. [CrossRef] [PubMed]
26. Ford, E.S.; Mokdad, A.H. Dietary magnesium intake in a national sample of U.S. adults. *J. Nutr.* **2003**, *133*, 2879–2882. [CrossRef]
27. Mensink, G.B.M.; Fletcher, R.; Gurinovic, M.; Huybrechts, I.; Lafay, L.; Serra-Majem, L.; Szponar, L.; Tetens, I.; Verkaik-Kloosterman, J.; Baka, A.; et al. Mapping low intake of micronutrients across Europe. *Br. J. Nutr.* **2013**, *110*, 755–773. [CrossRef]
28. King, D.E.; Mainous, A.G., 3rd; Geesey, M.E.; Woolson, R.F. Dietary magnesium and C-reactive protein levels. *J. Am. Coll. Nutr.* **2005**, *24*, 166–171. [CrossRef]
29. Rosanoff, A.; Dai, Q.; Shapses, S.A. Essential nutrient interactions: Does low or suboptimal magnesium status interact with vitamin D and/or calcium status? *Adv. Nutr.* **2016**, *7*, 25–43. [CrossRef]
30. National Institutes of Health, Magnesium, National Institutes of Health, Bethesda, Maryland, USA, 2018. Available online: https://ods.od.nih.gov/factsheets/Magnesium-HealthProfessional/ (accessed on 24 October 2020).
31. Veronese, N.; Demurtas, J.; Pesolillo, G.; Celotto, S.; Barnini, T.; Calusi, G.; Caruso, M.G.; Notarnicola, M.; Reddavide, R.; Stubbs, B.; et al. Magnesium and health outcomes: An umbrella review of systematic reviews and meta-analyses of observational and intervention studies. *Eur. J. Nutr.* **2019**, *59*, 263–272. [CrossRef]
32. Department of Health and Human Services. *US Department of Agriculture (2015) 2015–2020 Dietary Guidelines for Americans*, 8th ed.; Department of Health and Human Services: Washington, DC, USA, 2020.
33. Van Leer, E.M.; Seidell, J.C.; Kromhout, D. Dietary calcium, potassium, magnesium and blood pressure in the Netherlands. *Int. J. Epidemiol.* **1995**, *24*, 1117–1123. [CrossRef]
34. Ma, J.; Folsom, A.R.; Melnick, S.L.; Eckfeldt, J.H.; Sharrett, A.; Nabulsi, A.A.; Hutchinson, R.G.; Metcalf, P.A. Associations of serum and dietary magnesium with cardiovascular disease, hypertension, diabetes, insulin, and carotid arterial wall thickness: The aric study. *J. Clin. Epidemiol.* **1995**, *48*, 927–940. [CrossRef]
35. Kesteloot, H.; Joossens, J.V. Relationship of dietary sodium, potassium, calcium, and magnesium with blood pressure. Belgian interuniversity research on nutrition and health. *Hypertension* **1988**, *12*, 594–599. [CrossRef]
36. Witteman, J.C.; Willett, W.C.; Stampfer, M.J.; Colditz, G.A.; Sacks, F.M.; Speizer, F.E.; Rosner, B.; Hennekens, C.H. A prospective study of nutritional factors and hypertension among US women. *Circulation* **1989**, *80*, 1320–1327. [CrossRef] [PubMed]
37. Ascherio, A.; Hennekens, C.; Willett, W.C.; Sacks, F.; Rosner, B.; Manson, J.; Witteman, J.; Stampfer, M.J. Prospective study of nutritional factors, blood pressure, and hypertension among US women. *Hypertension* **1996**, *27*, 1065–1072. [CrossRef]
38. Ascherio, A.; Rimm, E.B.; Giovannucci, E.L.; Colditz, G.A.; Rosner, B.A.; Willett, W.C.; Sacks, F.; Stampfer, M.J. A prospective study of nutritional factors and hypertension among US men. *Circulation* **1992**, *86*, 1475–1484. [CrossRef]
39. He, K.; Liu, K.; Daviglus, M.L.; Morris, S.J.; Loria, C.M.; Van Horn, L.; Jacobs, D.R.; Savage, P.J. Magnesium intake and incidence of metabolic syndrome among young adults. *Circulation* **2006**, *113*, 1675–1682. [CrossRef] [PubMed]
40. Song, Y.; Sesso, H.D.; Manson, J.E.; Cook, N.R.; Buring, J.E.; Liu, S. Dietary magnesium intake and risk of incident hypertension among middle-aged and older US women in a 10-year follow-up study. *Am. J. Cardiol.* **2006**, *98*, 1616–1621. [CrossRef]
41. Peacock, J.M.; Folsom, A.R.; Arnett, D.K.; Eckfeldt, J.H.; Szklo, M. Relationship of serum and dietary magnesium to incident hypertension: The Atherosclerosis Risk in Communities (ARIC) Study. *Ann. Epidemiol.* **1999**, *9*, 159–165. [CrossRef]
42. Charlton, E.; Steyn, K.; Levitt, N.S.; Zulu, J.V.; Jonathan, D.; Veldman, F.J.; Nel, J.H. Diet and blood pressure in South Africa: Intake of foods containing sodium, potassium, calcium, and magnesium in three ethnic groups. *Nutrition* **2005**, *21*, 39–50. [CrossRef]
43. Townsend, M.S.; Fulgoni, V.L., 3rd; Stern, J.S.; Adu-Afarwuah, S.; McCarron, D.A. Low mineral intake is associated with high systolic blood pressure in the Third and Fourth National Health and Nutrition Examination Surveys: Could we all be right? *Am. J. Hypertens.* **2005**, *18*, 261–269. [CrossRef]
44. Verma, H.; Garg, R. Effect of magnesium supplementation on type 2 diabetes associated cardiovascular risk factors: A systematic review and meta-analysis. *J. Hum. Nutr. Diet.* **2017**, *30*, 621–633. [CrossRef] [PubMed]
45. Jee, S.H.; Miller, E.R., 3rd; Guallar, E.; Singh, V.K.; Appel, L.J.; Klag, M.J. The effect of magnesium supplementation on blood pressure: A meta-analysis of randomized clinical trials. *Am. J. Hypertens.* **2002**, *15*, 691–696. [CrossRef]
46. Quamme, G.A. Recent developments in intestinal magnesium absorption. *Curr. Opin. Gastroenterol.* **2008**, *24*, 230–235. [CrossRef] [PubMed]
47. Saris, N.E.; Mervaala, E.; Karppanen, H.; Khawaja, J.A.; Lewenstam, A. Magnesium. An update on physiological, clinical and analytical aspects. *Clin. Chim. Acta* **2000**, *294*, 1–26. [CrossRef]
48. Shils, M.E. Experimental production of magnesium deficiency in man*. *Ann. N. Y. Acad. Sci.* **1969**, *162*, 847–855. [CrossRef]
49. Quamme, G.A. Renal magnesium handling: New insights in understanding old problems. *Kidney Int.* **1997**, *52*, 1180–1195. [CrossRef]
50. Barbagallo, M.; Dominguez, L.J. Magnesium metabolism in type 2 diabetes mellitus, metabolic syndrome and insulin resistance. *Arch. Biochem. Biophys.* **2007**, *458*, 40–47. [CrossRef]
51. Monteiro, C.A.; Cannon, G.; Levy, R.B.; Moubarac, J.-C.; Louzada, M.L.; Rauber, F.; Khandpur, N.; Cediel, G.; Neri, D.; Martinez-Steele, E.; et al. Ultra-processed foods: What they are and how to identify them. *Public Health Nutr.* **2019**, *22*, 936–941. [CrossRef]

52. Schnabel, L.; Kesse-Guyot, E.; Allès, B.; Touvier, M.; Srour, B.; Hercberg, S.; Buscail, C.; Julia, C. Association between ultraprocessed food consumption and risk of mortality among middle-aged adults in France. *JAMA Intern. Med.* **2019**, *179*, 490–498. [CrossRef]
53. Machado, P.P.; Steele, E.M.; Levy, R.B.; Sui, Z.; Rangan, A.; Woods, J.; Gill, T.; Scrinis, G.; Monteiro, C.A. Ultra-processed foods and recommended intake levels of nutrients linked to non-communicable diseases in Australia: Evidence from a nationally representative cross-sectional study. *BMJ Open* **2019**, *9*, e029544. [CrossRef]
54. Martinez Steele, E.; Baraldi, L.G.; Louzada, M.L.; Moubarac, J.C.; Mozafarian, D.; Monteiro, C.A. Ultra-processed foods and added sugars in the US diet: Evidence from a nationally representative cross-sectional study. *BMJ Open* **2016**, *6*, e009892. [CrossRef] [PubMed]
55. World Health Organization. Noncommunicable Diaseases. Available online: https://www.who.int/news-room/fact-sheets/detail/noncommunicable-diseases (accessed on 26 October 2020).
56. Rico-Campà, A.; AMartínez-González, M.; Alvarez-Alvarez, I.; Mendonça, R.D.D.; De La Fuente-Arrillaga, C.; Gómez-Donoso, C.; Bes-Rastrollo, M. Association between consumption of ultra-processed foods and all cause mortality: SUN prospective cohort study. *BMJ* **2019**, *365*, l1949. [CrossRef] [PubMed]
57. Kim, H.; AHu, E.; Rebholz, C.M. Ultra-processed food intake and mortality in the USA: Results from the Third National Health and Nutrition Examination Survey (NHANES III, 1988–1994). *Public Health Nutr.* **2019**, *22*, 1777–1785. [CrossRef] [PubMed]
58. Eicher-Miller, H.A.; Fulgoni, V.L., III; Keast, D.R. Contributions of processed foods to dietary intake in the US from 2003–2008: A report of the food and nutrition science solutions joint task force of the academy of nutrition and dietetics, american society for nutrition, institute of food technologists, and international food information council. *J. Nutr.* **2012**, *142*, 2065–2072.
59. Slimani, N.; Deharveng, G.; Southgate, D.A.T.; Biessy, C.; Chajès, V.; Van Bakel, M.M.E.; Boutron-Ruault, M.C.; McTaggart, A.; Grioni, S.; Verkaik-Kloosterman, J.; et al. Contribution of highly industrially processed foods to the nutrient intakes and patterns of middle-aged populations in the European Prospective Investigation into Cancer and Nutrition study. *Eur. J. Clin. Nutr.* **2009**, *63*, S206–S225. [CrossRef]
60. Serra-Majem, L.; Bes-Rastrollo, M.; Román-Viñas, B.; Pfrimer, K.; Sánchez-Villegas, A.; Martínez-González, M.A. Dietary patterns and nutritional adequacy in a Mediterranean country. *Br. J. Nutr.* **2009**, *101*, S21–S28. [CrossRef]
61. Altura, B.M. Magnesium ions and contraction of vascular smooth muscles: Relationship to some vascular diseases. *Fed. Proc.* **1981**, *40*, 2672–2679.
62. Altura, B.M.; Gebrewold, A.; Ising, H.; Gunther, T. Magnesium deficiency and hypertension: Correlation between magnesium-deficient diets and microcirculatory changes in situ. *Science* **1984**, *223*, 1315–1317. [CrossRef]
63. Turlapaty, P.; Altura, B. Magnesium deficiency produces spasms of coronary arteries: Relationship to etiology of sudden death ischemic heart disease. *Science* **1980**, *208*, 198–200. [CrossRef]
64. Machado, A.R.D.C.; Umbelino, B.; Correia, M.L.; Neves, M.F. Magnesium and vascular changes in hypertension. *Int. J. Hypertens.* **2012**, *2012*, 1–7. [CrossRef]
65. Iseri, L.T.; French, J.H. Magnesium: Nature's physiologic calcium blocker. *Am. Heart J.* **1984**, *108*, 188–193. [CrossRef]
66. Agus, Z.S.; Kelepouris, E.; Dukes, I.; Morad, M. Cytosolic magnesium modulates calcium channel activity in mammalian ventricular cells. *Am. J. Physiol. Physiol.* **1989**, *256*, C452–C455. [CrossRef] [PubMed]
67. Louvet, L.; Bazin, D.; Büchel, J.; Steppan, S.; Passlick-Deetjen, J.; Massy, Z. Characterisation of calcium phosphate crystals on calcified human aortic vascular smooth muscle cells and potential role of magnesium. *PLoS ONE* **2015**, *10*, e0115342. [CrossRef] [PubMed]
68. Jahnen-Dechent, W.; Ketteler, M. Magnesium basics. *Clin. Kidney J.* **2012**, *5*, i3–i14. [CrossRef]
69. Kolte, D.; Vijayaraghavan, K.; Khera, S.; Sica, D.A.; Frishman, W.H. Role of magnesium in cardiovascular diseases. *Cardiol. Rev.* **2014**, *22*, 182–192. [CrossRef] [PubMed]
70. Houston, M. The Role of Magnesium in Hypertension and Cardiovascular Disease. *J. Clin. Hypertens.* **2011**, *13*, 843–847. [CrossRef]
71. Belin, R.J.; He, K. Magnesium physiology and pathogenic mechanisms that contribute to the development of the metabolic syndrome. *Magnes. Res.* **2007**, *20*, 107–129.
72. Altura, B.M.; Altura, B.T. Cardiovascular risk factors and magnesium: Relationships to atherosclerosis, ischemic heart disease and hypertension. *Magnes. Trace Elements* **1991**, *10*, 182–192.
73. Maier, J.A.; Bernardini, D.; Rayssiguier, Y.; Mazur, A. High concentrations of magnesium modulate vascular endothelial cell behaviour in vitro. *Biochim. Biophys. Acta* **2004**, *1689*, 6–12. [CrossRef]
74. Satake, K.; Lee, J.-D.; Shimizu, H.; Uzui, H.; Mitsuke, Y.; Yue, H.; Ueda, T. Effects of magnesium on prostacyclin synthesis and intracellular free calcium concentration in vascular cells. *Magnes. Res.* **2004**, *17*, 20–27.
75. Soltani, N.; Keshavarz, M.; Sohanaki, H.; Asl, S.Z.; Dehpour, A.R. Relaxatory effect of magnesium on mesenteric vascular beds differs from normal and streptozotocin induced diabetic rats. *Eur. J. Pharmacol.* **2005**, *508*, 177–181. [CrossRef]
76. Laurant, P.; Berthelot, A. Endothelin-1-induced contraction in isolated aortae from normotensive and DOCA-salt hypertensive rats: Effect of magnesium. *Br. J. Pharmacol.* **1996**, *119*, 1367–1374. [CrossRef]
77. Ferrè, S.; Baldoli, E.; Leidi, M.; Maier, J.A. Magnesium deficiency promotes a pro-atherogenic phenotype in cultured human endothelial cells via activation of NFkB. *Biochim. Biophys. Acta (BBA) Mol. Basis Dis.* **2010**, *1802*, 952–958. [CrossRef] [PubMed]
78. Maier, J.A. Endothelial cells and magnesium: Implications in atherosclerosis. *Clin. Sci.* **2011**, *122*, 397–407. [CrossRef] [PubMed]

79. Marques, B.C.A.A.; Klein, M.R.S.T.; Da Cunha, M.R.; Mattos, S.D.S.; Nogueira, L.D.P.; De Paula, T.; Corrêa, F.M.; Oigman, W.; Neves, M.F. Effects of Oral Magnesium Supplementation on Vascular Function: A Systematic Review and Meta-analysis of Randomized Controlled Trials. *High Blood Press. Cardiovasc. Prev.* **2019**, *27*, 19–28. [CrossRef] [PubMed]
80. Laurant, P.; Dalle, M.; Berthelot, A.; Rayssiguier, Y. Time-course of the change in blood pressure level in magnesium-deficient Wistar rats. *Br. J. Nutr.* **1999**, *82*, 243–251. [CrossRef]
81. Cantin, M. Relationship of juxtaglomerular apparatus and adrenal cortex to biochemical and extracellular fluid volume changes in magnesium deficiency. *Lab. Investig.* **1970**, *22*, 558–568.
82. Nadler, J.L.; Buchanan, T.; Natarajan, R.; Antonipillai, I.; Bergman, R.; Rude, R. Magnesium deficiency produces insulin resistance and increased thromboxane synthesis. *Hypertension* **1993**, *21*, 1024–1029. [CrossRef]
83. DeLalio, L.J.; Sved, A.F.; Stocker, S.D. Sympathetic nervous system contributions to hypertension: Updates and therapeutic relevance. *Can. J. Cardiol.* **2020**, *36*, 712–720. [CrossRef]
84. James, M.M.F.M. Use of magnesium sulphate in the anaesthetic management of phaeochromocytoma: A review of 17 anaesthetics. *Br. J. Anaesth.* **1989**, *62*, 616–623. [CrossRef]
85. James, M.F.M.; Cronje, L. Pheochromocytoma Crisis: The Use of Magnesium Sulfate. *Anesthesia Analg.* **2004**, *99*, 680–686. [CrossRef] [PubMed]
86. James, M.F.; Beer, R.E.; Esser, J.D. Intravenous magnesium sulfate inhibits catecholamine release associated with tracheal intubation. *Anesth. Analg.* **1989**, *68*, 772–776. [CrossRef] [PubMed]
87. Torshin, I.I.; Gromova, O.A.; Gusev, E.I. Mechanisms of antistress and antidepressive effects of magnesium and pyridoxine. *Zhurnal Nevrol. i psikhiatrii im. S.S. Korsakova* **2009**, *109*, 107–111.
88. Caddell, J.; Kupiecki, R.; Proxmire, D.L.; Satoh, P.; Hutchinson, B. Plasma catecholamines in acute magnesium deficiency in weanling rats. *J. Nutr.* **1986**, *116*, 1896–1901. [CrossRef]
89. Shimosawa, T.; Takano, K.; Ando, K.; Fujita, T. Magnesium inhibits norepinephrine release by blocking N-type calcium channels at peripheral sympathetic nerve endings. *Hypertension* **2004**, *44*, 897–902. [CrossRef]
90. Greenwood, J.; Nygard, B.; Brickey, D. Effectiveness of intravenous magnesium sulfate to attenuate hemodynamic changes in laparoscopic surgery: A systematic review and meta-analysis. *JBI Evid. Synth.* **2020**. [CrossRef] [PubMed]
91. Kalra, S.S.; Shanahan, C.M. Vascular calcification and hypertension: Cause and effect. *Ann. Med.* **2012**, *44*, S85–S92. [CrossRef]
92. Gorgels, T.G.M.F.; Waarsing, J.H.; De Wolf, A.; Brink, J.B.T.; Loves, W.J.P.; Bergen, A.A.B. Dietary magnesium, not calcium, prevents vascular calcification in a mouse model for pseudoxanthoma elasticum. *J. Mol. Med.* **2010**, *88*, 467–475. [CrossRef]
93. Turgut, F.H.; Kanbay, M.; Metin, M.R.; Uz, E.; Akcay, A.; Covic, A. Magnesium supplementation helps to improve carotid intima media thickness in patients on hemodialysis. *Int. Urol. Nephrol.* **2008**, *40*, 1075–1082. [CrossRef]
94. Louvet, L.; Büchel, J.; Steppan, S.; Passlick-Deetjen, J.; Massy, Z. Magnesium prevents phosphate-induced calcification in human aortic vascular smooth muscle cells. *Nephrol. Dial. Transplant.* **2012**, *28*, 869–878. [CrossRef]
95. Kircelli, F.; Peter, M.E.; Ok, E.S.; Celenk, F.G.; Yilmaz, M.; Steppan, S.; Asci, G.; Passlick-Deetjen, J. Magnesium reduces calcification in bovine vascular smooth muscle cells in a dose-dependent manner. *Nephrol. Dial. Transplant.* **2011**, *27*, 514–521. [CrossRef] [PubMed]
96. Montes de Oca, A.; Guerrero, F.; Martinez-Moreno, J.M.; Madueno, J.A.; Herencia, C.; Peralta, A.; Almaden, Y.; Lopez, I.; Aguilera-Tejero, E.; Gundlach, K.; et al. Magnesium inhibits Wnt/beta-catenin activity and reverses the osteogenic transformation of vascular smooth muscle cells. *PLoS ONE* **2014**, *9*, e89525. [CrossRef] [PubMed]
97. Hruby, A.; O'Donnell, C.J.; Jacques, P.F.; Meigs, J.B.; Hoffmann, U.; McKeown, N.M. Magnesium intake is inversely associated with coronary artery calcification: The Framingham Heart Study. *JACC Cardiovasc. Imaging* **2014**, *7*, 59–69. [CrossRef] [PubMed]
98. de Boer, I.H.; Bangalore, S.; Benetos, A.; Davis, A.M.; Michos, E.D.; Muntner, P.; Rossing, P.; Zoungas, S.; Bakris, G. Diabetes and hypertension: A position statement by the american diabetes association. *Diabetes Care* **2017**, *40*, 1273–1284. [CrossRef]
99. Tsimihodimos, V.; Gonzalez-Villalpando, C.; Meigs, J.B.; Ferrannini, E. Hypertension and diabetes mellitus: Coprediction and time trajectories. *Hypertension* **2018**, *71*, 422–428. [CrossRef]
100. Lopez-Ridaura, R.; Willett, W.C.; Rimm, E.B.; Liu, S.; Stampfer, M.J.; Manson, J.E.; Hu, F.B. Magnesium intake and risk of type 2 diabetes in men and women. *Diabetes Care* **2004**, *27*, 134–140. [CrossRef]
101. Barbagallo, M.; Dominguez, L. Ligia, J. Magnesium intake in the pathophysiology and treatment of the cardiometabolic syndrome: Where are we in 2006? *J. CardioMetabolic Syndr.* **2006**, *1*, 356–357. [CrossRef]
102. Guerrero-Romero, F.; Rodríguez-Morán, M. Low serum magnesium levels and metabolic syndrome. *Acta Diabetol.* **2002**, *39*, 209–213. [CrossRef]
103. Song, Y.; Ridker, P.M.; Manson, J.E.; Cook, N.R.; Buring, J.E.; Liu, S. Magnesium Intake, C-reactive protein, and the prevalence of metabolic syndrome in middle-aged and older, U.S. Women. *Diabetes Care* **2005**, *28*, 1438–1444. [CrossRef]
104. Corica, F.; Corsonello, C.P.A.R.A.I.A.; Ientile, R.; Cucinotta, D.; Di Benedetto, A.; Perticone, F.; Dominguez, L.J.; Barbagallo, M. Serum Ionized Magnesium Levels in Relation to Metabolic Syndrome in Type 2 Diabetic Patients. *J. Am. Coll. Nutr.* **2006**, *25*, 210–215. [CrossRef]
105. Barbagallo, M.; Dominguez, L.J. Magnesium and type 2 diabetes. *World J. Diabetes.* **2015**, *6*, 1152–1157. [CrossRef] [PubMed]
106. Mather, H.; Levin, G. Magnesium status in diabetes. *Lancet* **1979**, *313*, 924. [CrossRef]
107. Schnack, C.; Bauer, I.; Pregant, P.; Hopmeier, P.; Schernthaner, G. Hypomagnesaemia in Type 2 (non-insulin-dependent) diabetes mellitus is not corrected by improvement of long-term metabolic control. *Diabetologia* **1992**, *35*, 77–79. [CrossRef] [PubMed]

108. Resnick, L.M.; Barbagallo, M.; Gupta, R.K.; Laragh, J.H. Ionic basis of hypertension in diabetes mellitus. Role of hyperglycemia. *Am. J. Hypertens.* **1993**, *6*, 413–417. [CrossRef]
109. Resnick, L.M.; Altura, B.T.; Gupta, R.K.; Laragh, J.H.; Alderman, M.H. Intracellular and extracellular magnesium depletion in Type 2 (non-insulin-dependent) diabetes mellitus. *Diabetologia* **1993**, *36*, 767–770. [CrossRef]
110. Barbagallo, M.; Di Bella, G.; Brucato, V.; D'Angelo, D.; Damiani, P.; Monteverde, A.; Belvedere, M.; Dominguez, L.J. Serum ionized magnesium in diabetic older persons. *Metabolism* **2014**, *63*, 502–509. [CrossRef]
111. Wälti, M.K.; Zimmermann, M.B.; Walczyk, T.; Spinas, G.A.; Hurrell, R.F. Measurement of magnesium absorption and retention in type 2 diabetic patients with the use of stable isotopes. *Am. J. Clin. Nutr.* **2003**, *78*, 448–453. [CrossRef]
112. McNair, P.; Christensen, M.S.; Christiansen, C.; Madsbad, S.; Transbøl, I. Renal hypomagnesaemia in human diabetes mellitus: Its relation to glucose homeostasis. *Eur. J. Clin. Investig.* **1982**, *12*, 81–85. [CrossRef]
113. Djurhuus, M.; Skøtt, P.; Hother-Nielsen, O.; Klitgaard, N.; Beck-Nielsen, H. Insulin increases renal magnesium excretion: A possible cause of magnesium depletion in hyperinsulinaemic states. *Diabet. Med.* **1995**, *12*, 664–669. [CrossRef]
114. Banting, F.G.; Best, C.H.; Collip, J.B.; Campbell, W.R.; Fletcher, A. Pancreatic extracts in the treatment of diabetes mellitus. *Can. Med. Assoc. J.* **1922**, *12*, 141–146.
115. Atchley, D.W.; Loeb, R.F.; Richards, D.W.; Benedict, E.M.; Driscoll, M.E. On diabetic acidosis: A detailed study of electrolyte balances following the withdrawal and reestablishment of insulin therapy. *J. Clin. Investig.* **1933**, *12*, 297–326. [CrossRef] [PubMed]
116. Aikaws, J.K. Effect of glucose and insulin on magnesium metabolism in rabbits. A study with Mg28. *Proc. Soc. Exp. Biol. Med.* **1960**, *103*, 363–366. [CrossRef]
117. Mandon, B.; Siga, E.; Chabardes, D.; Firsov, D.; Roinel, N.; De Rouffignac, C. Insulin stimulates Na+, Cl−, Ca2+, and Mg2+ transports in TAL of mouse nephron: Cross-potentiation with AVP. *Am. J. Physiol. Physiol.* **1993**, *265*, F361–F369. [CrossRef] [PubMed]
118. Dai, L.-J.; Ritchie, G.; Bapty, B.W.; Kerstan, D.; Quamme, G.A. Insulin stimulates Mg2+ uptake in mouse distal convoluted tubule cells. *Am. J. Physiol. Content* **1999**, *277*, F907–F913. [CrossRef]
119. Nair, A.V.; Hocher, B.; Verkaart, S.; Van Zeeland, F.; Pfab, T.; Slowinski, T.; Chen, Y.-P.; Schlingmann, K.P.; Schaller, A.; Gallati, S.; et al. Loss of insulin-induced activation of TRPM6 magnesium channels results in impaired glucose tolerance during pregnancy. *Proc. Natl. Acad. Sci. USA* **2012**, *109*, 11324–11329. [CrossRef]
120. Hruby, A.; Ngwa, J.S.; Renström, F.; Wojczynski, M.K.; Ganna, A.; Hallmans, G.; Houston, D.K.; Jacques, P.F.; Kanoni, S.; Lehtimäki, T.; et al. Higher magnesium intake is associated with lower fasting glucose and insulin, with no evidence of interaction with select genetic loci, in a meta-analysis of 15 charge consortium studies. *J. Nutr.* **2013**, *143*, 345–353. [CrossRef]
121. Lee, C.-T.; Lien, Y.-H.; Lai, L.-W.; Chen, J.-B.; Lin, C.-R.; Chen, H.-C. Increased renal calcium and magnesium transporter abundance in streptozotocin-induced diabetes mellitus. *Kidney Int.* **2006**, *69*, 1786–1791. [CrossRef]
122. Takayanagi, K.; Shimizu, T.; Tayama, Y.; Ikari, A.; Anzai, N.; Iwashita, T.; Asakura, J.; Hayashi, K.; Mitarai, T.; Hasegawa, H. Downregulation of transient receptor potential M6 channels as a cause of hypermagnesiuric hypomagnesemia in obese type 2 diabetic rats. *Am. J. Physiol. Physiol.* **2015**, *308*, F1386–F1397. [CrossRef]
123. Groenestege, W.M.T.; Hoenderop, J.G.; Heuvel, L.V.D.; Knoers, N.; Bindels, R.J. The epithelial Mg2+ channel transient receptor potential melastatin 6 is regulated by dietary Mg^{2+} content and estrogens. *J. Am. Soc. Nephrol.* **2006**, *17*, 1035–1043. [CrossRef]
124. Chávez-Canales, M.; Arroyo, J.P.; Ko, B.; Vázquez, N.; Bautista, R.; Castañeda-Bueno, M.; Bobadilla, N.A.; Hoover, R.S.; Gamba, G. Insulin increases the functional activity of the renal NaCl cotransporter. *J. Hypertens.* **2013**, *31*, 303–311. [CrossRef]
125. Komers, R.; Rogers, S.; Oyama, T.T.; Xu, B.; Yang, C.-L.; McCormick, J.; Ellison, D.H. Enhanced phosphorylation of Na+–Cl− co-transporter in experimental metabolic syndrome: Role of insulin. *Clin. Sci.* **2012**, *123*, 635–647. [CrossRef] [PubMed]
126. Nishida, H.; Sohara, E.; Nomura, N.; Chiga, M.; Alessi, D.R.; Rai, T.; Sasaki, S.; Uchida, S. Phosphatidylinositol 3-kinase/Akt signaling pathway activates the WNK-OSR1/SPAK-NCC phosphorylation cascade in hyperinsulinemic db/db mice. *Hypertension* **2012**, *60*, 981–990. [CrossRef] [PubMed]
127. Sohara, E.; Rai, T.; Yang, S.-S.; Ohta, A.; Naito, S.; Chiga, M.; Nomura, N.; Lin, S.-H.; Vandewalle, A.; Ohta, E.; et al. Acute insulin stimulation induces phosphorylation of the Na-Cl cotransporter in cultured distal mpkDCT cells and mouse kidney. *PLoS ONE* **2011**, *6*, e24277. [CrossRef] [PubMed]
128. Song, Y.; Manson, J.E.; Buring, J.E.; Liu, S. Dietary magnesium intake in relation to plasma insulin levels and risk of type 2 diabetes in women. *Diabetes Care* **2003**, *27*, 59–65. [CrossRef]
129. Barbagallo, M.; Dominguez, L.; Ligia, J. Magnesium and aging. *Curr. Pharm. Des.* **2010**, *16*, 832–839. [CrossRef]
130. Suarez, A.; Pulido, N.; Casla, A.; Casanova, B.; Arrieta, F.J.; Rovira, A. Impaired tyrosine-kinase activity of muscle insulin receptors from hypomagnesaemic rats. *Diabetologia* **1995**, *38*, 1262–1270. [CrossRef] [PubMed]
131. Matsunobu, S.; Terashima, Y.; Senshu, T.; Sano, H.; Itoh, H. Insulin secretion and glucose uptake in hypomagnesemic sheep fed a low magnesium, high potassium diet. *J. Nutr. Biochem.* **1990**, *1*, 167–171. [CrossRef]
132. Balon, T.W.; Gu, J.L.; Tokuyama, Y.; Jasman, A.P.; Nadler, J.L. Magnesium supplementation reduces development of diabetes in a rat model of spontaneous NIDDM. *Am. J. Physiol. Content* **1995**, *269*, 745–752. [CrossRef]
133. Fung, T.T.; Manson, J.E.; Solomon, C.G.; Liu, S.; Willett, W.C.; Hu, F.B. The association between magnesium intake and fasting insulin concentration in healthy middle-aged women. *J. Am. Coll. Nutr.* **2003**, *22*, 533–538. [CrossRef]

34. Humphries, S.; Kushner, H.; Falkner, B. Low dietary magnesium is associated with insulin resistance in a sample of young, nondiabetic Black Americans. *Am. J. Hypertens.* **1999**, *12*, 747–756. [CrossRef]
35. Von Ehrlich, B.; Barbagallo, M.; Classen, H.G.; Guerrero-Romero, F.; Mooren, F.C.; Rodriguez-Moran, M.; Vierling, W.; Vormann, J.; Kisters, K. The significance of magnesium in insulin resistance, metabolic syndrome and diabetes—Recommendations of the association of magnesium research. V. I die bedeutung von magnesium für insulinresistenz, metabolisches sindrom un diabetes mellitus—Empfehlungen der gesellschaft für magnesium forschung e.V. *Diabetol. Stoffwechs.* **2014**, *9*, 96–100.
36. Veronese, N.; Watutantrige-Fernando, S.; Luchini, C.; Solmi, M.; Sartore, G.; Sergi, G.; Manzato, E.; Barbagallo, M.; Maggi, S.; Stubbs, B. Effect of magnesium supplementation on glucose metabolism in people with or at risk of diabetes: A systematic review and meta-analysis of double-blind randomized controlled trials. *Eur. J. Clin. Nutr.* **2016**, *70*, 1354–1359. [CrossRef] [PubMed]
37. Dustan, H.P. Irvine Page lecture. Legacies of Irvine, H. Page. *J. Hypertens. Suppl.* **1990**, *8*, S29–S34. [PubMed]
38. Harrison, D.G. The Mosaic Theory revisited: Common molecular mechanisms coordinating diverse organ and cellular events in hypertension. *J. Am. Soc. Hypertens* **2013**, *7*, 68–74. [CrossRef]
39. Ross, R. The pathogenesis of atherosclerosis: A perspective for the 1990s. *Nat. Cell Biol.* **1993**, *362*, 801–809. [CrossRef]
40. Barrows, I.R.; Ramezani, A.; Raj, D.S. Inflammation, immunity, and oxidative stress in hypertension—Partners in crime? *Adv. Chronic Kidney Dis.* **2019**, *26*, 122–130. [CrossRef]
41. Carbone, F.; Elia, E.; Casula, M.; Bonaventura, A.; Liberale, L.; Bertolotto, M.; Artom, N.; Minetti, S.; Dallegri, F.; Contini, P.; et al. Baseline hs-CRP predicts hypertension remission in metabolic syndrome. *Eur. J. Clin. Investig.* **2019**, *49*, e13128. [CrossRef]
42. Schüler, R.; Efentakis, P.; Wild, J.; Lagrange, J.; Garlapati, V.; Molitor, M.; Kossmann, S.; Oelze, M.; Stamm, P.; Li, H.; et al. T cell-derived IL-17A induces vascular dysfunction via perivascular fibrosis formation and dysregulation of ·NO/cGMP signaling. *Oxid. Med. Cell. Longev.* **2019**, *2019*. [CrossRef]
43. Tomiyama, H.; Shiina, K.; Matsumoto-Nakano, C.; Ninomiya, T.; Komatsu, S.; Kimura, K.; Chikamori, T.; Yamashina, A. The Contribution of Inflammation to the Development of Hypertension Mediated by Increased Arterial Stiffness. *J. Am. Heart Assoc.* **2017**, *6*, e005729. [CrossRef]
44. Kramer, J.H.; Mak, I.T.; Phillips, T.M.; Weglicki, W.B. Dietary Magnesium Intake Influences Circulating Pro-Inflammatory Neuropeptide Levels and Loss of Myocardial Tolerance to Postischemic Stress. *Exp. Biol. Med.* **2003**, *228*, 665–673. [CrossRef]
45. Mazur, A.; Maier, J.A.; Rock, E.; Gueux, E.; Nowacki, W.; Rayssiguier, Y. Magnesium and the inflammatory response: Potential physiopathological implications. *Arch. Biochem. Biophys.* **2007**, *458*, 48–56. [CrossRef] [PubMed]
46. Malpuech-Brugère, C.; Nowacki, W.; Daveau, M.; Gueux, E.; Linard, C.; Rock, E.; Lebreton, J.-P.; Mazur, A.; Rayssiguier, Y. Inflammatory response following acute magnesium deficiency in the rat. *Biochim. Biophys. Acta (BBA) Mol. Basis Dis.* **2000**, *1501*, 91–98. [CrossRef]
47. Galland, L. Magnesium and immune function: An overview. *Magnesium* **1988**, *7*, 290–299. [PubMed]
48. Bussière, F.; Tridon, A.; Zimowska, W.; Mazur, A.; Rayssiguier, Y. Increase in complement component C3 is an early response to experimental magnesium deficiency in rats. *Life Sci.* **2003**, *73*, 499–507. [CrossRef]
49. Maier, J.A.; Malpuech-Brugere, C.; Zimowska, W.; Rayssiguier, Y.; Mazur, A. Low magnesium promotes endothelial cell dysfunction: Implications for atherosclerosis, inflammation and thrombosis. *Biochim. Biophys. Acta* **2004**, *1689*, 13–21. [CrossRef]
50. Guerrero-Romero, F.; Bermudez-Peña, C.; Rodríguez-Morán, M. Severe hypomagnesemia and low-grade inflammation in metabolic syndrome. *Magnes. Res.* **2011**, *24*, 45–53. [CrossRef]
51. Kim, D.J.; Xun, P.; Liu, K.; Loria, C.; Yokota, K.; Jacobs, D.R.; He, K. Magnesium intake in relation to systemic inflammation, insulin resistance, and the incidence of diabetes. *Diabetes Care* **2010**, *33*, 2604–2610. [CrossRef]
52. Konstari, S.; Sares-Jäske, L.; Heliövaara, M.; Rissanen, H.; Knekt, P.; Arokoski, J.; Sundvall, J.; Karppinen, J. Dietary magnesium intake, serum high sensitivity C-reactive protein and the risk of incident knee osteoarthritis leading to hospitalization—A cohort study of 4953 Finns. *PLoS ONE* **2019**, *14*, e0214064. [CrossRef]
53. Weglicki, W.B.; Mak, I.T.; Kramer, J.H.; Dickens, B.F.; Cassidy, M.M.; Stafford, R.E.; Phillips, T.M. Role of free radicals and substance P in magnesium deficiency. *Cardiovasc. Res.* **1996**, *31*, 677–682. [CrossRef]
54. Kolisek, M.; Launay, P.; Beck, A.; Sponder, G.; Serafini, N.; Brenkus, M.; Froschauer-Neuhauser, E.; Martens, H.; Fleig, A.; Schweigel, M. SLC41A1 is a novel mammalian Mg^{2+} carrier. *J. Biol. Chem.* **2008**, *283*, 16235–16247. [CrossRef]
55. Yamanaka, R.; Tabata, S.; Shindo, Y.; Hotta, K.; Suzuki, K.; Soga, T.; Oka, K. Mitochondrial Mg^{2+} homeostasis decides cellular energy metabolism and vulnerability to stress. *Sci. Rep.* **2016**, *6*, 30027. [CrossRef] [PubMed]
56. Mastrototaro, L.; Smorodchenko, A.; Aschenbach, J.R.; Kolisek, M.; Sponder, G. Solute carrier 41A3 encodes for a mitochondrial $Mg(2+)$ efflux system. *Sci. Rep.* **2016**, *6*, 27999. [CrossRef] [PubMed]
57. Liu, M.; Jeong, E.-M.; Liu, H.; Xie, A.; So, E.Y.; Shi, G.; Jeong, G.E.; Zhou, A.; Dudley, J.S.C. Magnesium supplementation improves diabetic mitochondrial and cardiac diastolic function. *JCI Insight* **2019**, *4*. [CrossRef] [PubMed]
58. Liu, M.; Liu, H.; Xie, A.; Kang, G.-J.; Feng, F.; Zhou, X.; Zhao, Y.; Dudley, S.C. Magnesium deficiency causes reversible diastolic and systolic cardiomyopathy. *Biophys. J.* **2020**, *118*, 245. [CrossRef]
59. Gout, E.; Rébeillé, F.; Douce, R.; Bligny, R. Interplay of Mg^{2+}, ADP, and ATP in the cytosol and mitochondria: Unravelling the role of Mg^{2+} in cell respiration. *Proc. Natl. Acad. Sci. USA* **2014**, *111*, E4560–E4567. [CrossRef]
60. Panov, A.; Scarpa, A. Mg^{2+} Control of Respiration in Isolated Rat Liver Mitochondria†. *Biochemistry* **1996**, *35*, 12849–12856. [CrossRef]

161. Rodríguez-Zavala, J.; Moreno-Sánchez, R.; Rodriguez-Zavala, J.S. Modulation of oxidative phosphorylation by Mg^{2+} in rat heart mitochondria. *J. Biol. Chem.* **1998**, *273*, 7850–7855. [CrossRef]
162. Kramer, J.H.; Mišík, V.; Weglicki, W.B. Magnesium-deficiency potentiates free radical production associated with postischemic injury to rat hearts: Vitamin E affords protection. *Free Radic. Biol. Med.* **1994**, *16*, 713–723. [CrossRef]
163. Morais, J.B.; Severo, J.S.; Santos, L.R.; de Sousa Melo, S.R.; de Oliveira Santos, R.; de Oliveira, A.R.S.; Cruz, K.J.; do Nascimento Marreiro, D. Role of magnesium in oxidative stress in individuals with obesity. *Biol. Trace. Elem. Res.* **2017**, *176*, 20–26. [CrossRef]
164. Calviello, G.; Ricci, P.; Lauro, L.; Palozza, P.; Cittadini, A. Mg deficiency induces mineral content changes and oxidative stress in rats. *Biochem. Mol. Biol. Int.* **1994**, *32*, 903–911.
165. Shah, N.C.; Liu, J.-P.; Iqbal, J.; Hussain, M.; Jiang, X.-C.; Li, Z.; Li, Y.; Zheng, T.; Li, W.; Sica, A.C.; et al. Mg deficiency results in modulation of serum lipids, glutathione, and NO synthase isozyme activation in cardiovascular tissues: Relevance to de novo synthesis of ceramide, serum Mg^{2+} and atherogenesis. *Int. J. Clin. Exp. Med.* **2011**, *4*, 103–118. [PubMed]
166. Kumar, B.P.; Shivakumar, K. Depressed antioxidant defense in rat heart in experimental magnesium deficiency implications for the pathogenesis of myocardial lesions. *Biol. Trace Element Res.* **1997**, *60*, 139–144. [CrossRef] [PubMed]
167. Racay, P. Effect of magnesium on calcium-induced depolarisation of mitochondrial transmembrane potential. *Cell Biol. Int.* **2008**, *32*, 136–145. [CrossRef] [PubMed]
168. Blomeyer, C.A.; Bazil, J.N.; Stowe, D.F.; Dash, R.K.; Camara, A.K. Mg^{2+} differentially regulates two modes of mitochondrial Ca^{2+} uptake in isolated cardiac mitochondria: Implications for mitochondrial Ca^{2+} sequestration. *J. Bioenerg. Biomembr.* **2016**, *48*, 175–188. [CrossRef]
169. Chen, Y.; Wei, X.; Yan, P.; Han, Y.; Sun, S.; Wu, K.-C.; Fan, D. Human mitochondrial Mrs2 protein promotes multidrug resistance in gastric cancer cells by regulating p27, cyclin D1 expression and cytochrome C release. *Cancer Biol. Ther.* **2009**, *8*, 607–614. [CrossRef]
170. Salvi, M.; Bozac, A.; Toninello, A. Gliotoxin induces Mg^{2+} efflux from intact brain mitochondria. *Neurochem. Int.* **2004**, *45*, 759–764. [CrossRef]
171. Sponder, G.; Abdulhanan, N.; Fröhlich, N.; Mastrototaro, L.; Aschenbach, J.R.; Röntgen, M.; Pilchova, I.; Cibulka, M.; Racay, P.; Kolisek, M. Overexpression of $Na+/Mg^{2+}$ exchanger SLC41A1 attenuates pro-survival signaling. *Oncotarget* **2017**, *9*, 5084–5104. [CrossRef]
172. Bednarczyk, P.; Dołowy, K.; Szewczyk, A. Matrix Mg^{2+} regulates mitochondrial ATP-dependent potassium channel from heart. *FEBS Lett.* **2005**, *579*, 1625–1632. [CrossRef]
173. Beavis, A.D.; Powers, M.F. On the regulation of the mitochondrial inner membrane anion channel by magnesium and protons. *J. Biol. Chem.* **1989**, *264*, 17148–17155.
174. Zoratti, M.; Szabò, I. The mitochondrial permeability transition. *Biochim. Biophys. Acta (BBA) Rev. Biomembr.* **1995**, *1241*, 139–176. [CrossRef]
175. Gorgoglione, V.; Laraspata, D.; La Piana, G.; Marzulli, D.; Lofrumento, N.E. Protective effect of magnesium and potassium ions on the permeability of the external mitochondrial membrane. *Arch. Biochem. Biophys.* **2007**, *461*, 13–23. [CrossRef] [PubMed]
176. La Piana, G.; Gorgoglione, V.; Laraspata, D.; Marzulli, D.; Lofrumento, N.E. Effect of magnesium ions on the activity of the cytosolic NADH/cytochrome c electron transport system. *FEBS J.* **2008**, *275*, 6168–6179. [CrossRef] [PubMed]
177. Seo, Y.-W.; Na Shin, J.; Ko, K.H.; Cha, J.H.; Park, J.Y.; Lee, B.R.; Yun, C.-W.; Kim, Y.M.; Seol, D.-W.; Kim, D.-W.; et al. The Molecular Mechanism of Noxa-induced Mitochondrial Dysfunction in p53-Mediated Cell Death. *J. Biol. Chem.* **2003**, *278*, 48292–48299. [CrossRef]
178. Sharikabad, M.N.; Ostbye, K.M.; Brors, O. Increased $[Mg^{2+}]o$ reduces Ca^{2+} influx and disruption of mitochondrial membrane potential during reoxygenation. *Am. J. Physiol. Heart Circ. Physiol.* **2001**, *281*, H2113–H2123. [CrossRef] [PubMed]
179. Huang, C.Y.; Hsieh, Y.L.; Ju, D.T.; Lin, C.C.; Kuo, C.H.; Liou, Y.-F.; Ho, T.-J.; Tsai, C.-H.; Lin, J.-Y. Attenuation of magnesium sulfate on $CoCl_2$—Induced cell death by activating ERK1/2/MAPK and inhibiting HIF-1alpha via mitochondrial apoptotic signaling suppression in a neuronal cell line. *Chin. J. Physiol.* **2015**, *58*, 244–253. [CrossRef] [PubMed]
180. Ferrari, R.; Albertini, A.; Curello, S.; Ceconi, C.; Di Lisa, F.; Raddino, R.; Visioli, O. Myocardial recovery during post-ischaemic reperfusion: Effects of nifedipine, calcium and magnesium. *J. Mol. Cell. Cardiol.* **1986**, *18*, 487–498. [CrossRef]
181. Boelens, A.D.; Pradhan, R.K.; Blomeyer, C.A.; Camara, A.K.S.; Dash, R.K.; Stowe, D.F. Extra-matrix Mg^{2+} limits Ca^{2+} uptake and modulates Ca^{2+} uptake–independent respiration and redox state in cardiac isolated mitochondria. *J. Bioenerg. Biomembr.* **2013**, *45*, 203–218. [CrossRef] [PubMed]
182. Li, Y.; Wang, J.; Yue, J.; Wang, Y.; Yang, C.; Cui, Q. High magnesium prevents matrix vesicle-mediated mineralization in human bone marrow-derived mesenchymal stem cells via mitochondrial pathway and autophagy. *Cell Biol. Int.* **2018**, *42*, 205–215. [CrossRef]
183. Franceschi, C.; Garagnani, P.; Vitale, G.; Capri, M.; Salvioli, S. Inflammaging and 'garb-aging'. *Trends Endocrinol. Metab.* **2017**, *28*, 199–212. [CrossRef]
184. Weglicki, W.B.; Bloom, S.; Cassidy, M.M.; Freedman, A.M.; Atrakchi, A.H.; Dickens, B.F. Antioxidants and the cardiomyopathy of Mg-deficiency. *Am. J. Cardiovasc. Pathol.* **1992**, *4*, 210–215.
185. AlGhatrif, M.; Wang, M.; Fedorova, O.V.; Bagrov, A.Y.; Lakatta, E.G. The pressure of aging. *Med. Clin. N. Am.* **2017**, *101*, 81–101. [CrossRef] [PubMed]

186. Vasan, R.S.; Beiser, A.; Seshadri, S.; Larson, M.G.; Kannel, W.B.; D'Agostino, R.B.; Levy, D. Residual lifetime risk for developing hypertension in middle-aged women and men: The framingham heart study. *JAMA* **2002**, *287*, 1003–1010. [CrossRef] [PubMed]
187. Lakatta, E.G. Arterial and cardiac aging: Major shareholders in cardiovascular disease enterprises: Part III: Cellular and molecular clues to heart and arterial aging. *Circulation* **2003**, *107*, 490–497. [CrossRef]
188. Lakatta, E.G.; Levy, D. Arterial and cardiac aging: Major shareholders in cardiovascular disease enterprises: Part II: The aging heart in health: Links to heart disease. *Circulation* **2003**, *107*, 346–354. [CrossRef] [PubMed]
189. Lakatta, E.G.; Levy, D. Arterial and cardiac aging: Major shareholders in cardiovascular disease enterprises: Part I: Aging arteries: A "set up" for vascular disease. *Circulation* **2003**, *107*, 139–146. [CrossRef] [PubMed]
190. Safar, M.E.; Levy, B.I.; Struijker-Boudier, H. Current perspectives on arterial stiffness and pulse pressure in hypertension and cardiovascular diseases. *Circulation* **2003**, *107*, 2864–2869. [CrossRef]
191. Mitchell, G.F.; Lacourciere, Y.; Ouellet, J.P.; Izzo, J.L., Jr.; Neutel, J.; Kerwin, L.J.; Block, A.J.; Pfeffer, M.A. Determinants of elevated pulse pressure in middle-aged and older subjects with uncomplicated systolic hypertension: The role of proximal aortic diameter and the aortic pressure-flow relationship. *Circulation* **2003**, *108*, 1592–1598. [CrossRef]
192. Lakatta, E.G. The reality of aging viewed from the arterial wall. *Artery Res.* **2013**, *7*, 73–80. [CrossRef]
193. Laurant, P.; Hayoz, D.; Brunner, H.; Berthelot, A. Dietary magnesium intake can affect mechanical properties of rat carotid artery. *Br. J. Nutr.* **2000**, *84*, 757–764. [CrossRef]
194. Adrian, M.; Chanut, E.; Laurant, P.; Gaume, V.; Berthelot, A. A long-term moderate magnesium-deficient diet aggravates cardiovascular risks associated with aging and increases mortality in rats. *J. Hypertens.* **2008**, *26*, 44–52. [CrossRef]
195. Hirohama, D.; Fujita, T. Evaluation of the pathophysiological mechanisms of salt-sensitive hypertension. *Hypertens. Res.* **2019**, *42*, 1848–1857. [CrossRef] [PubMed]
196. Resnick, L.M.; Gupta, R.K.; DiFabio, B.; Barbagallo, M.; Mann, S.; Marion, R.; Laragh, J.H. Intracellular ionic consequences of dietary salt loading in essential hypertension. Relation to blood pressure and effects of calcium channel blockade. *J. Clin. Investig.* **1994**, *94*, 1269–1276. [CrossRef] [PubMed]
197. Yang, X.Y.; Hosseini, J.M.; Ruddel, M.E.; Elin, R.J. Blood magnesium parameters do not differ with age. *J. Am. Coll. Nutr.* **1990**, *9*, 308–313. [CrossRef] [PubMed]
198. Gullestad, L.; Midtvedt, K.; Dolva, L.Ø.; Norseth, J.; Kjekshus, J. The magnesium loading test: Reference values in healthy subjects. *Scand. J. Clin. Lab. Investig.* **1994**, *54*, 23–31. [CrossRef]
199. Barbagallo, M.; Gupta, R.K.; Dominguez, L.J.; Resnick, L.M. Cellular ionic alterations with age: Relation to hypertension and diabetes. *J. Am. Geriatr. Soc.* **2000**, *48*, 1111–1116. [CrossRef]
200. Galan, P.; Preziosi, P.; Durlach, V.; Valeix, P.; Ribas, L.; Bouzid, D.; Favier, A.; Hercberg, S. Dietary magnesium intake in a French adult population. *Magnes. Res.* **1997**, *10*, 321–328.
201. Dominguez, L.; Ligia, J.; Barbagallo, M. The multidomain nature of malnutrition in older persons. *J. Am. Med. Dir. Assoc.* **2017**, *18*, 908–912. [CrossRef]
202. Morley, J.E. Anorexia, weight loss, and frailty. *J. Am. Med. Dir. Assoc.* **2010**, *11*, 225–228. [CrossRef]
203. O'Shea, E.; Trawley, S.; Manning, E.; Barrett, A.; Browne, V.; Timmons, S. Malnutrition in hospitalised older adults: A multicentre observational study of prevalence, associations and outcomes. *J. Nutr. Health Aging* **2016**, *21*, 830–836. [CrossRef]
204. Kaiser, M.J.; Bauer, J.; Ms, R.P.S.A.; Uter, W.; Guigoz, Y.; Cederholm, T.; Thomas, D.R.; Anthony, P.S.; Charlton, K.E.; Maggio, M.; et al. Frequency of malnutrition in Older Adults: A multinational perspective using the mini nutritional assessment. *J. Am. Geriatr. Soc.* **2010**, *58*, 1734–1738. [CrossRef]
205. Thomas, A.J.; Bunker, V.W.; Sodha, N.; Clayton, B.E. Calcium, magnesium and phosphorus status of elderly inpatients: Dietary intake, metabolic balance studies and biochemical status. *Br. J. Nutr.* **1989**, *62*, 211–219. [CrossRef] [PubMed]
206. Löwik, M.R.; Van Dokkum, W.; Kistemaker, C.; Schaafsma, G.; Ockhuizen, T. Body composition, health status and urinary magnesium excretion among elderly people (Dutch Nutrition Surveillance System). *Magnes. Res.* **1993**, *6*, 223–232. [PubMed]
207. Costello, R.B.; Moser-Veillon, P.B. A review of magnesium intake in the elderly. A cause for concern? *Magnes. Res.* **1992**, *5*, 61–67. [PubMed]
208. McIntosh, W.; Kubena, K.S.; Walker, J.; Smith, D.; Landmann, W.A. The relationship between beliefs about nutrition and dietary practices of the elderly. *J. Am. Diet. Assoc.* **1990**, *90*, 671–676.
209. Rosanoff, A.; Weaver, C.M.; Rude, R.K. Suboptimal magnesium status in the United States: Are the health consequences underestimated? *Nutr. Rev.* **2012**, *70*, 153–164. [CrossRef] [PubMed]
210. Hunt, C.D.; Johnson, L.K. Magnesium requirements: New estimations for men and women by cross-sectional statistical analyses of metabolic magnesium balance data. *Am. J. Clin. Nutr.* **2006**, *84*, 843–852. [CrossRef] [PubMed]
211. Gámez, C.; Artacho, R.; Ruiz-López, M.-D.; Navarro, M.; Puerta, A.; López, M. Serum concentration and dietary intake of Mg and Ca in institutionalized elderly people. *Sci. Total Environ.* **1997**, *203*, 245–251. [CrossRef]
212. Lipski, P.S.; Torrance, A.; Kelly, P.J.; James, O.F.W. A study of nutritional deficits of long-stay geriatric patients. *Age Ageing* **1993**, *22*, 244–255. [CrossRef]
213. Aghdassi, E.; McArthur, M.; Liu, B.; McGeer, A.; Simor, A.; Allard, J.P.; McGeer, A. Dietary intake of elderly living in Toronto long-term care facilities: Comparison to the dietary reference intake. *Rejuvenation Res.* **2007**, *10*, 301–310. [CrossRef]
214. Iuliano-Burns, S.; Olden, A.; Woods, J. Meeting the nutritional needs of elderly residents in aged-care: Are we doing enough? *J. Nutr. Health Aging* **2013**, *17*, 503–508. [CrossRef]

215. Lengyel, C.O.; Whiting, S.J.; Zello, G.A. Nutrient inadequacies among elderly residents of long-term care facilities. *Can. J. Diet. Pract. Res.* **2008**, *69*, 82–88. [CrossRef] [PubMed]
216. Lammes, E.; Törner, A.; Akner, G. Nutrient density and variation in nutrient intake with changing energy intake in multimorbid nursing home residents. *J. Hum. Nutr. Diet.* **2009**, *22*, 210–218. [CrossRef] [PubMed]
217. Vaquero, M.P. Magnesium and trace elements in the elderly: Intake, status and recommendations. *J. Nutr. Health Aging* **2002**, *6*, 147–153. [PubMed]
218. Coudray, C.; Feillet-Coudray, C.; Rambeau, M.; Tressol, J.C.; Gueux, E.; Mazur, A.; Rayssiguier, Y. The effect of aging on intestinal absorption and status of calcium, magnesium, zinc, and copper in rats: A stable isotope study. *J. Trace Elements Med. Biol.* **2006**, *20*, 73–81. [CrossRef]
219. Chrysant, S.G.; Chrysant, G.S. Adverse cardiovascular and blood pressure effects of drug-induced hypomagnesemia. *Expert Opin. Drug Saf.* **2019**, *19*, 59–67. [CrossRef]
220. Hansen, B.-A.; Bruserud, Ø. Hypomagnesemia in critically ill patients. *J. Intensive Care* **2018**, *6*, 1–11. [CrossRef]
221. Almoussa, M.; Goertzen, A.; Brauckmann, S.; Fauser, B.; Zimmermann, C.W. Posterior reversible encephalopathy syndrome due to hypomagnesemia: A case report and literature review. *Case Rep. Med.* **2018**, *2018*, 1–6. [CrossRef]
222. Koiwai, K.; Takemi, Y.; Hayashi, F.; Ogata, H.; Matsumoto, S.; Ozawa, K.; Machado, P.P.; Monteiro, C.A. Consumption of ultra-processed foods decreases the quality of the overall diet of middle-aged Japanese adults. *Public Health Nutr.* **2019**, *22*, 2999–3008. [CrossRef]
223. Guo, W.; Nazim, H.; Liang, Z.; Yang, D. Magnesium deficiency in plants: An urgent problem. *Crop J.* **2016**, *4*, 83–91. [CrossRef]
224. Cakmak, I.; Yazıcı, M.A.; Tutus, Y.; Ozturk, L. Glyphosate reduced seed and leaf concentrations of calcium, manganese, magnesium, and iron in non-glyphosate resistant soybean. *Eur. J. Agron.* **2009**, *31*, 114–119. [CrossRef]
225. Griffiths, A.M.; Cook, D.M.; Eggett, D.L.; Christensen, M.J. A retail market study of organic and conventional potatoes (Solanum tuberosum): Mineral content and nutritional implications. *Int. J. Food Sci. Nutr.* **2012**, *63*, 393–401. [CrossRef] [PubMed]
226. Dickinson, H.O.; Nicolson, D.; Campbell, F.; Cook, J.V.; Beyer, F.R.; Ford, G.A.; Mason, J. Magnesium supplementation for the management of primary hypertension in adults. *Cochrane Database Syst. Rev.* **2006**, CD004640. [CrossRef] [PubMed]
227. Rosanoff, A.; Plesset, M.R. Oral magnesium supplements decrease high blood pressure (SBP > 155mmHg) in hypertensive subjects on anti-hypertensive medications: A targeted meta-analysis. *Magnes. Res.* **2013**, *26*, 93–99. [CrossRef] [PubMed]
228. Wu, J.; Xun, P.; Tang, Q.; Cai, W.; He, K. Circulating magnesium levels and incidence of coronary heart diseases, hypertension, and type 2 diabetes mellitus: A meta-analysis of prospective cohort studies. *Nutr. J.* **2017**, *16*, 1–13. [CrossRef]
229. Altman, D.; Carroli, G.; Duley, L.; Farrell, B.; Moodley, J.; Neilson, J.; Smith, D.; Magpie Trial Collaboration Group. Do women with pre-eclampsia, and their babies, benefit from magnesium sulphate? The Magpie Trial: A randomised placebo-controlled trial. *Lancet* **2002**, *359*, 1877–1890.
230. Fishel Bartal, M.; Sibai, B.M. Eclampsia in the 21(st) century. *Am. J. Obstet. Gynecol.* **2020**, S0002-9378(20)31128-5. [CrossRef]
231. Fang, X.; Wang, H.; Liu, Z.; Chen, J.; Tan, H.; Liang, Y.; Chen, D. Posterior reversible encephalopathy syndrome in preeclampsia and eclampsia: The role of hypomagnesemia. *Seizure* **2020**, *76*, 12–16. [CrossRef]
232. Pollock, W.; Peek, M.J.; Wang, A.; Li, Z.; Ellwood, D.; Homer, C.; Pulver, L.J.; McLintock, C.; Vaughan, G.; Knight, M.; et al. Eclampsia in Australia and New Zealand: A prospective population-based study. *Aust. N. Z. J. Obstet. Gynaecol.* **2019**, *60*, 533–540. [CrossRef]
233. Winkler, A.W.; Smith, P.K.; Hoff, H.E. Intravenous magnesium sulfate in the treatment of nephritic convulsions in adults. *J. Clin. Investig.* **1942**, *21*, 207–216. [CrossRef]
234. Joffres, M.R.; Reed, D.M.; Yano, K. Relationship of magnesium intake and other dietary factors to blood pressure: The Honolulu heart study. *Am. J. Clin. Nutr.* **1987**, *45*, 469–475. [CrossRef]
235. Schwingshackl, L.; Chaimani, A.; Schwedhelm, C.; Toledo, E.; Pünsch, M.; Hoffmann, G.; Boeing, H. Comparative effects of different dietary approaches on blood pressure in hypertensive and pre-hypertensive patients: A systematic review and network meta-analysis. *Crit. Rev. Food Sci. Nutr.* **2018**, *59*, 2674–2687. [CrossRef] [PubMed]
236. Busch, V.; Van Stel, H.F.; Schrijvers, A.J.P.; De Leeuw, J.R.J. Clustering of health-related behaviors, health outcomes and demographics in Dutch adolescents: A cross-sectional study. *BMC Public Health* **2013**, *13*, 1118. [CrossRef] [PubMed]

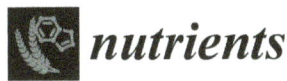

Article

Effect of Magnesium Supplementation on Circulating Biomarkers of Cardiovascular Disease

Alvaro Alonso [1,*], Lin Y. Chen [2], Kyle D. Rudser [3], Faye L. Norby [4], Mary R. Rooney [5] and Pamela L. Lutsey [4]

1. Department of Epidemiology, Rollins School of Public Health, Emory University, Atlanta, GA 30322, USA
2. Cardiovascular Division, Department of Medicine, University of Minnesota, Minneapolis, MN 55455, USA; chenx484@umn.edu
3. Division of Biostatistics, School of Public Health, University of Minnesota, Minneapolis, MN 55455, USA; rudser@umn.edu
4. Division of Epidemiology and Community Health, School of Public Health, University of Minnesota, Minneapolis, MN 55454, USA; flopez@umn.edu (F.L.N.); lutsey@umn.edu (P.L.L.)
5. Department of Epidemiology, Johns Hopkins Bloomberg School of Public Health, Baltimore, MD 21287, USA; mroone12@jhu.edu
* Correspondence: alvaro.alonso@emory.edu; Tel.: +1-404-727-8714

Received: 3 May 2020; Accepted: 2 June 2020; Published: 6 June 2020

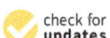

Abstract: (1) Background: Magnesium supplementation may be effective for the prevention of cardiometabolic diseases, but the mechanisms are unclear. Proteomic approaches can assist in identifying the underlying mechanisms. (2) Methods: We collected repeated blood samples from 52 individuals enrolled in a double-blind trial which randomized participants 1:1 to oral magnesium supplementation (400 mg magnesium/day in the form of magnesium oxide) or a matching placebo for 10 weeks. Plasma levels of 91 proteins were measured at baseline with follow-up samples using the Olink Cardiovascular Disease III proximity extension assay panel and were modeled as arbitrary units in a $\log_2$ scale. We evaluated the effect of oral magnesium supplementation for changes in protein levels and the baseline association between serum magnesium and protein levels. The Holm procedure was used to adjust for multiple comparisons. (3) Results: Participants were 73% women, 94% white, and had a mean age of 62. Changes in proteins did not significantly differ between the two intervention groups after correction for multiple comparisons. The most statistically significant effects were on myoglobin [difference −0.319 $\log_2$ units, 95% confidence interval (CI) (−0.550, −0.088), $p = 0.008$], tartrate-resistant acid phosphatase type 5 (−0.187, (−0.328, −0.045), $p = 0.011$), tumor necrosis factor ligand superfamily member 13B (−0.181, (−0.332, −0.031), $p = 0.019$), ST2 protein (−0.198, (−0.363, −0.032), $p = 0.020$), and interleukin-1 receptor type 1 (−0.144, (−0.273, −0.015), $p = 0.029$). Similarly, none of the associations of baseline serum magnesium with protein levels were significant after correction for multiple comparisons. (4) Conclusions: Although we did not identify statistically significant effects of oral magnesium supplementation in this relatively small study, this study demonstrates the value of proteomic approaches for the investigation of mechanisms underlying the beneficial effects of magnesium supplementation. Clinical Trials Registration: ClinicalTrials.gov NCT02837328.

Keywords: magnesium; proteomics; randomized trial

1. Introduction

Mounting evidence suggests that moderately elevated concentrations of circulating magnesium may reduce the risk of coronary heart disease and atrial fibrillation. This evidence comes from prospective observational studies [1,2], Mendelian randomization studies [3,4], and studies of magnesium supplementation in secondary prevention [5], even though observational studies do not support an effect of dietary magnesium on cardiovascular disease [6]. Mechanisms underlying this potential protective effect are unclear, but may include antiarrhythmic effects, improved glucose homeostasis, better vascular tone and endothelial function, and reduced oxidative stress and inflammation [1,7–9].

Recent advances in the field of proteomics allow the efficient evaluation of multiple proteins in biological tissues. This provides an opportunity to assess simultaneous multiple markers of distinct mechanistic pathways [10]; however, this approach has rarely been applied to the study of the effects of oral magnesium supplementation [11].

To provide novel insights into the pathways linking magnesium and cardiovascular risk, we evaluated the effect of oral magnesium supplementation on multiple cardiovascular-related circulating proteins measured using a novel proteomic assay. This analysis was done using repeated blood samples collected from 52 participants in a double-blind randomized trial testing efficacy and tolerability of 400 mg/day of magnesium oxide compared to placebo for the prevention of supraventricular arrhythmias.

2. Methods

2.1. Study Population

Between March and June 2017, we recruited and randomized 59 men and women to receive 400 mg/daily of oral magnesium in the form of magnesium oxide or a matching placebo for 12 weeks to determine the effect of oral magnesium supplementation on supraventricular arrhythmias (ClinicalTrials.gov #NCT02837328). Details about recruitment, inclusion and exclusion criteria, and study procedures have been published elsewhere [12]. Briefly, we included men and women 55 years of age or older without a prior history of heart disease (coronary heart disease, heart failure, atrial fibrillation), stroke, or kidney disease, not using magnesium supplements, and living in the Minneapolis/St. Paul, MN area. Eligible participants attended a baseline visit where they underwent a basic physical exam, blood collection, and had a heart rhythm monitor applied (Zio® XT, iRhythm Technologies, Inc., San Francisco, CA, USA). After wearing the monitor for two weeks, participants were randomized 1:1 to 400 mg/daily of magnesium or a matching placebo and the study intervention was mailed. Twelve weeks after the baseline exam (10 weeks after starting study intervention), participants underwent a follow-up visit, which included blood collection. For this analysis, we included 52 trial participants with blood samples available for proteomic analysis at baseline (pre-randomization) and the follow-up visit. The University of Minnesota Institutional Review Board approved the study protocol and all participants provided written informed consent.

2.2. Intervention

The University of Minnesota Institute for Therapeutics Discovery and Drug Development manufactured the study intervention (400 mg of magnesium in the form of magnesium oxide capsules) and the placebo (lactose) following Good Manufacturing Practices. The University of Minnesota Investigational Drug Service managed bottling. Participants and study staff were blinded to the treatment given. Compliance with the intervention was excellent. As previously reported, the magnesium group participants took 75% of tablets, whereas those in the placebo group took 83.4%, based on pill count. During the course of the trial, 50% of the participants who were assigned to magnesium and 7% who were assigned to the placebo commented on gastrointestinal changes at any point in the study, but only one participant in the magnesium arm discontinued the blinded study treatment [12].

2.3. Blood Biomarker Analysis

Participants were asked to fast for eight hours prior to blood draws at the baseline and follow-up visits. Serum and plasma samples were obtained and processed using standard procedures and stored in −80 °C freezers. Circulating magnesium was measured in serum samples using the Roche Cobas 6000 at the University of Minnesota Advanced Research and Diagnostic Laboratory.

2.4. Proteomic Measurements

Relative levels of 92 proteins were measured in never-thawed plasma samples using the Olink Cardiovascular III panel (www.olink.com, Olink Proteomics, Uppsala, Sweden). The Olink panel uses a proximity extension assay (PEA) to measure multiple protein biomarkers simultaneously [13]. Briefly, for each protein, a unique pair of oligonucleotide-labeled antibody probes bind to the targeted protein and if the two probes are brought into close proximity, the oligonucleotides will hybridize in a pairwise manner. The addition of a DNA polymerase leads to a proximity-dependent DNA polymerization event, generating a unique polymerase chain reaction target sequence. The resulting DNA sequence is subsequently detected and quantified using a microfluidic real-time polymerase chain reaction instrument (Biomark HD, Fluidigm, South San Francisco, CA, USA). Data are then quality controlled and normalized using an internal extension control and an interplate control to adjust for intra- and inter-run variation. The protein levels are given in Normalized Protein eXpression (NPX) units, which is an arbitrary measure on the $\log_2$-scale, with higher values corresponding to higher protein concentrations. All assay characteristics, including detection limits and measurements of assay performance and validations, are available from the manufacturer's webpage (http://www.olink.com). The analyses were based on 1 µL of plasma for each panel of 92 assays. To avoid batch effects, samples from the two intervention groups and the two visits were randomized across assay plates. Each plate included internal controls, as described previously, to adjust for technical variation and sample irregularities [13]. Due to technical issues, one of the protein assays (C-C motif chemokine 22) was not performed, resulting in measurements of 91 proteins.

2.5. Other Covariates

At the baseline and follow-up clinic visits, participants self-reported their age, sex, race, and smoking status. Trained technicians measured height, weight and blood pressure, and performed a phlebotomy. Anthropometric measures were obtained with the participant wearing light clothing and no shoes. Blood pressure was measured three times with the participant sitting after a five-minute rest.

2.6. Statistical Analysis

The primary goal of the analysis was to evaluate the effect of magnesium supplementation versus placebo for change in levels of multiple cardiovascular-related circulating proteins. Of the 91 measured proteins in the array, we excluded those with >25% values below the limit of detection across both groups combined as well as those with excessive within-person variability, for which an intervention effect would be unlikely to be detected. One protein [spondin-1 (SPON1)] was excluded due to a large number of values below the limit of detection. To evaluate within-person variability, we determined pairwise correlations between measurements from samples collected at the baseline and follow-up visits in the placebo group and excluded proteins with r <0.3. Three proteins were identified as having excessive variability and were subsequently excluded: ephrin type-B receptor 4 (EPHB4), azurocidin (AZU1), and kallikrein-6 (KLK6). Supplementary Table S1 presents complete results for the pairwise correlations and the proportion of samples with values below the limit of detection. All 87 proteins were available for analysis.

We used multiple linear regression with robust variance estimation to evaluate the effect of oral magnesium supplementation on change in levels of individual proteins (modeled as $\log_2$-transformed units). The dependent variable was the difference in protein levels (follow-up visit minus baseline visit). Models adjusted for randomization stratification factor (age <65 vs. ≥65) and baseline value of the protein. Since this was an exploratory hypothesis-free analysis, multiple comparisons were taken into account using the Holm procedure [14]. A secondary analysis was performed adjusting for sex. In an additional analysis, we assessed the baseline cross-sectional associations of serum magnesium with individual proteins considering baseline levels of the protein as the dependent variable and serum magnesium, modeled as a continuous variable, as the main independent variable, adjusting for age (continuous), sex, and race. The analyses were conducted using SAS version 9.4 (SAS Inc., Cary, NC, USA).

The sample size of the original trial ($n = 60$) was determined to detect a difference in the change of ectopic supraventricular beats (primary endpoint) between treatment groups of 0.79 standard deviation units with 80% power and 5% type I two-sided error and assuming that five participants would not complete the follow-up.

3. Results

Of 59 participants in the trial, 52 provided samples at baseline and follow-up visit and had available proteomic data. Of these, 24 were assigned to the magnesium intervention and 28 to the placebo group (Figure 1). The mean age of the two groups was similar (62 years), but the proportion of women was higher in the magnesium intervention group: 88% versus 61% in the placebo group (Table 1). Change in magnesium concentration was significantly higher for those assigned to magnesium supplementation compared to placebo (0.035 mmol/L, 95% confidence interval 0.015, 0.06, $p = 0.003$). This magnitude of change is equivalent to 0.6 standard deviations of baseline magnesium concentration.

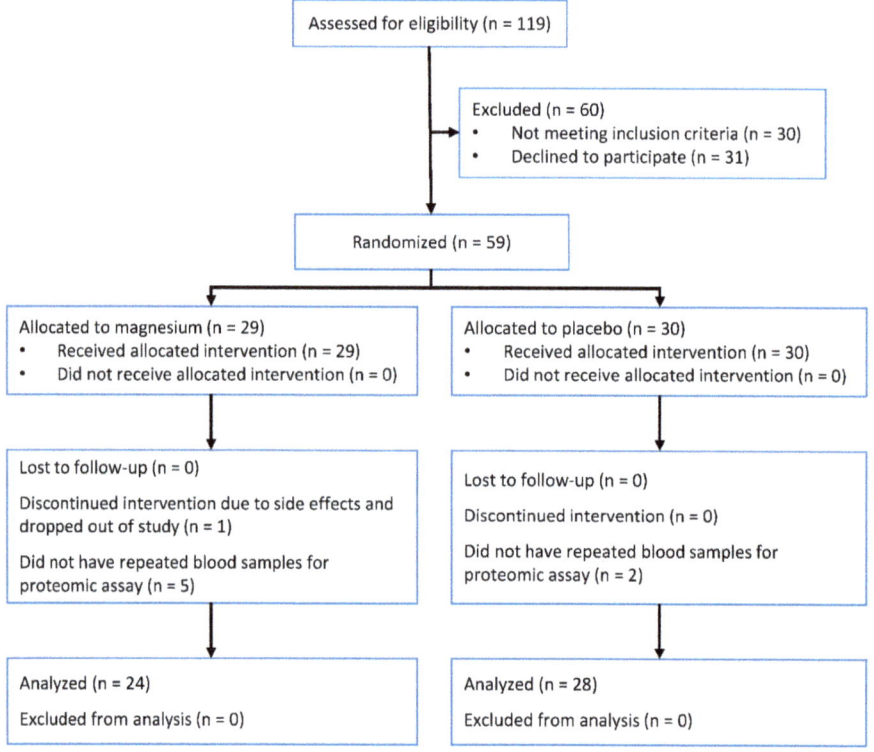

Figure 1. Participant flow diagram.

Table 1. Baseline characteristics of study participants by treatment assignment. Values presented are mean (SD) or frequency (%) where indicated.

	Magnesium (400 mg Daily)	Placebo
N	24	28
Age, years	62 (5)	62 (6)
Women, n (%)	21 (88)	17 (61)
Non-white, n (%)	2 (8)	1 (4)
Body mass index, kg/m^2	28.3 (5.1)	27.8 (4.2)
Systolic blood pressure, mmHg	118 (15)	119 (17)
Diastolic blood pressure, mmHg	73 (8)	71 (8)
Serum magnesium, mmol/L	0.86 (0.06)	0.84 (0.05)
Hypomagnesemia, n (%) *	2 (8.3)	2 (7.1)

* Hypomagnesemia defined as circulating magnesium <0.75 mmol/L.

An analysis of pairwise correlations between baseline protein levels showed most proteins were not strongly correlated to each other with three clusters, including a total of eleven proteins, correlated with r >0.8 (Figure 2). The first cluster included P-selectin (SELP), bleomycin (BLM) hydrolase, junctional adhesion molecule A (JAMA), caspase-3 (CASP3), platelet-derived growth factor (PDGF) subunit A, and platelet endothelial cell adhesion molecule (PECAM1). The second cluster included tumor necrosis factor receptor 1 (TNFR1), tumor necrosis factor receptor 2 (TNFR2), and interleukin-18-binding protein (IL18BP). Finally, the third cluster included carboxypeptidase A1 (CPA1) and carboxypeptidase B (CPB1).

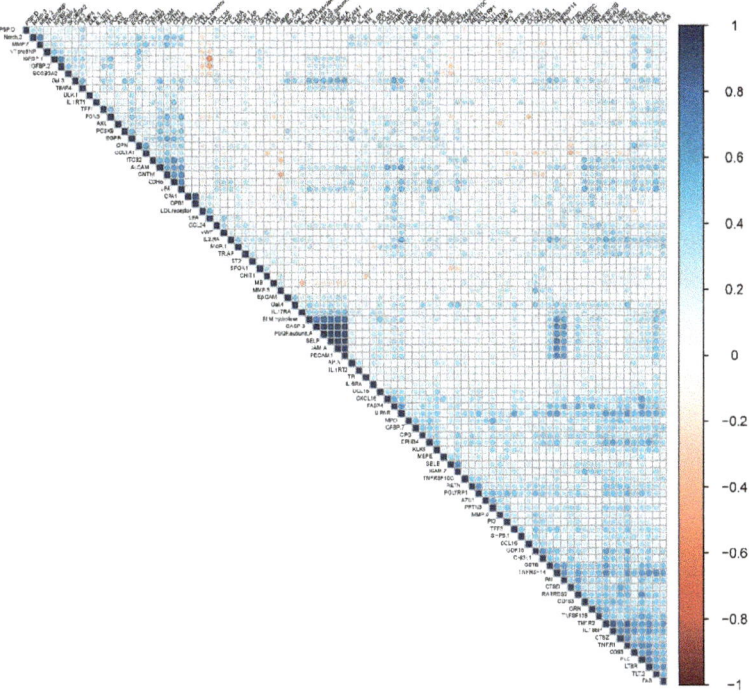

Figure 2. Pairwise correlations between baseline levels of individual proteins.

The effect of oral magnesium supplementation versus placebo on 87 circulating proteins is reported in Figure 3 and Supplementary Table S2. None of the associations were statistically significant after accounting for multiple comparisons with the Holm procedure. The strongest effect was on levels of myoglobin, with a difference of −0.319 NPX units (95% confidence interval −0.550, −0.088; $p = 0.008$) in the change over time between the intervention and placebo groups. Table 2 and Supplementary Figure S1 present results for the five proteins with between-group differences with p-value <0.05. Associations were of similar magnitude after adjustment for sex (Supplementary Table S3).

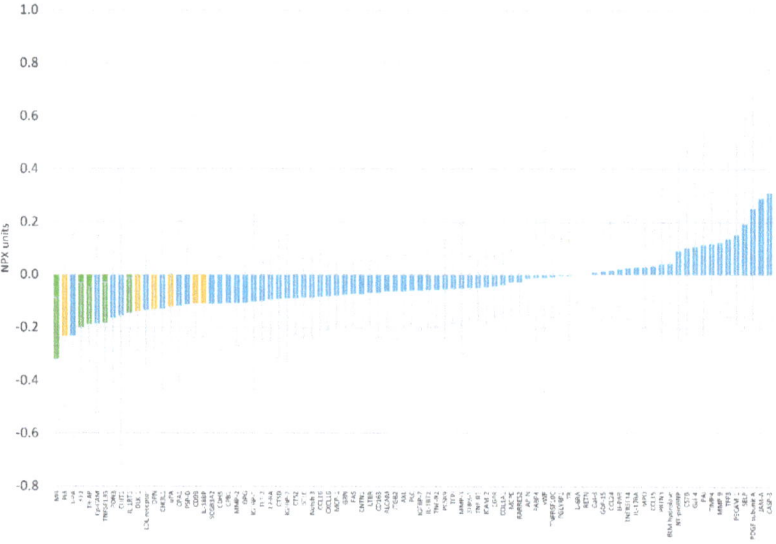

Figure 3. Mean difference in 12-week change of individual protein levels in Normalized Protein eXpression (NPX) units comparing oral magnesium supplementation to placebo. Error bars correspond to 95% confidence. Green bars indicate differences with p <0.05, yellow bars with p-value ≥0.05 and <0.10.

Table 2. Effect of magnesium supplementation on selected circulating proteins, expressed as a difference in change between magnesium and placebo group, in Normalized Protein eXpression (NPX) units. Results for effects with p-value <0.05.

	Protein	Difference in Change in Protein (NPX Units)	95% CI	p-Value
MB	Myoglobin	−0.319	−0.550, −0.088	0.008
TR-AP	Tartrate-resistant acid phosphatase type 5	−0.187	−0.328, −0.045	0.011
TNFSF13B	Tumor necrosis factor ligand superfamily member 13B	−0.181	−0.332, −0.031	0.019
ST2	ST2 protein	−0.198	−0.363, −0.032	0.020
IL-1RT1	Interleukin-1 receptor type 1	−0.144	−0.273, −0.015	0.029

Results from the general linear model with a difference in protein values between follow-up and baseline measurements in Normalized Protein eXpression (NPX) units as the dependent variable, treatment assignment as the main independent variable, adjusted for baseline levels of the protein and age stratum.

When evaluating the association of serum magnesium with circulating protein levels, we did not identify any statistically significant associations using the Holm procedure to account for multiple comparisons (Figure 4 and Supplementary Table S4). Four proteins had associations with a *p*-value <0.05 (Table 3). The strongest was the association between serum magnesium and epidermal growth factor receptor (beta = 0.053 NPX units, 95% CI 0.013, 0.093, *p* = 0.011, per 0.04 mmol/L difference in serum magnesium).

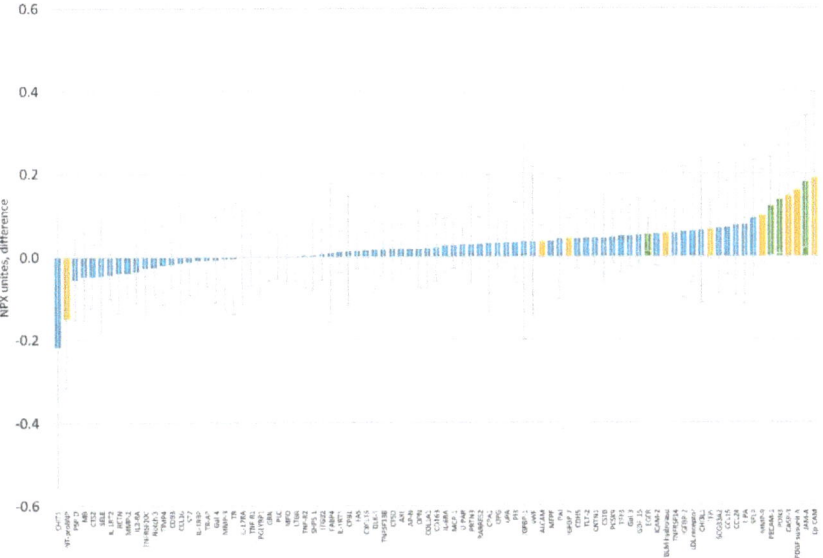

Figure 4. Baseline association of serum magnesium with individual protein levels in Normalized Protein eXpression (NPX) units. Coefficients correspond to the difference in protein levels per 0.04 mmol/L difference in serum magnesium. Error bars correspond to 95% confidence intervals. Green bars indicate differences with *p* <0.05, yellow bars with *p*-value ≥0.05 and <0.10.

Table 3. Association of baseline serum magnesium with levels of selected circulating proteins. Estimates correspond to a difference in protein levels, expressed in Normalized Protein eXpression (NPX) units, per 0.04 mmol/L difference in serum magnesium. Results for associations with *p*-value <0.05.

Protein		Difference in Protein Levels (NPX Units)	95% CI	*p*-Value
EGFR	Epidermal growth factor receptor	0.053	0.013, 0.093	0.011
JAM-A	Junctional adhesion molecule A	0.180	0.020, 0.339	0.028
PON3	Paraoxonase 3	0.137	0.039, 0.007	0.039
PECAM-1	Platelet endothelial cell adhesion molecule	0.121	0.002, 0.241	0.046

Results from general linear model with baseline levels of protein in Normalized Protein eXpression (NPX) units as the dependent variable, serum magnesium as the main independent variable, adjusted for age, sex, and race.

4. Discussion

In this analysis, we evaluated the effect of oral magnesium supplementation on the circulating levels of multiple proteins related to cardiovascular disease. We observed that, compared to placebo,

oral magnesium supplementation led to changes in levels of several proteins. For those with
p-values <0.05, all associations were in the hypothesized direction, with Mg supplementation versus
placebo associated with more advantageous levels of cardiovascular proteins. Similarly, we observed
associations between baseline serum magnesium and several circulating proteins. However, none of
the associations explored were statistically significant after correcting for multiple comparisons.

Growing observational evidence indicates that lower levels of circulating magnesium are associated
with increased risk of atrial fibrillation and coronary heart disease [1,2]. In addition, experimental
studies show that magnesium supplementation can be effective in the secondary prevention of cardiac
arrhythmias [5,15]. Mechanisms underlying these associations, however, are unknown. Though we
failed to identify significant effects of magnesium on circulating proteins, the magnitude of the protein
changes after a relatively short intervention supports the use of proteomic panels in future larger
studies of magnesium supplementation. These panels will facilitate the identification of biomarkers
and physiological pathways responsible for the potential effects of magnesium on cardiovascular risk.

To date, the use of proteomic approaches to evaluate effects of magnesium supplementation has
been extremely limited. In a crossover trial of 14 healthy overweight individuals, supplementation with
500 mg/day of magnesium (in the form of magnesium citrate) vs. placebo for 4 weeks did not result
in consistent changes in circulating inflammatory biomarkers. However, urine proteomic profiling
identified significant differences in the expression profiles of the proteome, but not specific proteins [11].
Similarly, a study of 52 overweight and obese individuals randomized to 350 mg/day of magnesium or
placebo for 24 weeks evaluated the effect of the intervention on multiple circulating biomarkers of
inflammation and endothelial dysfunction. No significant differences were reported between the two
intervention groups [16].

The proteins, for which we observed some evidence of effect (albeit not significant after multiple
correction), are involved in muscle structure and oxygen storage (myoglobin) [17], immune function
and inflammation (tumor necrosis factor ligand superfamily member 13B [18], ST2 protein [19],
interleukin-1 receptor type 1) [20], and bone metabolism (tartrate-resistant acid phosphatase type
5 [21]). Of interest, higher circulating levels of ST2 have been linked to adverse cardiovascular
outcomes [22]. Similarly, in our cross-sectional analysis, higher concentrations of serum magnesium
were associated with higher levels of proteins involved in multiple functions (epidermal growth factor
receptor) [23], cell adhesion (junctional adhesion molecule A [24], platelet endothelial cell adhesion
molecule [25]), and oxidative stress protection (paraoxonase 3) [26]. These effects were consistent with
some of the proposed effects of magnesium supplementation, including reductions in oxidative stress
and inflammation [7,8].

Our study had some strengths, including the randomized design, the demonstrated efficacy
of the intervention in increasing circulating magnesium [12,27], and the simultaneous assessment
of multiple circulating proteins. However, this analysis was hindered by the limited sample size
and absence of replication in an independent sample. The limited sample size precluded studying
specifically participants with hypomagnesemia. Also, we lacked information on kidney function,
which influences levels of numerous proteins. However, by including a healthy sample, this was
less likely to be an issue. Finally, we did not collect data on dietary magnesium and, among female
participants, menopausal status, use of hormone therapy, or circulating estrogens. We are uncertain of
the potential effect of these variables on our effect estimates. However, the randomized design would
contribute to balancing them across the control and intervention groups.

5. Conclusions

In summary, our study demonstrated the potential value of proteomic approaches for
the investigation of mechanisms underlying the beneficial effects of magnesium supplementation.
Future trials in larger samples are needed to establish with certainty the physiological impact
of magnesium and, therefore, inform the development of magnesium-based interventions for
the prevention of cardiovascular and metabolic diseases.

Supplementary Materials: The following are available online at http://www.mdpi.com/2072-6643/12/6/1697/s1, Figure S1: Mean levels of selected proteins at baseline and after 12 weeks by treatment group (oral magnesium supplementation vs placebo). Table S1. Quality control of proteomic measurements, Table S2. Effect of oral magnesium supplementation vs placebo on levels of circulating proteins, adjusted for baseline levels of the protein and age stratum, Table S3. Effect of oral magnesium supplementation vs placebo on levels of circulating proteins, adjusted for baseline levels of the protein, age stratum, and sex., Table S4. Association of baseline serum magnesium with levels of selected circulating proteins.

Author Contributions: Conceptualization: P.L.L. and A.A. Methodology: P.L.L., A.A. and K.D.R. Data collection: P.L.L., A.A. and L.Y.C. Formal analysis: A.A. Data interpretation: A.A., L.Y.C., K.D.R., F.L.N., M.R.R. and P.L.L. Writing—original draft: A.A. Writing—review and editing: L.Y.C., K.D.R., F.L.N., M.R.R. and P.L.L. All authors have read and agreed to the published version of the manuscript.

Funding: This work was supported by internal funds of the Division of Epidemiology and Community Health, University of Minnesota, the McKnight Land-Grant Professorship funds, the American Heart Association grant 16EIA26410001 (Alonso), the National Heart, Lung, And Blood Institute grants T32HL007779 and T32HL007024 (Rooney), the National Center for Advancing Translational Sciences award UL1TR002494. Dr. Alonso was additionally supported by the National Heart, Lung, And Blood Institute of the National Institutes of Health under award number K24HL148521. The content is solely the responsibility of the authors and does not necessarily represent the official views of the National Institutes of Health.

Acknowledgments: We thank the study participants, for taking part in this study.

Conflicts of Interest: The authors declare no conflicts of interest.

References

1. Del Gobbo, L.C.; Imamura, F.; Wu, J.H.; De Oliveira Otto, M.C.; Chiuve, S.E.; Mozaffarian, D. Circulating and dietary magnesium and risk of cardiovascular disease: A systematic review and meta-analysis of prospective studies. *Am. J. Clin. Nutr.* **2013**, *98*, 160–173. [CrossRef]
2. Misialek, J.R.; Lopez, F.L.; Lutsey, P.L.; Huxley, R.R.; Peacock, J.M.; Chen, L.Y.; Soliman, E.Z.; Agarwal, S.K.; Alonso, A. Serum and dietary magnesium and incidence of atrial fibrillation in whites and in African Americans–Atherosclerosis Risk in Communities (ARIC) Study. *Circ. J.* **2013**, *77*, 323–329. [CrossRef] [PubMed]
3. Larsson, S.C.; Burgess, S.; Michaëlsson, K. Serum magnesium levels and risk of coronary artery disease: Medelian randomisation study. *BMC Med.* **2018**, *16*, 68. [CrossRef] [PubMed]
4. Larsson, S.C.; Drca, N.; Michaëlsson, K. Serum magnesium and calcium levels and risk of atrial fibrillation. *Circ. Genom Precis Med.* **2019**, *12*, e002349. [CrossRef] [PubMed]
5. Arsenault, K.A.; Yusuf, A.M.; Crystal, E.; Healey, J.S.; Morillo, C.A.; Nair, G.M.; Whitlock, R.P. Interventions for preventing post-operative atrial fibrillation in patients undergoing heart surgery. *Cochrane Database Syst. Rev.* **2013**, CD003611. [CrossRef] [PubMed]
6. Veronese, N.; Demurtas, J.; Pesolillo, G.; Celotto, S.; Barnini, T.; Calusi, G.; Caruso, M.G.; Notarnicola, M.; Reddavide, R.; Stubbs, R.; et al. Magnesium and health outcomes: An umbrella review of systematic reviews and meta-analyses of observational and intervention studies. *Eur. J. Nutr.* **2020**, *59*, 263–272. [CrossRef]
7. Nielsen, F.H. Magnesium deficiency and increased inflammation: Current perspectives. *J. Inflamm. Res.* **2018**, *11*, 25–34. [CrossRef]
8. Morais, J.B.; Severo, J.S.; Santos, L.R.; De Sousa Melo, S.R.; De Oliveira Santos, R.; De Oliveira, A.R.; Cruz, K.J.; Do Nascimento Marreiro, D. Role of magnesium in oxidative stress in individuals with obesity. *Biol. Trace Elem. Res.* **2017**, *176*, 20–26. [CrossRef]
9. Barbagallo, M.; Dominguez, L.J.; Galioto, A.; Pineo, A.; Belvedere, M. Oral magnesium supplementation improves vascular function in elderly diabetic patients. *Magnes. Res.* **2010**, *23*, 131–137.
10. Lindsey, M.L.; Mayr, M.; Gomes, A.V.; Delles, C.; Arrell, D.K.; Murphy, A.M.; Lange, R.A.; Costello, C.E.; Jin, Y.F.; Laskowitz, D.T.; et al. Transformative impact of proteomics on cardiovascular health and disease: A scientific statement from the American Heart Association. *Circulation* **2015**, *132*, 852–872. [CrossRef]
11. Chacko, S.A.; Sul, J.; Song, Y.; Li, X.; LeBlanc, J.; You, Y.; Butch, A.; Liu, S. Magnesium supplementation, metabolic and inflammatory markers, and global genomic and proteomic profiling: A randomized, double-blind, controlled, crossover trial in overweight individuals. *Am. J. Clin. Nutr.* **2011**, *93*, 463–473. [CrossRef] [PubMed]

12. Lutsey, P.L.; Chen, L.Y.; Eaton, A.; Jaeb, M.; Rudser, K.D.; Neaton, J.D.; Alonso, A. A pilot randomized trial of oral magnesium supplementation on supraventricular arrhythmias. *Nutrients* **2018**, *10*, 884. [CrossRef] [PubMed]
13. Assarsson, E.; Lundberg, M.; Holmquist, G.; Björkesten, J.; Bucht Thorsen, S.; Ekman, D.; Eriksson, A.; Rennel Dickens, E.; Ohlsson, S.; Edfeldt, G.; et al. Homogenous 96-plex PEA immunoassay exhibiting high sensitivity, specificity, and excellent scalability. *PLoS ONE* **2014**, *9*, e95192. [CrossRef] [PubMed]
14. Holm, S. A simple sequentially rejective multiple test procedure. *Scand. J. Statist* **1979**, *6*, 65–70.
15. Salaminia, S.; Sayehmiri, F.; Angha, P.; Sayehmiri, K.; Motedayen, M. Evaluating the effect of magnesium supplementation and cardiac arrhythmias after acute coronary syndrome: A systematic review and meta-analysis. *BMC Cardiovasc. Disord* **2018**, *18*, 129. [CrossRef]
16. Joris, P.J.; Plat, J.; Bakker, S.J.; Mensink, R.P. Effects of long-term magnesium supplementation on endothelial function and cardiometabolic risk markers: A randomized controlled trial in overweight/obese adults. *Sci. Rep.* **2017**, *7*, 106. [CrossRef]
17. Ordway, G.A.; Garry, D.J. Myoglobin: An essential hemoprotein in striated muscle. *J. Exp. Biol.* **2004**, *207*, 3441–3446. [CrossRef]
18. Schneider, P.; MacKay, F.; Steiner, V.; Hofmann, K.; Bodmer, J.L.; Holler, N.; Ambrose, C.; Lawton, P.; Bixler, S.; Acha-Orbea, H.; et al. BAFF, a novel ligand of the tumor necrosis family, stimulates B cell growth. *J. Exp. Med.* **1999**, *189*, 1747–1756. [CrossRef]
19. Schmitz, J.; Owyang, A.; Oldham, E.; Song, Y.; Murphy, E.; McClanahan, T.K.; Zurawski, G.; Moshrefi, M.; Qin, J.; Li, X.; et al. IL-33, an interleukin-1-like cytokine that signals via the IL-1 receptor-related protein ST2 and induces T helper type 2-associated cytokines. *Immunity* **2005**, *23*, 479–490. [CrossRef]
20. Tominaga, K.; Yoshimoto, T.; Torigoe, K.; Kurimoto, M.; Matsui, K.; Hada, T.; Okamura, H.; Nakanishi, K. IL-12 synergizes with IL-18 or IL-1beta for IFN-gamma production from human T cells. *Int. Immunol.* **2000**, *12*, 151–160. [CrossRef]
21. Halleen, J.M.; Ylipahkala, H.; Alatalo, S.L.; Janckila, A.J.; Heikkinen, J.E.; Suominen, H.; Cheng, S.; Väänänen, H.K. Serum tartrate-resistant acid phosphatase 5b, but not 5a, correlates with other markers of bone turnover and bone mineral density. *Calcif. Tissue Int.* **2002**, *71*, 20–25. [CrossRef] [PubMed]
22. Pascual-Figal, D.A.; Januzzi, J.L. The biology of ST2: The International ST2 Consensus Panel. *Am. J. Cardiol.* **2015**, *115*, 3B–7B. [CrossRef] [PubMed]
23. Seshacharyulu, P.; Ponnusamy, M.P.; Haridas, D.; Jain, M.; Ganti, A.K.; Batra, S.K. Targeting the EGFR signaling pathway in cancer therapy. *Expert. Opin. Ther. Targets* **2012**, *16*, 15–31. [CrossRef] [PubMed]
24. Steinbacher, T.; Kummer, D.; Ebnet, K. Junctional adhesion molecule-A: Functional diversity through molecular promiscuity. *Cell Mol. Life Sci.* **2018**, *75*, 1393–1409. [CrossRef] [PubMed]
25. Lertkiatmongkol, P.; Liao, D.; Mei, H.; Hu, Y.; Newman, P.J. Endothelial functions of platelet/endothelial cell adhesion molecule-1 (CD31). *Curr. Opin. Hematol.* **2016**, *23*, 253–259. [CrossRef] [PubMed]
26. Précourt, L.P.; Amre, D.; Denis, M.C.; Lavoie, J.C.; Delvin, E.; Seidman, E.; Levy, E. The three-gene paraoxonase family: Physiologic roles, actions and regulation. *Atherosclerosis* **2011**, *214*. [CrossRef]
27. Zhang, X.; Del Gobbo, L.C.; Hruby, A.; Rosanoff, A.; He, K.; Dai, Q.; Costello, R.B.; Zhang, W.; Song, Y. The circulating concentration and 24-h urine excretion of magnesium dose- and time-dependently respond to oral magnesium supplementation in a meta-analysis of randomized controlled trials. *J. Nutr.* **2016**, *146*, 595–602. [CrossRef]

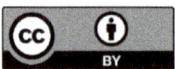

© 2020 by the authors. Licensee MDPI, Basel, Switzerland. This article is an open access article distributed under the terms and conditions of the Creative Commons Attribution (CC BY) license (http://creativecommons.org/licenses/by/4.0/).

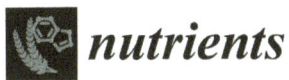

Article

Response of Vitamin D after Magnesium Intervention in a Postmenopausal Population from the Province of Granada, Spain

Héctor Vázquez-Lorente [1,*], Lourdes Herrera-Quintana [1], Jorge Molina-López [2], Yenifer Gamarra-Morales [1,*], Beatriz López-González [1], Claudia Miralles-Adell [1] and Elena Planells [1]

[1] Department of Physiology, School of Pharmacy, Institute of Nutrition and Food Technology "José Mataix", University of Granada, 18071 Granada, Spain; lourdesherra@ugr.es (L.H.-Q.); beatrizlogo@yahoo.es (B.L.-G.); cmirallesadell@gmail.com (C.M.-A.); elenamp@ugr.es (E.P.)
[2] Department of Physical Education and Sports, Faculty of Education, Psychology and Sports Sciences, University of Huelva, 21007 Huelva, Spain; jorge.molina@ddi.uhu.es
* Correspondence: hectorvazquez@ugr.es (H.V.-L.); jennifer_gamo@hotmail.com (Y.G.-M.); Tel.: +34-958241000 (ext. 20313) (H.V.-L. & Y.G.-M.)

Received: 25 June 2020; Accepted: 28 July 2020; Published: 30 July 2020

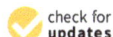

Abstract: Menopause is a stage of hormonal imbalance in women which, in addition to other physiopathological consequences, poses a risk of deficiency of key micronutrients such as magnesium and vitamin D. A study was made of the influence of a magnesium intervention upon vitamin D status in a postmenopausal population from the province of Granada (Spain). Fifty-two healthy postmenopausal women between 44–76 years of age were included. Two randomized groups—placebo and magnesium (500 mg/day)—were treated during eight weeks. Nutrient intake was assessed using questionnaires based on 72-h recall. Vitamin D was analyzed by liquid chromatography—tandem mass spectrometry. Baseline vitamin D proved deficient in over 80% of the subjects. The administration of magnesium resulted in significantly increased vitamin D levels in the intervention group versus the controls ($p < 0.05$). Magnesium supplementation improved vitamin D status in the studied postmenopausal women.

Keywords: vitamin D; magnesium; liquid chromatography—tandem mass spectrometry; post-menopause

1. Introduction

Menopause is characterized by physiological changes with important variations in hormone levels. If left unchecked, this situation can lead to disease [1], including an increased risk of different types of cancer, cardiovascular disorders, osteoporosis and type 2 diabetes, among other conditions [2,3]. During this stage of life, women may experience weight gain and a redistribution of fat mass. Added to the hormonal alteration, this could adversely affect the status of different key micronutrients such as magnesium (Mg) and vitamin D in this population [4,5].

Magnesium is necessary for most reactions in the human body, and is a cofactor of more than 300 enzymes [6]. Mg is essential for the functioning of parathyroid hormone (PTH) and vitamin D. Hypomagnesemia during postmenopause needs to be monitored together with the status of those minerals closely related to phosphorus-calcium metabolism, in order to optimize homeostatic equilibrium and bone health. Magnesium supplementation may offer benefits in this regard [7,8]. The inclusion of Mg supplementation in postmenopausal women in the event of deficiency has been suggested by a number of authors, as it seems to improve postmenopausal symptoms, avoiding long-term systemic consequences [9–11]. In recent years, the interest in vitamin D has increased, due to the high prevalence of vitamin D deficiency worldwide [12]. Vitamin D plays a key role in phosphorus-calcium metabolism, improving the intestinal absorption of Ca, and regulating bone mineralization and the renal excretion of Ca [13,14]. To prevent poor vitamin D status, the monitoring of risk populations such as postmenopausal women is recommended with a view to preserving bone health [15]. However, new studies have also addressed the role of vitamin D in non-skeletal diseases [16,17].

Nowadays, the routine analytical determination of vitamin D is recommended in healthy risk groups such as postmenopausal women. However, such determinations are characterized by variability of the results obtained—thus suggesting the need to standardize the laboratory test protocol employed [18]. One of the methods currently used to measure vitamin D is enzyme immunoassay (EIA), which is the most widely used method in hospitals [19,20]. Use is currently also made of chromatography, which yields stable and reproducible results, and distinguishes between 25-OH-D_3 and 25-OH-D_2 [12]. In this respect, Liquid Chromatography—Tandem Mass Spectrometry (LC-MS/MS) is regarded as the gold standard, offering greater sensitivity, flexibility and specificity [18]. Unfortunately, LC-MS/MS cannot always be used, due to its high cost [20,21]. The technique of choice is therefore conditioned by the availability of resources [22,23]. In general, all techniques measure mainly 25-hydroxy-vitamin D (25-OH-D), because of its long half-life (one month) in plasma. Plasma vitamin D concentrations are conditioned not only by homeostatic regulation but also by lifestyle, environmental and sociocultural factors such as the use of sunscreens, the female gender, postmenopausal status and fat mass [24–28]. During postmenopause, vitamin D supplementation could be recommended in women with confirmed vitamin D deficiency, since it seems to be associated with an increase in bone mineral density and could improve future quality of life [29].

Therefore, the postmenopausal period could be associated with a genuine risk of deficiency of various minerals and vitamins, particularly Mg and vitamin D [30,31]. The present study was carried out to assess vitamin D status in a population of postmenopausal women in the province of Granada (Spain), with evaluation of the influence of a magnesium intervention.

2. Materials and Methods

2.1. Study Design and Intervention

This is an eight-week, double-blinded, placebo-controlled, randomized intervention trial (Figure 1). Participants were randomly assigned to one of two treatment groups: Placebo group (PG: 25 women) and Magnesium Group—500 mg/day of Mg (MG: 27 women). Randomization was performed in a 1:1 ratio using a table of random numbers, prepared by a researcher who did not participate in the data collection. Allocation concealment was ensured, as the referred researcher did not release the randomization code until the participants were recruited into the trial after all baseline measurements were completed. Mg supplements were supplied by Botánica Nutrients SL, Seville, Spain (Number B91070797), following the period of eight weeks recommended. Placebo capsules were made of the same size and color as Mg supplements for identical appearance and taste. The intervention was carried out in winter from January 15th to March 15th. The study was registered at the US National Institutes of Health (ClinicalTrials.gov) NCT03672513.

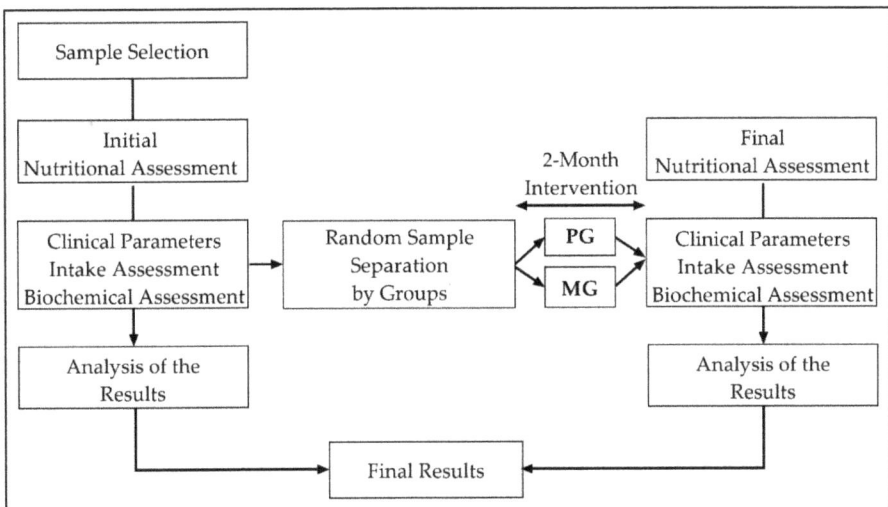

Figure 1. Study design. MG = Magnesium Group. PG = Placebo Group.

2.2. Study Participants

Fifty-two healthy postmenopausal women volunteers from the province of Granada, Spain aged between 44 and 76 years were recruited once they had been informed about the protocol. Inclusion criteria were (i) to present postmenopausal status (with at least 12 months of amenorrhea), (ii) to present low status in Mg obtained in a previous biochemical assessment, (iii) not present any pathology that could affect their nutritional status, (iv) not to be subjected to hormone replacement therapy (HRT), (v) not to take vitamin and mineral supplements. Women were excluded if they were unwilling to accept the randomization procedure. Written informed consent was obtained from all patients taking into account the approval of the Ethics Committee and the Research Committee of the Centre. The present study was conducted according to the principles of the Declaration of Helsinki and the approval by the Ethics Committee of the University of Granada (149/CEIH/2016), in accordance with the International Conference on Harmonization/Good Clinical Practice Standards.

Eligible participants of this study were 121 participants. Of these, 39 menopausal women were excluded because 18 women did not meet the inclusion criteria and 21 women declined to participle in the study after the initial interview, and so, 82 menopausal women were enrolled in the study and randomly assigned to the two arms (Figure 2). Of the 41 postmenopausal women that were allocated to intervention in the PG, a total of 16 women withdrew the study due time and supplementation commitment. In reference to the 41 postmenopausal women allocated into MG, a total of 13 postmenopausal women withdrew due to time and supplementation commitment, illness severity or not giving any reason. Of the 28 women included in the data analysis, one woman was excluded from the analysis because of insufficient blood sample was collected. Thus, 25 women in PG and 27 women in MG were enrolled in the present study.

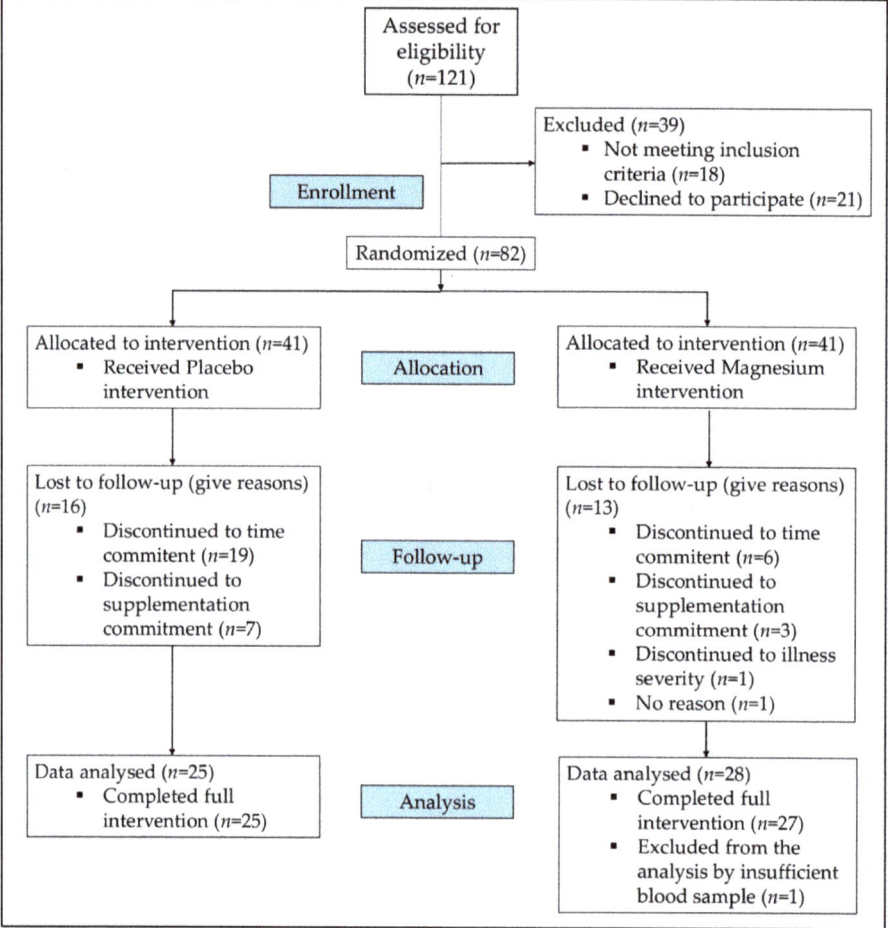

Figure 2. Flowchart of participants recruited, enrolled and involved in the clinical study.

2.3. Randomization and Blinding

Women were randomly assigned (simple randomization) to study groups (parallel design). In order to ensure comparable distribution across the treatment arms, women were stratified to balance baseline covariates. Both study participants and investigators were blinded to the group allocation. Initial and follow-up visits for evaluating dietary intake, body composition, biochemical and hormonal determination and antioxidant status parameters were performed at baseline and after two months of intervention.

2.4. Sample Size

We performed sample size calculation for our primary aim of a randomized controlled trial based on the influence of a Mg supplementation on vitamin D status. The number of participants to be included in the study was calculated on the basis of the change in vitamin D status after Mg intervention. To the best of our knowledge there were no available information regarding group difference changes on vitamin D in Mg intervened postmenopausal women. Therefore, we assumed a difference of 2.63 ng/mL as clinically meaningful based on previous observations in our group (unpublished data). A total of 68 participants were needed to detect a mean group difference of 2.63 ng/mL and a standard deviation of 3.85 ng/mL in vitamin D with a power of 80% and an alpha of 0.05, and assuming a maximum loss of 20% of participants ($n = 82$).

2.5. Compliance Evaluation

Adherence/compliance to nutritional intervention was determined as the percentage of all of the supplement capsules ingested throughout the study period. In addition, subjects were asked to keep daily records about side effects or other problems related to the supplements. Moreover, biochemical and clinical-nutritional parameters were taken at baseline and follow-up to evaluate the safety of the product and to verify the adverse effects.

2.6. Data Collection

All recorded data were obtained through the use of manual questionnaires administered by the interviewer that reflected information on personal data, sociodemographic aspects, an adequate diagnosis of the postmenopausal situation, smoking habits and physical activity [30].

2.7. Body Composition Analysis

Anthropometric recorded data were height (SECA® Model 274), waist circumference (SECA® Model 201), and body composition by bioelectrical impedance (Tanita MC-980 Body Composition Analyzer MA Multifrequency Segmental, Barcelona, Spain). The analyzer complied with the applicable European standards (93/42EEC, 90/384EEC) for use in the medical industry. Participants were informed in advance of the required conditions prior to the measurement: no alcohol less than 24 h before the measurement, no vigorous exercise less than 12 h prior to the measurement, no food or drink less than three h prior to the measurement, and no urination immediately before the measurement. All measurements were taken simultaneously during the morning in fasting conditions. Weight and BMI measurements were calculated and the compartmental analysis measured fat mass, fat free mass and muscle mass. The following measurements were taken: age, height, weight, BMI and fat percentage.

2.8. Intake Rating

Dietary nutrient intake was assessed using a manual 72 h-recall [30], taking into account a holiday and two non-holidays days, both at baseline and follow-up, which was administered by the interviewer. Recall accuracy was recorded with a set of photographs of prepared foods and dishes that are frequently consumed in Spain. The food intake assessment was converted to both energy and nutrients, determining the adequacy of the macronutrient and micronutrient intake according to the Recommended Dietary Allowance (RDA) for the female Spanish population within the age range included in our study [32] using Nutriber® software (1.1.5. version, Barcelona, Spain).

2.9. Sample Treatment

A blood extraction in the morning in fasting conditions was performed at baseline and follow-up, being centrifuged at 4 °C for 15 min at 3000 rpm to extract the plasma. Once the plasma was removed from the tube, it was frozen at −80 °C until the analytical determination of the different parameters. All samples were measured in one run, in the same assay batch and blinded quality control samples were included in the assay batches to assess laboratory error in the measurements.

Measurement of Biochemical Parameters

PTH and osteocalcin levels were measured using EIA by colorimetric method (ECLIA, Elecsys 2010 and Modular Analytics E170, Roche Diagnostics, Mannheim, Germany). Vitamin D levels were measured by LC-MS/MS (Acquity UHPLC System I-Class Waters, Milford, USA) [33]. The biochemical values of vitamin D obtained were classified according to the reference values of 25-OH-D in plasma, being sufficiency >30 ng/mL, insufficiency 20–30 ng/mL and deficiency <20 ng/mL for total vitamin D [33]. The remaining biochemical parameters such as glucose, urea, uric acid, creatinine, triglycerides, total cholesterol, high density lipoprotein (HDL) and low density lipoprotein (LDL) cholesterol, total proteins, transferrin, albumin, homocysteine, bilirubin and transaminases levels, were determined in the Analysis Unit at the Virgen de las Nieves Hospital, Granada (ECLIA, Elecsys 2010 and Modular Analytics E170, Roche Diagnostics, Mannheim, Germany).

2.10. Statistical Analysis

The statistical analysis was performed using the SPSS 22.0 Software for MAC (SPSS Inc. Chicago, IL, USA). Descriptive analysis has been used for data expression, indicating the results of the numerical variables such as arithmetical mean, standard deviation (X ± SD) and standard error of the mean (SEM), and the results of the categorical variables were expressed in frequencies (%). As a previous step to the execution of a parametric model or not, the hypothesis of normal distribution was accepted using the Kolmogorov-Smirnov test. For the comparative analysis based on categorical variables, chi square test was used. For the comparative analysis based on baseline and follow-up, the paired t-test for parametric samples was used. For the comparative analysis based on groups, the unpaired t-test for parametric samples was used. Correlation analyses and partial correlation coefficients were performed with Pearson test. A p value less than 0.05 was considered statistically significant.

3. Results

The mean levels of plasma and erythrocyte Mg were 1.85 ± 0.25 (1.70–2.60) and 4.03 ± 0.71 (4.20–6.70) respectively. Our results showed that 27% of the postmenopausal women were deficient in plasma Mg and 67% were deficient in erythrocyte Mg at the beginning of the study. Given the deficiency justified here, the study population was randomly supplemented with Mg.

Table 1 shows the general characteristics of the study population by groups. In both study groups, body mass index (BMI) was above and energy intake was below the reference values. Regarding Ca, 16.7% and 10.7% of the postmenopausal women in PG and MG did not reach two-thirds of the RDA at baseline. After the intervention, 20.0% of the women in PG and 11.1% of those in MG did not reach two-thirds of the RDA referred to Ca intake. With regard to Mg intake, 41.7% and 46.4% of the women in PG and MG, respectively, were below two-thirds of the RDA at baseline. Nevertheless, after Mg supplementation, 30% of the postmenopausal women in PG and 100% of those in MG reached two-thirds of the RDA for Mg. In the case of vitamin D intake, our results showed that 87.5% and 81.5% of the postmenopausal women in PG and MG, respectively, were below two-thirds of the vitamin D recommendations. After Mg supplementation, these figures were 75% and 92.6%.

Table 2 shows the biochemical parameters by group. In both groups, total cholesterol was above its reference values, and prealbumin significantly decreased in PG ($p < 0.05$) after the intervention. When using the LC-MS/MS method, the 25-OH-D levels were seen to have increased significantly after the intervention comparing baseline and follow-up ($p < 0.05$), though the levels were still below the recommended values. However, although an increase in 25-OH-D$_3$ and 25-OH-D$_2$ levels was also seen intra (MG) and inter-groups, the results were not statistically significant.

Table 1. General characteristics of the study population by group.

Features	Reference Values	PG (n = 25) Baseline (Mean ± SD)	PG (n = 25) Follow-Up (Mean ± SD)	MG (n = 27) Baseline (Mean ± SD)	MG (n = 27) Follow-Up (Mean ± SD)	p Value PG Follow-Up	p Value MG Follow-Up	p Value Inter-Groups
Age (Years)	-	59.7 ± 9.15	59.7 ± 9.15	57.7 ± 7.58	57.7 ± 7.58	-	-	-
Weight (Kg)	-	69.1 ± 11.0	67.8 ± 11.2	69.3 ± 14.2	69.7 ± 13.6	0.23	0.43	0.62
Height (cm)	-	157.2 ± 6.01	157.2 ± 6.01	160.2 ± 6.11	160.2 ± 6.11	-	-	-
BMI (Kg/m²)	22.0–27.0	28.0 ± 4.30	27.7 ± 4.41	26.9 ± 4.88	27.7 ± 4.41	0.21	0.49	0.65
Blood pressure n (%)								
Normal blood pressure	-	10 (40)	-	14 (51)	-	-	-	-
High blood pressure	-	15 (60)	-	13 (49)	-	-	-	-
Physical exercise n (%)								
Sedentary	-	9 (36)	-	6 (23)	-	-	-	-
Non-sedentary	-	16 (64)	-	21 (77)	-	-	-	-
Smoking habit n (%)								
Non-smoker	-	18 (75)	-	23 (82)	-	-	-	-
Smoker	-	6 (25)	-	5 (18)	-	-	-	-
Educational level n (%)								
Basic educational level	-	10 (40)	-	11 (40)	-	-	-	-
Secondary or high educational level	-	15 (60)	-	16 (60)	-	-	-	-
Energy intake (Kcal)	2000.0	1339.5 ± 283.1	1232.9 ± 285.5	1307.1 ± 323.3	1323.4 ± 264.5	0.17	0.66	0.27
CHO intake (g/day)	275.0	146.6 ± 40.3	146.5 ± 33.4	149.5 ± 48.2	150.5 ± 48.5	0.84	0.89	0.75
Protein intake (g/day)	50.0	59.7 ± 14.2	57.1 ± 10.4	61.1 ± 17.6	63.4 ± 15.6	0.47	0.42	0.12
Fat intake (g/day)	70.0	56.1 ± 17.2	47.9 ± 18.5	53.2 ± 14.7	51.8 ± 12.7	0.15	0.66	0.41
Cholesterol intake (mg/day)	<300.0	150.6 ± 61.6	151.7 ± 64.4	154.1 ± 64.6	158.3 ± 76.8	0.87	0.81	0.75
Fiber intake (g/day)	>25.0	17.1 ± 10.6	16.2 ± 4.07	15.7 ± 7.72	16.5 ± 7.50	0.42	0.53	0.88
P intake (mg/day)	800.0	996.1 ± 257.7	993.9 ± 219.1	1002.6 ± 318.9	1038.8 ± 282.5	0.86	0.57	0.55
Ca intake (mg/day)	800.0–1000.0	728.2 ± 223.1	679.9 ± 168.6	873.5 ± 250.2	832.5 ± 210.6	0.69	0.56	0.01
Mg intake (mg/day)	320.0	237.4 ± 87.0	232.7 ± 55.8	219.3 ± 71.1	726.4 ± 59.9	0.99	0.001	0.001
Vitamin D intake (µg/day)	10.0	3.36 ± 3.00	4.34 ± 2.91	3.89 ± 3.62	3.62 ± 2.57	0.35	0.72	0.57

n = 52. BMI = Body Mass Index. CHO = Carbohydrates. P = Phosphorous. Ca = Calcium. Mg = Magnesium. Baseline and follow-up values are expressed as mean ± standard deviation. Both for intra-group and inter-groups p-value, paired and unpaired t-student test was used. Categorial variables are expressed as continuous as sample size (n) and percentage of subjects (%), and chi-square test was used. PG = Placebo Group. MG = Magnesium Group.

Table 2. Biochemical parameters of the study population by group.

Features	Reference Values	PG (n = 25) Baseline (Mean ± SD)	PG (n = 25) Follow-Up (Mean ± SD)	MG (n = 27) Baseline (Mean ± SD)	MG (n = 27) Follow-Up (Mean ± SD)	p Value PG Follow-Up	p Value MG Follow-Up	p Value Inter-Groups
Glucose (mg/dL)	70.0–110.0	96.0 ± 19.8	95.8 ± 19.9	90.1 ± 11.1	95.8 ± 18.9	0.63	0.25	0.047
Transferrin (mg/dL)	200.0–360.0	285.9 ± 39.7	272.8 ± 43.4	284.2 ± 47.7	272.8 ± 43.4	0.89	0.18	0.71
Prealbumin (mg/dL)	20.0–40.0	26.6 ± 5.03	24.7 ± 5.01	24.8 ± 6.45	24.7 ± 5.01	0.001	0.06	0.62
Albumin (mg/dL)	3.50–5.20	4.50 ± 0.20	4.45 ± 0.27	4.50 ± 0.21	4.45 ± 0.27	0.62	0.055	0.57
Homocysteine (μmol/L)	<13.0	12.5 ± 6.45	12.7 ± 4.78	11.5 ± 4.25	12.7 ± 4.78	0.27	0.66	0.46
Creatinine (mg/dl)	0.50–0.90	0.75 ± 0.16	0.75 ± 0.16	0.68 ± 0.11	0.75 ± 0.16	0.31	0.81	0.08
Total bilirubin (mg/dL)	0.10–1.20	0.49 ± 0.13	0.55 ± 0.21	0.47 ± 0.11	0.55 ± 0.21	0.13	0.95	0.26
LDH (U/L)	110.0–295.0	182.8 ± 29.3	181.1 ± 26.1	192.5 ± 26.7	181.1 ± 26.1	0.96	0.41	0.81
Urea (mg/dL)	10.0–50.0	36.2 ± 10.2	36.7 ± 9.35	34.3 ± 8.98	36.7 ± 9.35	0.87	0.65	0.44
Uric acid (mg/dL)	2.40–5.70	4.51 ± 0.98	4.70 ± 1.02	4.43 ± 1.23	4.70 ± 1.02	0.21	0.26	0.21
Triglycerides (mg/dL)	50.0–200.0	115.8 ± 68.9	112.3 ± 62.2	111.1 ± 50.6	112.3 ± 62.2	0.79	0.41	0.80
HDL (mg/dL)	40.0–60.0	62.6 ± 11.2	64.1 ± 12.3	66.6 ± 14.4	64.1 ± 12.3	0.04	0.06	0.95
LDL (mg/dL)	70.0–190.0	134.5 ± 35.3	137.6 ± 30.5	130.4 ± 26.4	137.6 ± 30.5	0.76	0.06	0.19
Total cholesterol (mg/dL)	110.0–200.0	224.1 ± 39.7	221.4 ± 31.4	224.7 ± 30.1	221.4 ± 31.4	0.86	0.09	0.64
Osteocalcin (ng/mL)	15.0–46.0	17.4 ± 9.45	18.1 ± 7.21	16.8 ± 10.4	18.1 ± 7.21	0.69	0.22	0.91
PTH (pg/mL)	20.0–70.0	50.7 ± 15.8	53.3 ± 34.4	52.9 ± 17.2	53.3 ± 34.4	0.46	0.07	0.29
Ca (mg/dL)	8.60–10.2	9.31 ± 0.31	9.14 ± 0.44	9.27 ± 0.51	9.13 ± 0.49	0.31	0.07	0.98
P (mg/dL)	2.70–4.50	3.45 ± 0.45	3.57 ± 0.55	3.42 ± 0.53	3.60 ± 0.49	0.49	0.07	0.88
25-OH-D LC-MS/MS (ng/mL)	30.0–100.0	23.0 ± 8.99	24.2 ± 7.71	23.6 ± 5.70	27.8 ± 7.56	0.81	0.049	0.14
25-OH-D$_3$ LC-MS/MS (ng/mL)	>20	18.0 ± 8.37	19.7 ± 8.00	17.7 ± 6.25	21.1 ± 7.40	0.52	0.13	0.57
25-OH-D$_2$ LC-MS/MS (ng/mL)	>10	4.99 ± 2.11	4.55 ± 2.74	5.86 ± 3.05	6.80 ± 7.16	0.31	0.41	0.22

n = 52. LDH = Lactate dehydrogenase. HDL = High density lipoprotein. LDL = Low density lipoprotein. PTH = Parathyroid hormone. Ca = Calcium. P = Phosphorous. LC-MS/MS = Liquid chromatography—tandem mass spectrometry. Baseline and follow-up values are expressed as mean ± standard deviation. For intra-group and inter-groups p-value, paired and unpaired t-student test were used respectively. PG = Placebo Group. MG = Magnesium Group.

Figure 3a shows the distribution of 25-OH-D in the study population at baseline and after Mg intervention. Lesser data dispersion of the 25-OH-D levels was obtained after Mg supplementation when compared with baseline. Figure 3b shows the percentage of postmenopausal women with different vitamin D statuses by group. We found 80.8% of the study population to initially have vitamin D deficiency as established by LC-MS/MS. After the Mg intervention, the percentage of women in MG lacking in vitamin D decreased by about 20%.

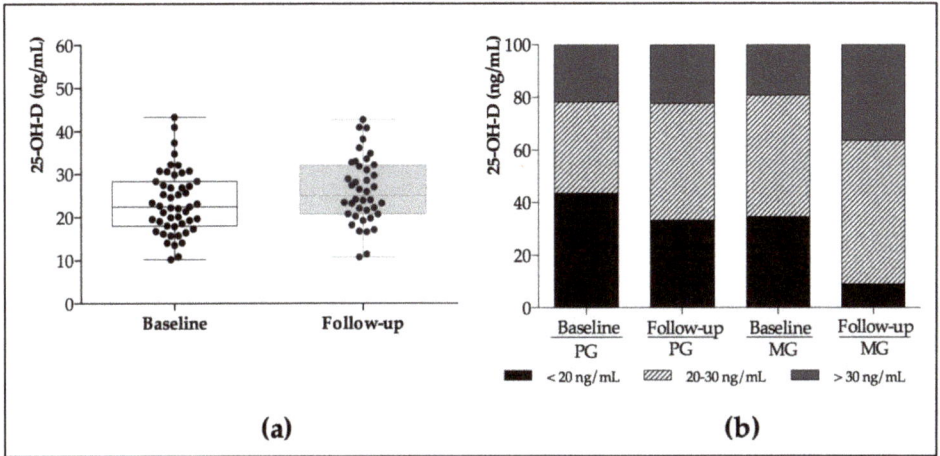

Figure 3. (a) Data distribution of 25-OH-D levels at baseline and follow-up. (b) Vitamin D status in the study population by groups. PG = Placebo Group. MG = Magnesium Group.

4. Discussion

Previous scientific evidence indicates that postmenopausal women are at risk of suffering numerous micronutrient deficiencies. However, although vitamin D and Mg could be candidates for deficiency in this population, there is currently not enough evidence of the interaction between them. On the other hand, a large part of our study population was deficient in vitamin D as evidenced by LC-MS/MS and the vitamin D status was seen to improve in MG after the Mg intervention.

Authors such as Rosanoff et al. [34] have affirmed that western populations (including Spain) are characterized by a low intake of Mg, since the latter is a predominant mineral in vegetables, and current consumption trends are towards an increased intake of animal products. Our results evidenced a pattern of low Mg consumption below the RDAs, with the exception of the MG population following the Mg intervention. In our study, Ca intake was seen to be within the recommended range for postmenopausal women. This is in contradiction to the findings of another study conducted in Spanish postmenopausal women, in which Ca intake fell short of the RDA. However, the data coincided with our own observation of vitamin D intakes below 50% of the RDA [35]. Another study involving a sample of 144 African women, in which dairy product consumption was lower, found that over 90% of the menopausal women analyzed failed to reach the RDA for Ca [36]. On the other hand, it should be noted that vitamin D intake in menopause is very low, as evidenced by studies such as that published by Rizzoli et al. [37], in which vitamin D intake among most postmenopausal women was seen to be very low in nine European countries. This is consistent with our own study, where most of the women failed to reach the RDA corresponding to vitamin D.

In the present study, Mg intake showed a significant correlation ($r = 0.451$; $p = 0.03$) to the 25-OH-D levels. Authors such as Deng et al. [38] have argued that Mg intake is inversely proportional to 25-OH-D deficiency, independently of whether Mg is administered alone or in combination with vitamin D. This association was suggested to be due to the close relationship between Mg and vitamin

D metabolism. Moreover, in our population, Mg and Ca intake were correlated ($r = 0.689$; $p = 0.001$). Authors such as Olza et al. [39] have mentioned the fact that Mg and Ca intake is based fundamentally on two food groups, namely cereals and dairy products, which are among the most widely consumed products in the Spanish population. Other authors such as Al-Musharaf et al. [40] have found vitamin D status to improve with the intake of Ca, as many food rich in Ca also have high a content of vitamin D. Nevertheless, we found no significant association between them, as well as no correlation to vitamin D intake, as this was too low—presenting high deficiency levels in almost all the women analyzed. These results could be explained by the data from studies such as that of Harris et al. [41], indicating that such correlations with vitamin D intake cannot be made, since its contribution depends on other elements such as genetic factors, as well as on exposure to the sun.

Vitamin D levels are deficient in a large percentage of the population (Figure 3), and this pattern is observed in all parts of the world and at any latitude [42]. In our study, a large percentage of the population presented 25-OH-D levels below the reference values when analyzed by LC-MS/MS. Authors such as Park et al. [43] analyzed 25-OH-D levels by LC-MS/MS in a population of postmenopausal women, and recorded the same high prevalence of vitamin D deficiency (82%) as in our study. This confirmed that despite use of the gold standard for the analytical determination of vitamin D, the levels of this vitamin were low. Schmitt et al. [44] studied 25-OH-levels by EIA among 463 postmenopausal women and found only 32% of them to have sufficient levels. Vitamin D deficiency therefore is a generalized finding in the postmenopausal population, with high deficiency levels being reported by both chromatographic and immunological laboratory test methods.

Several authors [38,45–47] have reported Mg to exert synergic action with vitamin D, placing special emphasis on the effect of Mg upon the vitamin D binding protein (DBP), as well as on the enzymes that mediate in the hydroxylation of vitamin D in the liver and kidney. Thus, a high intake of either dietary or supplemented Mg could lessen the risk of vitamin D deficiency. According to our results, there was a significant increase in 25-OH-D levels after Mg supplementation ($p < 0.05$) when analyzed by LC-MS/MS. However, authors such as Melamed et al. [48] have pointed out that the administration of Mg supplements does not increase the 25-OH-D levels, despite the fact that Mg has a direct relationship with vitamin D metabolism. This could be explained by considering that if a population has very low vitamin D levels, the supplemented Mg might not be able to mediate the hydroxylation of enough vitamin D to improve vitamin D status. Hence, Mg supplementation is usually recommended together with vitamin D, advising Mg in greater proportion than vitamin D, in order to prevent all the Mg from being depleted by the hydroxylation of vitamin D [49].

On considering the results referred to vitamin D obtained with LC-MS/MS when comparing baseline with follow-up, different values were observed (Figure 3) according to the level of deficiency with respect to the reference values. The LC-MS/MS technique provided data indicating higher vitamin D deficiency at baseline compared with the data obtained ($p < 0.05$) in MG after the intervention. Granado-Lorencio et al. [50] studied the 25-OH-D levels of 32,363 general population samples using the EIA method, and suggested that the results obtained were unable to predict vitamin D deficiency, since the technique usually underestimates vitamin status, and even more so when 25-OH-D is present in low amounts. Other authors such as Klapkova et al. [51] consider that different methods other than LC-MS/MS likewise underestimate vitamin D status, thus affecting clinical decision making. Nikooyeb et al. [26] analyzed 275 general population serum samples using different methods, and argued that although the chromatographic techniques are the gold standard for the laboratory test determination of vitamin D, the results are comparable, since there are no major differences among the techniques. However, other authors such as Garg et al. [52] stated that although the differences in results obtained by the various vitamin D analytical methods have been reduced in recent years, it is advisable to use chromatographic techniques until full harmonization of the analytical methods for vitamin D is achieved. To date, the immunochemical methods have not been able to match the precision and specificity of the chromatographic techniques [53]. Accordingly, LC-MS/MS would be a more appropriate method in this scenario, since the results exhibit less dispersion, and do not usually underestimate the values, in coincidence with Atef et al., [12] who found the LC-MS/MS technique to estimate within normality ranges in the studied adult subjects.

In addition to described findings, the present study has some strengths and limitations. As strength, the study is a randomized, placebo-controlled study in which nutritional intake of energy, macronutrients and related Mg and vitamin D minerals were controlled at baseline and follow-up. In this regard, we found that nutritional intake and high compliance to supplementation remained stable during the nutritional intervention. The present study used LC-MS/MS which is the gold standard analytical method, offering greater sensitivity, flexibility and specificity [18]. Despite it, this study has some limitations that should be considered as the small sample size. Although initially 82 women were randomly assigned to be supplemented, a total of 52 postmenopausal women completed the study (Figure 2). Although the primary outcome of the trial was to assess the influence of a Mg diet strategy on vitamin D status in postmenopausal women, the sample size in each group would allow us to preliminarily obtain significant results, although the results should be carefully considered. Clinical trials of the same nature and a similar sample size have shown a positive effect of different interventions on some parameters status in postmenopausal women [54–56]. Likewise, the sample size limitation did not allow us to make a more complex statistical approach since we did not have enough power to perform multivariate analyses and to be able to adjust our model based on possible confounding variables such as previously described age or BMI.

5. Conclusions

Magnesium supplementation in the postmenopausal women of our study had a significant positive impact upon their vitamin D status. Most of the postmenopausal population presented inadequate plasma 25-OH-D levels. Future studies are needed to shed light on the vitamin D status of this risk population and to define protocols and strategies such as Mg intervention in postmenopausal women, with a view to improving their health and quality of life.

Author Contributions: Conceptualization, E.P., B.L.-G. and L.H.-Q.; Methodology, J.M.-L. and C.M.-A.; Software, J.M.-L. and E.P.; Validation, Y.G.-M. and B.L.-G.; Formal Analysis, B.L.-G., C.M.-A. and H.V.-L.; Investigation, H.V.-L. and L.H.-Q.; Resources, E.P and H.V.-L.; Data Curation, J.M.-L.; Writing-Original Draft Preparation, H.V.-L. and E.P.; Writing-Review & Editing, H.V.-L. and J.M.-L.; Visualization, L.H.-Q. and H.V.-L.; Supervision, J.M.-L. and E.P.; Project Administration, E.P. and J.M.-L.; Funding Acquisition, E.P. All authors have read and agreed to the published version of the manuscript.

Funding: This research received external funding by FIS Carlos III (REF. PI10/1993). Héctor Vázquez-Lorente and Lourdes Herrera-Quintana are under a FPU fellowship from the Spanish Ministry of Education.

Acknowledgments: Thanks are due to all the postmenopausal women who participated in the present study.

Conflicts of Interest: The authors declare no conflict of interest.

References

1. López-González, B.; Florea, D.; García-Ávila, M.; Millan, E.; Saez, L.; Molina, J.; Planells, E.M. Calcic and hormonal levels in postmenopausal women of the province of Granada. *Ars Pharm.* **2010**, *51*, 685–696.
2. LeBlanc, E.S.; Desai, M.; Perrin, N.; Watctawski-Wende, J.; Manson, J.E.; Cauley, J.A.; Michael, Y.L.; Tang, J.; Womacl, C.; Song, Y.; et al. Vitamin D levels and menopause-related symptoms. *Menopause* **2014**, *21*, 1197–1203. [CrossRef] [PubMed]
3. Karlamangla, A.S.; Burnett-Bowie, S.-A.M.; Crandall, C.J. Bone health during the menopause transition and beyond. *Obstet. Gynecol. Clin. N. Am.* **2018**, *45*, 695–708. [CrossRef] [PubMed]
4. Pavón de Paz, I.; Alameda Hernando, C.; Olivar Roldán, J. Obesity and menopause. *Nutr. Hosp.* **2006**, *21*, 633–637. [PubMed]
5. Robinson, D.; Cardozo, L. The menopause and HRT. Urogenital effects of hormone therapy. *Best Pr. Res. Clin. Endocrinol. Metab.* **2003**, *17*, 91–104. [CrossRef]
6. Barbagallo, M.; Belvedere, M.; Dominguez, L.J. Magnesium homeostasis and aging. *Magnes. Res.* **2009**, *22*, 235–246. [CrossRef]

7. Loupy, A.; Ramakrishnan, S.K.; Wootla, B.; Chambrey, R.; de la Faille, R.; Bourgeois, S.; Bruneval, P.; Mandet, C.; Christensen, E.I.; Faure, H.; et al. PTH-independent regulation of blood calcium concentration by the calcium-sensing receptor. *J. Clin. Investig.* **2012**, *122*, 3355–3367. [CrossRef]
8. Zofková, I.; Kancheva, R.L. The relationship between magnesium and calciotropic hormones. *Magnes. Res.* **1995**, *8*, 77–84.
9. Agus, Z.S. Mechanisms and causes of hypomagnesemia. *Curr. Opin. Nephrol. Hypertens.* **2016**, *25*, 301–307. [CrossRef]
10. Ayuk, J.; Gittoes, N.J. Contemporary view of the clinical relevance of magnesium homeostasis. *Ann. Clin. Biochem.* **2014**, *51*, 179–188. [CrossRef]
11. Parazzini, F.; Martino, M.D.; Pellegrino, P. Magnesium in the gynecological practice: A literature review. *Magnes. Res.* **2017**, *30*, 1–7. [CrossRef] [PubMed]
12. Atef, S.H. Vitamin D assays in clinical laboratory: Past, present and future challenges. *J. Steroid. Biochem. Mol. Biol.* **2018**, *175*, 136–137. [CrossRef] [PubMed]
13. Jolfaie, N.R.; Rouhani, M.H.; Onvani, S.; Azadbakht, L. The association between Vitamin D and health outcomes in women: A review on the related evidence. *J. Res. Med. Sci.* **2016**, *21*, 76. [PubMed]
14. Wranicz, J.; Szostak-Węgierek, D. Health outcomes of vitamin D.; Part, I. characteristics and classic role. *Rocz. Panstw. Zakl. Hig.* **2014**, *65*, 179–184. [PubMed]
15. Palacios, C.; Gonzalez, L. Is vitamin D deficiency a major global public health problem? *J. Steroid. Biochem. Mol. Biol.* **2014**, *144*, 138–145. [CrossRef]
16. Van den Ouweland, J.M.W. Analysis of vitamin D metabolites by liquid chromatography-tandem mass spectrometry. *Trac Trend. Anal. Chem.* **2016**, *84*, 117–130. [CrossRef]
17. Hart, G.R.; Furniss, J.L.; Laurie, D.; Durham, S.K. Measurement of vitamin D status: Background, clinical use, and methodologies. *Clin. Lab.* **2006**, *52*, 335–343.
18. Babić, N. Analytical methods and performance of the immunoassay methods for determination of vitamin D in comparison to mass spectrometry. *J. Med. Biochem.* **2012**, *31*, 333–338.
19. Begum Azmathullah, A.; Kirubharan, S.; Jeyasubramanian, L.; Anbarasan, P.; Kandasamy, V.; Natesan, S. Study of vitamin D levels in postmenopausal women. *J. Evol. Med. Dent.* **2016**, *5*, 4740–4744.
20. Kasalová, E.; Aufartová, J.; Krčmová, L.K.; Solichová, D.; Solich, P. Recent trends in the analysis of vitamin D and its metabolites in milk–A review. *Food Chem.* **2015**, *171*, 177–190. [CrossRef]
21. Karaźniewicz-Łada, M.; Główka, A. A review of chromatographic methods for the determination of water- and fat-soluble vitamins in biological fluids. *J. Sep. Sci.* **2016**, *39*, 132–148. [CrossRef] [PubMed]
22. Romagnoli, E.; Carnevale, V.; Biondi, P.; Minisola, S. Vitamin D supplementation: When and how? *J. Endocrinol. Investig.* **2014**, *37*, 603–607. [CrossRef] [PubMed]
23. Romagnoli, E.; Pepe, J.; Piemonte, S.; Cipriani, C.; Minisola, S. Management of endocrine disease: Value and limitations of assessing vitamin D nutritional status and advised levels of vitamin D supplementation. *Eur. J. Endocrinol.* **2013**, *169*, R59–R69. [CrossRef] [PubMed]
24. Siggelkow, H. Vitamin-D-Analytic. *Diabetol* **2016**, *12*, 248–253. [CrossRef]
25. Delchiaro, A.; Oliveira, F.d.J.; Bonacordi, C.L.; Chedid, B.L.; Annicchino, G.; Fernandes, C.E.; Strufaldi, R.; Pompei, L.M.; Steiner, M.L. Evaluation of quality of life, physical activity and nutritional profile of postmenopausal women with and without vitamin D deficiency. *Rev. Bras. Ginecol. Obstet.* **2017**, *39*, 337–343. [CrossRef]
26. Bahareh, N.; Samiee, M.S.; Farzami, R.M.; Alavimajd, H.; Zahedirad, M.; Kalayi, A.; Shariatzadeh, N.; Boroumand, N.; Golshekan, E.; Gholamian, Y.; et al. Harmonization of serum 25-hydroxycalciferol assay results from high-performance liquid chromatography, enzyme immunoassay, radioimmunoassay, and immunochemiluminescence systems: A multicenter study. *J. Clin. Lab. Anal.* **2017**, *31*, e22117.
27. Cheng, T.-Y.D.; Millen, A.E.; Wactawski-Wende, J.; Beresford, S.A.A.; LaCroix, A.Z.; Zheng, Y.; Goodman, G.E.; Thornquist, M.D.; Neuhouser, M.L. Vitamin D intake determines vitamin D status of postmenopausal women, particularly those with limited sun exposure. *J. Nutr.* **2014**, *144*, 681–689. [CrossRef]
28. Damaso, E.L.; Albuquerque de Paula, F.J.; Franceschini, S.A.; Vieira, C.S.; Ferriani, R.A.; Silva de Sa, M.F.; Lara, L.A.d.S. Does the access to sun exposure ensure adequate levels of 25-Hydroxyvitamin D? *Rev. Bras. Ginecol. Obstet.* **2017**, *39*, 102–109. [CrossRef]
29. Watanabe, R.; Okazaki, R. Secondary osteoporosis or secondary contributors to bone loss in fracture. Vitamin D deficiency and fracture. *Clin. Calcium* **2013**, *23*, 1313–1319.

30. López-González, B.; Molina-López, J.; Florea, D.I.; Quintero-Osso, B. Association between magnesium-deficient status and anthropometric and clinical-nutritional parameters in posmenopausal women. *Nutr. Hosp.* **2014**, *29*, 658–664.
31. Holick, M.F. Vitamin D Deficiency. *N. Engl. J. Med.* **2007**, *357*, 266–281. [CrossRef] [PubMed]
32. Federation of Spanish Societies of Nutrition and Dietetics (FESNAD). Dietary Reference Intakes (DRI) for the Spanish Population—2010. *Act. Diet.* **2010**, *14*, 196–197.
33. Vázquez-Lorente, H.; Molina-López, J.; Herrera-Quintana, L.; Gamarra-Morales, Y.; López-González, B.; Planells, E. Association between Body Fatness and Vitamin D3 Status in a Postmenopausal Population. *Nutrients* **2020**, *12*, 667. [CrossRef] [PubMed]
34. Rosanoff, A.; Weaver, C.M.; Rude, R.K. Suboptimal magnesium status in the United States: Are the health consequences underestimated? *Nutr. Rev.* **2012**, *70*, 153–164. [CrossRef] [PubMed]
35. Ortega, R.M.; González, L.G.; Navia, B.; Sanchez, J.M.P.; Vizuete, A.A.; Sobaler, A.M.L. Calcium and vitamin D intakes in a representative sample of Spanish women; particular problem in menopause. *Nutr. Hosp.* **2013**, *28*, 306–313.
36. Wright, H.H.; Kruger, M.C.; Schutte, W.D.; Wentzel-Viljoen, E.; Kruger, I.M.; Kruger, H.S. Magnesium intake predicts bone turnover in postmenopausal black south African women. *Nutrients* **2019**, *11*, 2519. [CrossRef]
37. Rizzoli, R.; Bischoff-Ferrari, H.; Dawson-Hughes, B.; Weaver, C. Nutrition and bone health in women after menopause. *Womens Health (Lond. Engl.)* **2014**, *10*, 599–608. [CrossRef]
38. Deng, X.; Song, Y.; Manson, J.E.; Signorello, L.B.; Zhang, S.M.; Shrubsole, M.J.; Ness, R.M.; Seidner, D.L.; Dai, Q. Magnesium, vitamin D status and mortality: Results from US National Health and Nutrition Examination Survey (NHANES) 2001 to 2006 and NHANES III. *BMC Med.* **2013**, *11*, 187. [CrossRef]
39. Olza, J.; Aranceta-Bartrina, J.; González-Gross, M.; Ortega, R.M.; Serra-Majem, L.; Varela-Moreiras, G.; Gil, A. Reported dietary intake, disparity between the reported consumption and the level needed for adequacy and food sources of calcium, phosphorus, magnesium and vitamin D in the spanish population: Findings from the ANIBES study. *Nutrients* **2017**, *9*, 168. [CrossRef]
40. Al-Musharaf, S.; Al-Othman, A.; Al-Daghri, N.M.; Krishnaswamy, S.; Yusuf, D.; Alkharfy, K.M.; Al-Saleh, Y.; Al-Attas, O.S.; Alokail, M.S.; Moharram, O.; et al. Vitamin D deficiency and calcium intake in reference to increased body mass index in children and adolescents. *Eur. J. Pediatr.* **2012**, *171*, 1081–1086. [CrossRef]
41. Harris, H.R.; Chavarro, J.E.; Malspeis, S.; Willett, W.C.; Missmer, S.A. Dairy-food, calcium, magnesium, and vitamin D intake and endometriosis: A prospective cohort study. *Am. J. Epidemiol.* **2013**, *177*, 420–430. [CrossRef] [PubMed]
42. Cashman, K.D. Vitamin D deficiency: Defining, prevalence, causes, and strategies of addressing. *Calcif. Tissue. Int.* **2020**, *106*, 14–29. [CrossRef] [PubMed]
43. Park, E.J.; Lee, H.S.; Lee, S.H.; Shim, K.W.; Cho, C.; Yoo, B.-W. The level of vitamin D using the LC–MS/MS method and related factors in healthy Korean postmenopausal women. *J. Obstet. Gynaecol. Res.* **2018**, *44*, 1977–1984. [CrossRef] [PubMed]
44. Schmitt, E.B.; Nahas-Neto, J.; Bueloni-Dias, F.; Poloni, P.F.; Orsatti, C.L.; Petri Nahas, E.A. Vitamin D deficiency is associated with metabolic syndrome in postmenopausal women. *Maturitas* **2018**, *107*, 97–102. [CrossRef]
45. Erem, S.; Atfi, A.; Razzaque, M.S. Anabolic effects of vitamin D and magnesium in aging bone. *J. Steroid Biochem. Mol. Biol.* **2019**, *193*, 105400. [CrossRef]
46. Uwitonze, A.M.; Razzaque, M.S. Role of magnesium in vitamin D activation and function. *J. Am. Osteopath. Assoc.* **2018**, *118*, 181–189. [CrossRef]
47. Dai, Q.; Zhu, X.; Manson, J.E.; Song, Y.; Li, X.; Franke, A.A.; Costello, R.B.; Rosanoff, A.; Nian, H.; Fan, L.; et al. Magnesium status and supplementation influence vitamin D status and metabolism: Results from a randomized trial. *Am. J. Clin. Nutr.* **2018**, *108*, 1249–1258. [CrossRef]
48. Melamed, M.L.; Michos, E.D.; Post, W.; Astor, B. 25-hydroxyvitamin D levels and the risk of mortality in the general population. *Arch. Intern. Med.* **2008**, *168*, 1629–1637. [CrossRef]
49. Reddy, P.; Edwards, L.R. Magnesium supplementation in vitamin D deficiency. *Am. J. Ther.* **2019**, *26*, 124–132. [CrossRef]
50. Granado-Lorencio, F.; Blanco-Navarro, I.; Pérez-Sacristán, B. Criteria of adequacy for vitamin D testing and prevalence of deficiency in clinical practice. *Clin. Chem. Lab. Med.* **2016**, *54*, 791–798. [CrossRef]

51. Klapkova, E.; Cepova, J.; Pechova, M.; Dunovska, K.; Kotaska, K.; Prusa, R. A comparison of four Methods (Immunochemistry and HPLC) for determination of 25-(OH)-vitamin D in postmenopausal women. *Clin. Lab.* **2017**, *63*, 385–388. [CrossRef] [PubMed]
52. Garg, U. 25-Hydroxyvitamin D testing: Immunoassays versus tandem mass spectrometry. *Clin. Lab. Med.* **2018**, *38*, 439–453. [CrossRef] [PubMed]
53. Vázquez-Lorente, H.; Herrera-Quintana, L.; Quintero-Osso, B.; Molina-López, J.; Planells, E. Current trends in the analytical determination of vitamin D. *Nutr. Hosp.* **2019**, *36*, 1418–1423. [PubMed]
54. Catalano, A.; Morabito, N.; Basile, G.; Cucinotta, D.; Lasco, A. Calcifediol improves lipid profile in osteopenicatorvastatin-treated postmenopausal women. *Eur. J. Clin. Investig.* **2015**, *45*, 144–149. [CrossRef]
55. Pop, L.C.; Sukumar, D.; Schneider, S.H.; Sclussel, Y.; Stahl, T.; Gordon, C.; Wang, X.; Papathomas, T.V.; Shapses, S.A. Three doses of vitamin D, bone mineral density, and geometry in older women during modest weight control in a 1-year randomized controlled trial. *Osteoporos. Int.* **2017**, *28*, 377–388. [CrossRef]
56. Watcharanon, W.; Kaewrudeem, S.; Soontrapa, S.; Somboonporn, W.; Srisaenpang, P.; Panpanit, L.; Pongchaiyakul, C. Effects of sunlight exposure and vitamin D supplementation on vitamin D levels in postmenopausal women in rural Thailand: A randomized controlled trial. *Complement Ther. Med.* **2018**, *40*, 243–247. [CrossRef]

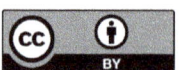

© 2020 by the authors. Licensee MDPI, Basel, Switzerland. This article is an open access article distributed under the terms and conditions of the Creative Commons Attribution (CC BY) license (http://creativecommons.org/licenses/by/4.0/).

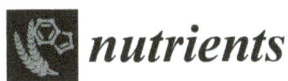

Article

Association between Changes in Nutrient Intake and Changes in Muscle Strength and Physical Performance in the SarcoPhAge Cohort

Laetitia Lengelé [1], Pauline Moehlinger [2], Olivier Bruyère [1,*], Médéa Locquet [1], Jean-Yves Reginster [1,3] and Charlotte Beaudart [1]

1. WHO Collaborating Centre for Public Health Aspects of Musculoskeletal Health and Aging, Division of Public Health, Epidemiology and Health Economics, University of Liège, CHU—Sart Tilman, Quartier Hôpital, Avenue Hippocrate 13 (Bât. B23), 4000 Liège, Belgium; llengele@uliege.be (L.L.); medea.locquet@uliege.be (M.L.); jyr.ch@bluewin.ch (J.-Y.R.); c.beaudart@uliege.be (C.B.)
2. Engineering and Health Field: People, Bioproducts, Environment, Paris Institute of Technology for Life, Food and Environmental Sciences, 16 Claude Bernard Street, CEDEX 05, F-75231 Paris, France; pauline.moehlinger@agroparistech.fr
3. Chair for Biomarkers of Chronic Diseases, Biochemistry Department, College of Science, King Saud. University, Riyadh 11451, Saudi Arabia
* Correspondence: olivier.bruyere@uliege.be; Tel.: +32-43-66-3230

Received: 15 October 2020; Accepted: 11 November 2020; Published: 13 November 2020

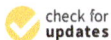

Abstract: Muscle weakness and physical performance impairment are common geriatric conditions that raise morbidity and mortality. They are known to be affected by nutrition, but only a few longitudinal studies exist. This study aims to fill this gap by exploring the association, over 3 years, between variations of nutrient intakes, as well as, on one side, the variations of handgrip strength, as a surrogate of muscle strength, and on the other side, the physical performance, assessed by gait speed. Participants from the SarcoPhAge study, a Belgian cohort of people aged 65 years and older, were asked to complete a self-administered food frequency questionnaire (FFQ) at the second (T2) and the fifth (T5) year of follow-up. Daily macro- and micronutrient intakes were measured and their changes in consumption over the three years of follow-up were then calculated. The association between changes in nutrients consumption and the variations in muscle parameters were investigated through multiple linear regressions. Out of the 534 participants included in the cohort, 238 had complete data at T2 and T5 (median age of 72.0 years (70.0–78.0 years), 60.9% women). In the cross-sectional analysis, calories, omega-3 fatty acids, potassium, and vitamins D, A, and K intakes were positively correlated with muscle strength. In the longitudinal analysis, neither the gait speed nor the muscle strength changes were significantly impacted by the variations. Other longitudinal investigations with longer follow-up are required to improve knowledge about these interrelations.

Keywords: malnutrition; SarcoPhAge; macronutrients; micronutrients; muscle strength; physical performance; gait speed

1. Introduction

Muscle function decline and impaired physical performance characterize, among others factors, the aging process [1,2]. These two parameters are significant indicators of muscle health as they are part of the definition of sarcopenia, a common muscle disease in older adults defined by a low muscle mass, a reduction in muscle strength, and/or a decrease in physical performance [3]. The age-associated decline in muscle strength is more rapid than muscle mass loss, with an annual rate decline varying from 1.9% to 5.0% [4,5], compared to a maximum of 1% for muscle mass in older adults [5]. Although the decline in muscle strength is associated with the decline in muscle mass in older adults, maintaining or increasing muscle mass does not prevent the loss of muscle strength [5]. Regarding the measure of the gait speed, it is a major indicator of the independence level of older adults in daily activities [6] and, therefore, provides a good predictive value for the onset of disability.

These two muscle health components are associated with real public health challenges. Indeed, their deterioration increases the risk of health-related adverse consequences such as longer hospital stays, higher risk of institutionalizations and falls, lower quality of life, and increased mortality [7–14]. In terms of costs, it is recognized that all these consequences significantly increase health care costs both for society and the patient [15,16]. The age-associated muscle wasting disorders are impacted by multiple factors, including biological (i.e., hormones, inflammation, insulin resistance), psychosocial (i.e., self-efficacy, fear of falling), and lifestyle factors like nutrition and exercise [17]. Since the lifestyle factors are modifiable, research focusing on these is essential to help to improve strategies in the prevention and treatment of impaired function and disabilities.

Malnutrition accentuates age-related physical function loss [18,19], furthermore raising disability, morbidity, and mortality [20–22]. It is frequent for older individuals to experience a loss of appetite and therefore decrease their food consumption [23–25]. This condition, called anorexia of aging, has multiple determinants including medical, social, environmental, and psychological factors [24–27]. The altered eating habits affect the amount of food intake, as older adults consume from 16% to 20% lower calories than younger adults [26,28], and worsen the risk of nutrient inadequacy in older adults [29]. There is now evidence that links nutrition to muscle health parameters [18,30–33], highlighting the relevance of appropriate nutritional strategies to limit the decline of muscle strength and physical performance. However, the literature mostly includes cross-sectional studies with inconsistent results. Indeed, some studies provide evidence that higher nutrient intake benefits muscle health, while others provide no findings [33]. A recent study, performed in the sarcopenia and physical impairment with advancing age (SarcoPhAge) cohort, has indicated a cross-sectional association between low nutrient consumption and sarcopenia [34].

Longitudinal analyses would be required to investigate the impact of dietary changes on muscle parameter changes. Longitudinal studies exist, such as those on protein [35,36], vitamin D [37,38], C, and E intakes [39], but they only measure the longitudinal change in muscle parameters according to baseline dietary intakes, and do not measure the change in dietary intakes during follow-up. This is important because there is a decline in energy consumption with advancing age that can compromise nutrient intake in older adults [40], due to several reasons mentioned above, especially regarding anorexia of aging. Additionally, the absorption of nutrients decreases with age [41]. Given the fact that dietary intake varies broadly with increasing age, measuring the change in dietary intake during the follow-up of the study therefore appears essential to establish a causal relationship with the decline in muscle health. This is exactly the aim of the present longitudinal study: To explore the effect of variations of macro- and micronutrient intakes on muscle parameters changes, specifically muscle strength and physical performance, in the SarcoPhAge cohort.

2. Materials and Methods

2.1. Participants' Characteristics

Participants from the SarcoPhAge study were included in the present analysis. The full methodology and protocol of the SarcoPhAge study have already been described in detail previously [34]. Briefly, the SarcoPhAge study is an observational study, which included 534 older adults in Liège, Belgium, followed up from June 2013 to September 2019. The cohort includes community-dwelling adults aged 65 years or older with an annual follow-up. No specific exclusion criteria related to health or demographic characteristics were applied, except for the exclusion criteria established for the Dual-energy X-ray Absorptiometry scan for individuals with an amputated limb or with a body mass index (BMI) above 50 kg/m^2. Written informed consent was provided by participants, and the study was approved by the ethics committee of our institution (reference 2012/277), with two amendments in 2015 and 2018.

During the second year of follow-up of the participants (T2), a food frequency questionnaire (FFQ) was self-administered to assess the macro- and micronutrient intakes of the participants. Although the questionnaire has not been validated in an older population, it has been developed by a group of experts in the field. The FFQ was self-administered for a second time during the last year of follow-up (T5). Thus, we have two full sets of data, separated by three years, which offer the possibility of prospective analyses. The present longitudinal study is based on the population still participating in the SarcoPhAge study at T5 and who completed the FFQs at both T2 and T5. Among the 534 participants included in the SarcoPhAge study, 238 met this condition.

2.2. Data Collection

Participants were seen in the Polyclinique Lucien Brull in Liège, Belgium, by one research assistant for a mean time of 1 h. During their follow-up visits, among a series of tests and evaluations, their muscle health was evaluated and they were asked to complete an FFQ.

2.3. Assessment of Physical and Muscle Parameters

Physical performance was assessed by the usual gait speed on a 4-m distance [42]. Muscle function was assessed by muscle strength using the hand-held hydraulic dynamometer (Saehan Corporation—MSD Europe BVBA, Belgium), calibrated each year for 10, 40, and 90 kg. For this test, participants had to squeeze the device as hard as possible, three times with each hand. The highest measure was recorded, as advised by the Southampton protocol [43].

2.4. Energy and Nutrient Intakes

The complete methodology and protocol for the treatment of FFQs and their analyses have already been described in detail elsewhere [34]. The same methodology of processing FFQs was applied for T2 and for T5, which is briefly recalled here.

Each participant was asked to complete a self-administered FFQ to assess their usual food intake over one month and to bring this completed questionnaire at the T2 and T5 follow-up visits. For each food in the FFQ, the daily amount consumed was calculated according to the following formula:

$$\text{Quantity consumed} = \text{Frequency} \times \text{portion size}$$

The quantity consumed, calculated from the FFQ data, was expressed in g/day for solid food and in mL/day for drinks. For non-standardized portions, a list of images representing seven different sizes of portions of various food was used. Participants had to choose between them the image that best represented, in their opinion, the size of their portions. Then, for each of the food items of the FFQ, a detailed nutrient composition was calculated using the NutriNet-Santé table [44]. This food composition table is used in the NutriNet-Santé study, a large prospective cohort followed across 10 years to collect information on nutrition and health. When items grouped several foods, such as the low-fat cheese item which includes several kinds of cheese, the nutritional composition was calculated as the mean composition of all the corresponding foods from the NutriNet-Santé table. The mean composition was then weighted by the frequency of sex-specific consumption of each food among the older participants of the NutriNet-Santé study. We then measured the total energy intake, and the consumption of micro- and macronutrients per day and per participant. The following macronutrients were selected for the study: Proteins, lipids, saturated fatty acids (AGS), polyunsaturated fatty acids (AGP), omega 3 and 6 fatty acids, monounsaturated fatty acids (AGM), and carbohydrates. For micronutrients, sodium, potassium, magnesium, phosphorus, iron, calcium, zinc, and vitamins D, A, E, C, and K were studied.

2.5. Covariate Data Collection

In this study, we also used the following information that had been collected for all participants during the annual follow-ups: Age, sex, body mass index (BMI), smoking status (yes/no), number of comorbidities, number of drugs consumed, and the level of physical activity based on the Minnesota leisure time activity questionnaire [45]. These covariates are known to significantly affect muscle health and dietary intake [46–50]. Furthermore, they have been identified as such in previous studies of the SarcoPhAge cohort [51].

2.6. Statistical Analyses

The data were processed using the SPSS Statistics 24 (IBM Corporation, Armonk, NY, USA) software package. The normality of the variables was checked by examining the histogram, the quantile–quantile plot, the Shapiro–Wilk test, and the difference between the mean and the median values. The characteristics of the population and the consumption of micronutrients and macronutrients were expressed as median (twenty-fifth to seventy-fifth percentile) because they did not follow a Gaussian distribution. Binary and categorical variables were described by absolute (n) and relative (%) frequencies. A global evaluation of all participants' baseline characteristics was performed.

Differences in socio-demographics and clinical characteristics, and in the consumption of micronutrients and macronutrients between T2 and T5 were investigated through Wilcoxon paired tests for skewed variables. Both the associations between nutrient consumption and either muscle strength or gait speed at T2 were studied by multiple linear regressions with one of the muscle parameters as a dependent variable and each nutrient as independent variable. The multiple covariates that were incorporated into the model are shown here at the bottom of each of the corresponding tables. In order to study the association between the evolution of nutrient consumption and the evolution of muscle parameters between T2 and T5, multiple linear regressions were performed including the confounding variables presented above. The evolution of muscle parameters was calculated by the absolute difference between the variables at T2 and T5. To calculate the evolution of nutritional parameters, macronutrient intakes were calculated as a percentage relative to the total caloric intake of the participant and for micronutrients, the amount was expressed per 1000 kcal. Both macro- and micronutrient changes correspond to the difference between T2 and T5. This method corresponds to an adjustment method called the density method. It uses the quotient of the nutrient intake over the total energy intake [52]. Indeed, because of the strong correlation between nutritional intake and caloric intake, it was essential to adjust the nutrient intake on the energy intake if we wanted to know the isolated effect of each nutrient. Other adjustment methods could have been applied, but the density method appeared to be the most easily interpretable, and nutrient densities are used in the Belgian national nutritional recommendations [53].

Sensibility analyses were performed to assess the robustness of our results, with the relative difference of muscle parameters between T2 and T5 instead of the absolute difference. The relative difference was obtained by dividing the absolute difference by the initial value (at T2) of the parameter.

The results were considered statistically significant at the 0.05 critical threshold.

3. Results

3.1. Characteristics of Participants

Out of the 534 older adults initially included in the SarcoPhAge study, a total of 238 individuals completed both FFQs at T2 and T5 and were included in the present study (median age of 72 years (70.0–78.0), 60.9% of women) (Figure 1). Sociodemographic and clinical characteristics of the whole population are presented in Table 1. As a summary, participants had good cognitive status (mini-mental state examination (MMSE) >24 points), a median of 4 concomitant diseases at T2 and T5, consumed daily 6 drugs at T2 and 7 drugs at T5, and 7.6% ($n = 18$) were smokers. The level of physical activity increased between the two time points for both men and women ($p < 0.001$), and the body mass index significantly decreased ($p = 0.01$). Included participants were compared to the patients who did not complete the FFQ to investigate the potential differences. Lost-to-follow-up patients were older (median age of 74.6 (69.6–79.7) vs. 70.4 (67.5–75.3), $p \leq 0.001$), had lower muscle strength (median of 25.0 (18.0–35.0) vs. 28.0 kg (22.0–39.0) $p \leq 0.001$) and were composed of more malnourished patients according to the mini-nutritional assessment questionnaire (18.5% vs. 9.3%, $p = 0.003$) than patients included in this study.

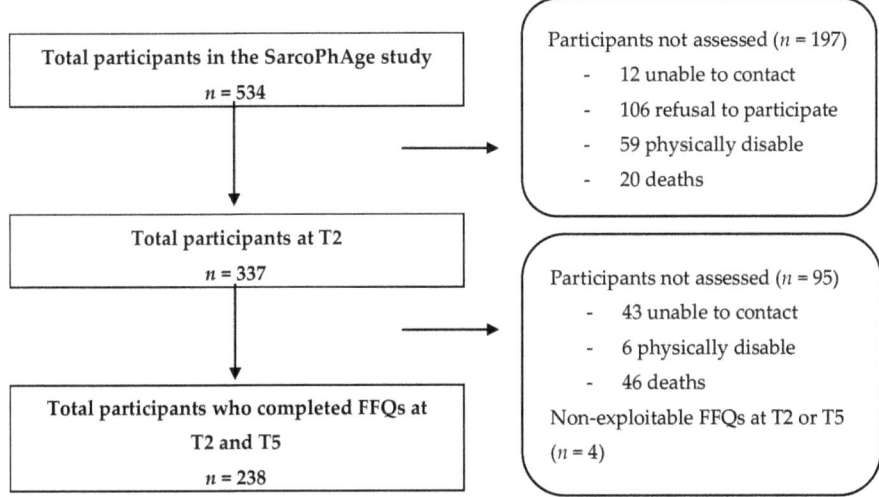

Figure 1. Flow chart.

Table 1. Socio-demographic and clinical characteristics of participants at inclusion (T2) and after three years of follow-up (T5).

	T2 (n = 238)	T5 (n = 238)	p-Value
Age (years)	72.0 (70.0–78.0)	76 (73.0–81.0)	<0.001
Sex			
Women	145 (60.9)	145 (60.9)	—
Number of drugs	6.0 (4.0–8.0)	7.0 (5.0–10.0)	<0.001
Number of concomitant diseases	4.0 (2.7–5.0)	4.0 (3.0–5.0)	0.001
MMSE (/30 points)			
25–30 points	231 (97.1)	222 (93.3)	0.04
21–24 points	2 (0.8)	13 (5.5)	
≤20 points	3 (1.2)	2 (0.8)	
Level of physical activity (kcal/day)			
Women	1323.0 (677.2–2527.2)	1484.5 (847.0–2697.0)	<0.001
Men	1687.0 (1011.5–2761.7)	1837.0 (847.0–3265.9)	<0.001
Smoking			
Yes	18 (7.6) *	18 (7.6) *	—
Body mass index (kg/m^2)	26.9 (23.9–29.4)	26.4 (23.6–29.5)	0.01
Gait speed (m/s)	1.2 (1.0–1.3)	1.2 (1.0–1.4)	0.01
Grip strength (kg)			
Women	21.0 (18.0–24.0)	16.0 (12.0–18.5)	<0.001
Men	39.5 (34.5–44.0)	32.0 (26.5–39.0)	<0.001

Quantitative variables were expressed as median (twenty-fifth to seventy-fifth percentile), and binary or categorical variables were described by absolute (*n*) and relative (%) frequencies. * Baseline data (T0).

3.2. Dietary Nutrient Consumption

The nutritional intakes of the population at T2 and T5 are displayed in Table 2. Overall, FFQ analyses revealed that participants had a lower total energy intake at T5 than at T2 (1615.4 versus 1767.9 kcal/day, p-value = 0.002). Regarding macronutrients, the volunteers at T5 consumed less carbohydrates than at T2 (32.68% at T5 and 34.76% at T2, difference of −2%, p-value < 0.001). The participants at T5 also consumed more saturated fatty acids than at T2 (+0.53%, p-value = 0.038). The following micronutrients were significantly less consumed by participants at T5 than at T2: Sodium, magnesium, iron, calcium, and zinc (all p-values < 0.05). No other significant difference between the consumption of micro- and macronutrients between T2 and T5 were observed. Absolute consumption of these macro- and micronutrients (in terms of quantity/day) is presented in the Appendix A Table A1).

Table 2. Dietary characteristics of participants at T2 and at T5 and mean change over a 3-year follow-up (studied sample n = 238).

	Median T2 (P25–P75)	Median T5 (P25–P75)	Diff [1]	p-Value
Total energy intake (kcal/day)	1767.9 (1439.0–2071.0)	1615.4 (1264.3–2050.2)	−159.4	0.002 [§]
Macronutrients (% in relation to the calorie intake)				
Proteins	18.3 (16.7–20.3)	18.6 (16.4–21.0)	0.3	0.124
Carbohydrates	34.8 (30.7–39.4)	32.7 (28.5–37.9)	−2.0	<0.001 [§]
Lipids	41.6 (37.7–45.5)	42.4 (37.7–46.5)	0.8	0.052
Saturated fatty acids	15.6 (14.2–17.5)	16.4 (14.1–18.6)	0.5	0.038 [§]
Polyunsaturated fatty acids	6.0 (5.1–7.2)	6.0 (4.9–8.0)	0.0	0.413
Omega 3 fatty acids	0.8 (0.7–1.0)	0.8 (0.6–1.0)	−0.0	0.065
Omega 6 fatty acids	4.7 (4.0–5.9)	4.8 (3.9–6.5)	0.0	0.238
Monounsaturated fatty acids	15.9 (13.9–18.3)	16.2 (13.8–18.5)	0.5	0.307
Micronutrients (per 1000 kcal)				
Vitamin D (µg/day)	1.3 (1.0–1.8)	1.3 (1.0–1.9)	0.0	0.226
Vitamin A (µg/day)	497.0 (409.6–565.3)	479.4 (391.9–569.1)	−13.4	0.530
Vitamin E (mg/day)	5.8 (4.9–7.0)	5.6 (4.7–7.2)	−0.0	0.770
Vitamin C (mg/day)	51.4 (37.2–71.7)	49.5 (35.8–65.7)	−0.6	0.768
Vitamin K (µg/day)	70.8 (54.9–85.6)	67.0 (52.5–88.5)	−2.7	0.176
Iron (mg/day)	8.3 (7.1–9.8)	7.8 (6.7–8.7)	−0.5	<0.001 [§]
Calcium (mg/day)	508.8 (435.6–602.6)	481.0 (390.0–572.1)	−33.5	0.005 [§]
Sodium (mg/day)	1512.8 (1360.1–1720.9)	1374.5 (1232.3–1514.8)	141.5	<0.001 [§]
Potassium (mg/day)	1823.7 (1620.1–2030.7)	1820.0 (1608.8–2047.0)	−11.4	0.975
Magnesium (mg/day)	263.0 (220.4–308.3)	236.3 (195.0–275.7)	−22.0	<0.001 [§]
Phosphorus (mg/day)	730.8 (653.1–782.7)	727.1 (643.0–794.4)	−2.3	0.834
Zinc (mg/day)	6.6 (5.9–7.4)	6.4 (5.6–7.2)	−0.2	0.004 [§]

[1] Median of the absolute difference between T2 and T5. [§] Results for which the p-value was statistically significant (<0.05).

Moreover, less than half of the participants met the Belgian national recommendations for the carbohydrates, saturated fatty acids, omega-3 and omega-6 fatty acids, vitamins D, C, and K, sodium, and potassium (Table A3) [53].

3.3. Association between Macro- and Micronutrients and Muscle Health Components

From the cross-sectional analyses on our baseline population (Table 3) at T2, it emerged that muscle strength seemed to be positively associated, after adjustment for potential confounding variables, with calorie intake (p = 0.003) and the consumption of omega-3 fatty acids (p = 0.03), potassium (p = 0.04), and vitamins D (p = 0.03), A (p = 0.045), and K (p = 0.01).

When we carried out further longitudinal analyses to assess the changes of nutritional consumption between T2 and T5 and their effect on changes of muscle parameters during the same period (Table 4), no association was found to be statistically significant between either changes in gait speed or muscle strength and changes in dietary intakes.

Table 3. Baseline associations between macro- and micronutrient consumption and muscle health components.

Muscle Parameters at T2	Gait Speed		Muscle Strength	
Intake at T2	β	p-Value *	β	p-Value *
Macronutrients				
Calorie	5.538×10^{-5}	0.122	0.003	0.003 §
Protein	0.003	0.606	0.26	0.098
Carbohydrate	0.000	0.898	−0.077	0.280
Lipid	0.000	0.882	0.046	0.524
Saturated fatty acids	0.002	0.666	−0.031	0.828
Polyunsaturated fatty acids	−0.006	0.480	0.116	0.599
Omega 3 fatty acids	−0.056	0.230	2.578	0.031 §
Omega 6 fatty acids	−0.006	0.562	0.015	0.951
Monounsaturated fatty acids	0.002	0.610	0.120	0.311
Micronutrients				
Vitamin D	−0.013	0.419	0.899	0.031 §
Vitamin A	0.000	0.291	0.006	0.045 §
Vitamin E	−0.009	0.373	0.119	0.630
Vitamin C	0.001	0.403	0.019	0.276
Vitamin K	0.001	0.247	0.042	0.013 §
Iron	−0.005	0.552	−0.179	0.427
Calcium	-9.261×10^{-5}	0.463	0.004	0.231
Sodium	6.525×10^{-5}	0.221	0.002	0.176
Potassium	5.335×10^{-5}	0.316	0.003	0.035 §
Magnesium	-3.843×10^{-5}	0.987	0.005	0.376
Phosphorus	-5.244×10^{-5}	0.744	0.005	0.207
Zinc	0.006	0.585	0.119	0.685

* p-values obtained from linear regression including age, sex, BMI, number of drugs, number of concomitant diseases, physical activity level, smoking status, and kcal consumed at T2 as covariates. § Results for which the p-value was statistically significant (<0.05).

Table 4. Association between longitudinal changes in macro- and micronutrient consumption and longitudinal changes in muscle health components.

Change of Muscle Health Components between T2 and T5	Gait Speed		Muscle Strength	
Change of Consumption between T2 and T5	β	p-Value *	β	p-Value *
Macronutrients				
Calorie	1.645×10^{-5}	0.506	4.612×10^{-6}	0.994
Protein	0.004	0.326	−0.112	0.245
Carbohydrate	-2.795×10^{-5}	0.988	−0.079	0.077
Lipid	0.001	0.513	0.077	0.077
Saturated fatty acids	0.003	0.375	0.183	0.051
Polyunsaturated fatty acids	0.001	0.875	0.013	0.927
Omega 3 fatty acids	−0.024	0.567	−0.206	0.838
Omega 6 fatty acids	0.001	0.814	0.024	0.873
Monounsaturated fatty acids	0.001	0.741	0.139	0.086
Micronutrients				
Vitamin D	−0.009	0.550	−0.485	0.164
Vitamin A	-7.567×10^{-5}	0.300	0.000	0.904
Vitamin E	−0.003	0.621	0.024	0.877
Vitamin C	0.000	0.789	0.016	0.141
Vitamin K	0.000	0.631	0.015	0.174
Iron	−0.011	0.122	−0.260	0.112
Calcium	0.000	0.158	−0.001	0.792
Sodium	-5.914×10^{-5}	0.230	−0.001	0.620
Potassium	-1.716×10^{-5}	0.655	0.001	0.445
Magnesium	0.000	0.212	−0.002	0.628
Phosphorus	0.000	0.066	−0.005	0.111
Zinc	0.003	0.789	−0.274	0.232

* p-values obtained from linear regression including age, sex, BMI, smoking status, number of drugs, number of concomitant diseases, physical activity level, kcal consumed at T2, and muscle parameters value at T2 as covariates.

In the sensitivity analysis, when we performed similar longitudinal analyses but with the relative difference of muscle parameters between T2 and T5 instead of the absolute difference, we found similar conclusions except for one nutrient: An increase in saturated fatty acids seemed to have a positive impact on the muscle strength evolution ($p = 0.039$) (Table A2 in the Appendix A).

4. Discussion

At the baseline, a higher consumption of calories, omega-3 fatty acids, potassium, and vitamins D, A, and K seemed to be positively associated with better muscle strength. However, when we analyzed the impact of the changes in nutrient intake across years on the muscle parameters changes, no nutrient was correlated with changes of gait speed or muscle strength between the baseline and the three-year follow-up. In our older population from the SarcoPhAge cohort, the absolute dietary intake had significantly decreased for almost every macro- and micronutrient over a period of three years (i.e., between T2 and T5). This was in line with the fact that the older adults from our cohort experienced a deficit in food consumption also called "anorexia of aging" [26]. People suffering from this condition are at high risk of protein-energy malnutrition, sarcopenia, and frailty, leading to higher morbidity and mortality [26,54]. Furthermore, adjusted on the calorie intake, the amount of carbohydrates, sodium, magnesium, iron, calcium, and zinc taken by the population of our sample has significantly declined. When we compared dietary intakes to Belgian national recommendations (Table A3) [53], less than half of the participants met these recommendations for the carbohydrates, saturated fatty acids, omega-3 and omega-6 fatty acids, vitamins D, C, and K, sodium, and potassium. Regarding the muscle parameters, both muscle strength and gait speed significantly decreased at the end of the three-year follow-up. The median decline in muscle strength after three years of follow-up reached the minimal clinical important difference (MCID) value ranged between 5.0 and 6.5 kg [55], but the median difference in gait speed between the two time points did not reach the MCID value of 1.0 m/s [56]. This could have impacted our analyses because this change in gait speed would have been too small to detect an influence of dietary intake on it.

Several studies, mentioned below, have already investigated the cross-sectional impact of macro- and micronutrients on muscle parameters. Some of them, like our study, investigated the dietary intake alone, while others studied the biochemical status with or without the nutrient consumption. Two reviews focusing on the relationship between muscle strength and, either or both, the biochemical status of nutrients and the dietary intake, corroborate our results regarding omega-3 fatty acids. Indeed, they concluded that omega-3 fatty acids were positively correlated to muscle strength among older adults in cross-sectional studies [57,58]. Regarding vitamin A, one of these reviews discussed the carotenoid status, where a lower blood concentration of carotenoids was associated with lower muscle strength in cross-sectional analyses including older adults [57]. Moreover, the carotenoid status was found to have a long-term impact on muscle strength in the InCHIANTI study, where older community-dwelling adults with lower plasma carotenoids levels were at higher risk of low grip strength (OR = 1.88, 95% CI, 0.93–3.56, $p = 0.07$) [59]. The anti-inflammatory and antioxidant potentials of these two nutrients, vitamin A and omega-3 fatty acids, could explain the effects observed [60,61]. Regarding vitamin D, several studies have investigated the biochemical status, the 25-hydroxyvitamin D blood concentration, and its association with muscle strength and physical performance in older adults. A first study of Houston et al. found a positive association between a low serum concentration of vitamin D and low handgrip strength ($p < 0.05$) and with poor physical performance too, measured by the short physical performance battery test ($p < 0.05$) [62]. While these results are in line with ours concerning the association with muscle strength, it is contrasting with our results concerning physical performance. These cross-sectional results were confirmed in a second study of Houston et al., and longitudinal associations were also explored in this study, where patients with a low blood serum concentration of 25-hydroxyvitamin D at the baseline had poorer physical performance at 2 and 4 years of follow-up ($p < 0.01$) but not lower grip strength ($p > 0.05$) [38]. Inconsistent longitudinal results were found in the study by Visser et al. regarding muscle strength, where participants with a low blood concentration of vitamin D at the baseline had 2.57 (95% CI 1.40–4.70) more risk of experiencing low muscle strength [37]. Evidence suggests that this vitamin can stimulate the proliferation and the differentiation of the skeletal muscle fibers, thus enhancing muscle strength [63]. Concerning vitamin K, one study, including 1089 community-dwelling older adults and investigating the biochemical status of this vitamin, found a statistically significant positive association both with muscle strength ($p < 0.04$) and gait speed cross-sectionally [64]. While these results are in line with ours concerning the association with muscle strength, it is contrasting with our results concerning gait speed. Nowadays, the role of vitamin K on muscle health is not yet fully understood, and more studies on its biological mechanisms and its impact on muscle function are needed [65]. To our knowledge, no research investigating the link between potassium and muscle strength has been performed, except for the study of Beaudart et al. in the same cohort as the one of the present study, where potassium intake was associated with lower risk of sarcopenia ($p = 0.04$) [34]. Potassium is necessary for nerve activity and therefore contributes to the contractibility of the muscle [66].

From a longitudinal perspective, we cannot confirm the relationships observed in the cross-sectional analyses. In fact, the muscle parameters changes did not seem to be impacted by the nutrient intake changes during the three years of follow-up. Several possible hypotheses could explain the different results between the cross-sectional and longitudinal analyses. Firstly, the length of follow-up, potentially too short, could have impacted the statistical power of our study and secondly, we can mention the biases inherent to the dietary assessment method like the recall bias. Moreover, these are two different investigations. Indeed, the cross-sectional analyses evaluated a precise value at a given time, while the longitudinal analyses measured a difference between T2 and T5. Therefore, the results and the conclusions are difficult to compare adequately. To our knowledge, no study exists on the longitudinal association between changes in dietary intake and changes in muscle parameters, in older adults aged over 65 years. Longitudinal research on this topic only studied food consumption at baseline and its impact on the muscle strength and physical performance changes over time. Therefore, we cannot compare our results regarding the longitudinal analysis since the nutritional data evaluated were not similar. Moreover, our conclusions were confirmed by the assessment of the robustness of our results, which were identical to the analyses performed on the relative variations instead of the absolute variations of muscle parameters. Only the saturated fatty acids became significantly positively associated with muscle strength. Yet, this relationship has not been investigated elsewhere. There is a real lack of research on the longitudinal effects of nutrient intake changes on muscle parameter changes. Nonetheless, food consumption of older adults can vary broadly over a period of only three years as described in this present study. This type of longitudinal research is therefore essential.

Strengths and Limitations

This study has an original design. It is one of the first studies to consider longitudinal changes in the intake of a large number of nutrients and to evaluate how those changes impact individual muscle parameter changes. Another strength of this study is the adjustment of the macro- and micronutrient intakes on the total energy intake according to the density method. This allowed us to avoid the impact of any existing correlation between the consumption of calories and nutrients on our results.

Several aspects must be taken into consideration when interpreting our results. Firstly, we measured the dietary intake but not the biochemical status of macro- and micronutrients. Dynamic factors could alter single nutrient absorption, when consumed with other nutrients [29], such as the known synergy between vitamin D and calcium. Moreover, the biochemical status of some micronutrients, such as calcium and magnesium, is complex to evaluate because they have no specific markers [29]. Secondly, we did not take into account the potential impact of a more global diet. In fact, we studied the impact of each specific nutrient, but it is a necessary first step before considering the overall nutritional quality. In addition, we adjusted our analyses on a large number of covariates, known to affect dietary intake and the muscle parameters, but other confounding factors could have been considered. Indeed, we took into account the level of physical activity of the participants but not the type of physical activity. It is now well established that resistance exercise training and aerobic exercise training are two types of exercise that have a positive effect on muscle and even help prevent a decline in mobility [67]. These exercises may enhance the myofibrillar protein synthesis, and it has been suggested that it was due to nutrient-stimulated vasodilatation and improvement in nutrient delivery to muscle [68]. Additionally, the results indicated that the effects of these types of physical activity, particularly resistance training, may be impacted by nutritional status [69] and nutrient supplementation [70]. Ethnicity is also known to influence muscle parameters and nutritional status [71,72], but we did not adjust our analyses on this variable since the included participants in our cohort were homogeneous in terms of ethnicity. The probability that this could predominantly have impacted our results remains low.

The FFQ entailed an inevitable reporting bias in the data reporting since it is based on participants' memory. This dietary assessment method was chosen for the following reasons: It does not require trained interviewers, it can be self-administered, and it can be used for large scale studies. Nevertheless, other methods to record daily dietary intake are available and could have been used. Moreover, a selection bias was brought by the constitution of our population that was composed of volunteers. Indeed, they were presumably in better health than the general population, and the evolution of their muscle parameters was therefore potentially better. Additionally, the decline observed for gait speed did not even reach the small detectable change threshold of 0.05 m/s [56], which could eventually partially explain why we did not find any association between nutrient consumption and gait speed. There was also a potential attrition bias because of the patients lost to follow-up. They possibly underwent a more important health decline than the participants interviewed throughout the entire follow-up. In fact, as presented in the results section, the volunteers included in the study had a better muscle strength and physical performance, were younger, and were composed of less malnourished patients than those lost to follow-up. Consequently, our results are probably not truly representative of the target population and they cannot be generalized to other populations or geriatric settings. Finally, we did not estimate one potential confounding factor, which is the consumption of nutritional supplements among participants. The intake of any supplemented nutrients could have been increased without being assessed in our analyses, and thus have an indirect positive impact on the muscle components, affecting the potential significant observations in our models. However, these data were not available.

5. Conclusions

Based on an FFQ dietary assessment method, muscle strength seems positively associated with caloric intake, omega-3 fatty acids, potassium, and vitamin D, A, and K consumption at a given time. When studying variations over a period of three years, no association was found between the evolution of nutrient intake and either gait speed or muscle strength. The longitudinal impact of dietary intake on muscle parameters needs further investigation to fill the gap in the current knowledge on this subject. Cohort studies with a longer follow-up and longitudinal investigations on dietary patterns and their impact on muscle health are needed to elaborate on our findings. It is important to better understand these interrelations to enable the implementation of optimal nutritional strategies for the prevention of age-related muscle disabilities.

Author Contributions: Conceptualization, C.B., O.B., and J.-Y.R.; methodology, L.L., P.M., and C.B.; software, L.L. and P.M.; validation, L.L., P.M., O.B., M.L., J.-Y.R., and C.B.; formal analysis, L.L. and P.M.; investigation, L.L., M.L., and C.B.; resources, O.B. and J-Y.R.; data curation, L.L., M.L., and C.B.; writing—original draft preparation, L.L.; writing—review and editing, L.L., M.L., O.B., and C.B.; supervision, O.B. and J.-Y.R. All authors have read and agreed to the published version of the manuscript.

Funding: This research received no external funding.

Acknowledgments: We would like to thank all participants from the SarcoPhAge study for their collaboration.

Conflicts of Interest: The authors declare no conflict of interest.

Appendix A

Table A1. Dietary consumption at T2 and T5 (absolute values of consumption).

	Median T2 (P25–P75)	Median T5 (P25–P75)	Median of the Difference between T2 and T5	p-Value
Total energy intake (kcal/day)	1767.88 (1439.02–2070.96)	1615.41 (1264.34–2050.16)	−151.97	0.002
Macronutrients				
Proteins (g/day)	80.95 (64.42–97.07)	73.88 (54.54–101.21)	−4.15	0.020
Carbohydrates (g/day)	151.41 (124.52–180.36)	133.15 (100.49–162.91)	−18.64	<0.001
Lipids (g/day)	80.25 (61.86–98.12)	75.78 (57.35–98.67)	−5.30	0.083
Saturated fatty acids (g/day)	29.84 (22.99–38.51)	29.20 (21.39–37.94)	−1.51	0.121
Polyunsaturated fatty acids (g/day)	11.70 (8.65–15.47)	11.17 (7.96–15.61)	−0.64	0.188
Omega 3 (g/day)	1.56 (1.17–2.08)	1.40 (1.04–1.96)	−0.17	0.004
Omega 6 (g/day)	9.30 (6.85–12.25)	9.12 (6.37–12.90)	−0.38	0.299
Monounsaturated fatty acids (g/day)	30.84 (25.14–38.63)	29.26 (21.84–39.11)	−2.57	0.048
Micronutrients				
Sodium (mg/day)	2686.85 (2148.48–3228.33)	2190.19 (1717.06–2711.49)	−467.19	<0.001
Potassium (mg/day)	3210.88 (2615.01–3857.28)	2964.15 (2328.73–3685.18)	−249.92	<0.001
Magnesium (mg/day)	449.30 (362.82–575.20)	385.85 (307.86–467.27)	−69.45	<0.001
Phosphorus (mg/day)	1249.66 (1027.50–1543.91)	1181.27 (871.23–1524.57)	−79.40	0.002
Iron (mg/day)	14.53 (11.30–18.34)	12.43 (9.93–15.68)	−1.80	<0.001
Calcium (mg/day)	884.41 (703.09–1122.55)	784.78 (575.14–1045.49)	−91.62	<0.001
Zinc (mg/day)	11.60 (9.04–14.56)	10.28 (7.80–13.08)	−1.20	<0.001
Vitamin D (µg/day)	2.32 (1.63–3.17)	2.29 (1.54–3.49)	−0.04	0.657
Vitamin A (µg/day)	880.88 (644.14–1097.42)	789.27 (550.44–1047.74)	−66.28	0.006
Vitamin E (mg/day)	10.04 (7.78–13.29)	9.43 (7.18–12.68)	−0.31	0.037
Vitamin C (mg/day)	87.79 (62.72–126.79)	83.44 (57.71–112.70)	−6.14	0.010
Vitamin K (µg/day)	120.08 (92.41–163.89)	104.02 (74.77–151.08)	−9.92	0.003

Table A2. Association between longitudinal changes in macro- and micronutrient consumption and longitudinal relative changes in muscle health components.

Change of Muscle Health Components between T2 and T5	Gait Speed		Muscle Strength	
Change of Consumption between T2 and T5	β	p-Value	β	p-Value
Calorie	1.621×10^{-5}	0.512	2.527×10^{-6}	0.997
Protein	0.004	0.343	−0.113	0.235
Carbohydrate	-9.7219×10^{-5}	0.961	−0.085	0.058
Lipid	0.001	0.481	0.083	0.059
Saturated fatty acids	0.004	0.356	0.195	0.039
Polyunsaturated fatty acids	0.001	0.846	0.024	0.864
Omega-3 fatty acids	−0.024	0.565	−2.220	0.826
Omega-6 fatty acids	0.002	0.784	0.037	0.806
Monounsaturated fatty acids	0.001	0.708	0.146	0.071
Vitamin D	−0.009	0.546	−0.486	0.162
Vitamin A	-7.492×10^{-5}	0.307	0.000	0.846
Vitamin E	−0.003	0.646	0.036	0.816
Vitamin C	0.000	0.797	0.015	0.146
Vitamin K	0.000	0.623	0.014	0.183
Iron	−0.011	0.110	−0.282	0.087
Calcium	0.000	0.154	−0.001	0.801
Sodium	-6.001×10^{-5}	0.224	−0.001	0.583
Potassium	-1.691×10^{-5}	0.660	0.001	0.444
Magnesium	0.000	0.199	−0.002	0.548
Phosphorus	0.000	0.068	−0.005	0.106
Zinc	0.002	0.816	−0.290	0.204

* p-values obtained from linear regression including age, sex, BMI, smoking status, number of drugs, number of concomitant diseases, physical activity (Minnesota), kcal consumed at T2, and muscle parameters value at T2.

Table A3. Adequation of the consumption of macro- and micronutrients at T2 and T5.

	Population with an Adequate Intake at T2 (%)	Population with an Adequate Intake at T5 (%)	p-Value
Macronutrients			
Proteins	90.3	79.4	0.001
Carbohydrates	1.3	0.8	0.625
Lipids	46.2	45.4	0.039
Saturated fatty acids	20.2	31.1	0.003
Polyunsaturated fatty acids	45.0	40.3	0.417
Omega-3 fatty acids	15.1	14.7	0.538
Omega-6 fatty acids	43.3	38.2	0.210
Monounsaturated fatty acids	69.7	55.9	0.006
Micronutrients			
Vitamin D	0.8	0.0	0.485
Vitamin A	85.7	79.8	0.059
Vitamin E	60.1	54.6	0.193
Vitamin C	46.2	42.4	0.391
Vitamin K	3.8	4.2	0.644
Iron	97.1	94.5	0.210
Calcium	69.3	56.7	0.001
Sodium	0.8	5.5	0.007
Potassium	29.8	30.7	0.002
Magnesium	95.8	85.7	<0.001
Phosphorus	97.5	94.5	0.092
Zinc	82.4	76.5	0.070

The prevalence of participants below the recommended daily allowance (RDA) for macronutrients, measured from the Belgian nutritional recommendations [53], and below the estimated average requirement (EAR) for micronutrients were computed. Since the EAR was not available in the Belgian nutritional recommendations, the following formulas were used [73,74]:

- For vitamins D, A, E, K, iron, calcium, sodium, potassium, phosphorus, and zinc: 0.77 * RDA
- For magnesium and vitamin C: 0.83 * RDA

It was established that the EAR is a reliable estimate of the usual intake requirements of a group of subjects [75].

RDA tailored to populations aged over 60 years where applied when available. Alternatively, recommendations for adults older than 18 years were used.

References

1. Ponti, F.; Santoro, A.; Mercatelli, D.; Gasperini, C.; Conte, M.; Martucci, M.; Sangiorgi, L.; Franceschi, C.; Bazzocchi, A. Aging and Imaging Assessment of Body Composition: From Fat to Facts. *Front. Endocrinol.* **2020**, *10*. [CrossRef] [PubMed]
2. Tangen, G.G.; Robinson, H.S. Measuring physical performance in highly active older adults: Associations with age and gender? *Aging Clin. Exp. Res.* **2020**, *32*, 229–237. [CrossRef] [PubMed]
3. Cruz-Jentoft, A.J.; Bahat, G.; Bauer, J.; Boirie, Y.; Bruyère, O.; Cederholm, T.; Cooper, C.; Landi, F.; Rolland, Y.; Sayer, A.A.; et al. Sarcopenia: Revised European consensus on definition and diagnosis. *Age Ageing* **2019**, *48*, 16–31. [CrossRef] [PubMed]
4. Auyeung, T.W.; Lee, S.W.J.; Leung, J.; Kwok, T.; Woo, J. Age-associated decline of muscle mass, grip strength and gait speed: A 4-year longitudinal study of 3018 community-dwelling older Chinese. *Geriatr. Gerontol. Int.* **2014**, *14*, 76–84. [CrossRef]
5. Goodpaster, B.H.; Park, S.W.; Harris, T.B.; Kritchevsky, S.B.; Nevitt, M.; Schwartz, A.V.; Simonsick, E.M.; Tylavsky, F.A.; Visser, M.; Newman, A.B. The Loss of Skeletal Muscle Strength, Mass, and Quality in Older Adults: The Health, Aging and Body Composition Study. *J. Gerontol.* **2006**, *61*, 1059–1064. [CrossRef]

6. Kuo, H.-K.; Leveille, S.G.; Yen, C.-J.; Chai, H.-M.; Chang, C.-H.; Yeh, Y.-C.; Yu, Y.-H.; Bean, J.F. Exploring How Peak Leg Power and Usual Gait Speed Are Linkedto Late-Life Disability: Data from the National Health and Nutrition Examination Survey (NHANES), 1999-2002. *Am. J. Phys. Med. Rehabil.* **2006**, *85*, 650–658. [CrossRef]
7. Hardy, S.E.; Perera, S.; Roumani, Y.F.; Chandler, J.M.; Studenski, S.A. Improvement in usual gait speed predicts better survival in older adults. *J. Am. Geriatr. Soc.* **2007**, *55*, 1727–1734. [CrossRef]
8. Roberts, H.C.; Syddall, H.E.; Cooper, C.; Aihie sayer, A. Is grip strength associated with length of stay in hospitalised older patients admitted for rehabilitation? Findings from the Southampton grip strength study. *Age Ageing* **2012**, *41*, 641–646. [CrossRef]
9. Leong, D.P.; Teo, K.K.; Rangarajan, S.; Lopez-Jaramillo, P.; Avezum, A.; Orlandini, A.; Seron, P.; Ahmed, S.H.; Rosengren, A.; Kelishadi, R.; et al. Prognostic value of grip strength: Findings from the Prospective Urban Rural Epidemiology (PURE) study. *Lancet* **2015**, *386*, 266–273. [CrossRef]
10. Schmid, A.; Duncan, P.W.; Studenski, S.; Lai, S.M.; Richards, L.; Perera, S.; Wu, S.S. Improvements in speed-based gait classifications are meaningful. *Stroke* **2007**, *38*, 2096–2100. [CrossRef]
11. De Rekeneire, N.; Visser, M.; Peila, R.; Nevitt, M.C.; Cauley, J.A.; Tylavsky, F.A.; Simonsick, E.M.; Harris, T.B. Is a Fall Just a Fall: Correlates of Falling in Healthy Older Persons. The Health, Aging and Body Composition Study. *J. Am. Geriatr. Soc.* **2003**, *51*, 841–846. [CrossRef] [PubMed]
12. Studenski, S.; Perera, S.; Wallace, D.; Chandler, J.M.; Duncan, P.W.; Rooney, E.; Fox, M.; Guralnik, J.M. Physical Performance Measures in the Clinical Setting. *J. Am. Geriatr. Soc.* **2003**, *51*, 314–322. [CrossRef] [PubMed]
13. Penninx, B.W.J.H.; Ferrucci, L.; Leveille, S.G.; Rantanen, T.; Pahor, M.; Guralnik, J.M. Lower Extremity Performance in Nondisabled Older Persons as a Predictor of Subsequent Hospitalization. *J. Gerontol.* **2000**, *55*, 691–697. [CrossRef]
14. Hajek, A.; Brettschneider, C.; Eisele, M.; Kaduszkiewicz, H.; Mamone, S.; Wiese, B.; Weyerer, S.; Werle, J.; Fuchs, A.; Pentzek, M.; et al. Correlates of hospitalization among the oldest old: Results of the AgeCoDe–AgeQualiDe prospective cohort study. *Aging Clin. Exp. Res.* **2020**, *32*, 1295–1301. [CrossRef]
15. Mijnarends, D.M.; Luiking, Y.C.; Halfens, R.J.G.; Evers, S.M.A.A.; Lenaerts, E.L.A.; Verlaan, S.; Wallace, M.; Schols, J.M.G.A.; Meijers, J.M.M. Muscle, Health and Costs: A Glance at their Relationship. *J. Nutr. Health Aging* **2018**, *22*, 766–773. [CrossRef] [PubMed]
16. Guerra, R.S.; Amaral, T.F.; Sousa, A.S.; Pichel, F.; Restivo, M.T.; Ferreira, S.; Fonseca, I. Handgrip strength measurement as a predictor of hospitalization costs. *Eur. J. Clin. Nutr.* **2015**, *69*, 187–192. [CrossRef]
17. Tieland, M.; Trouwborst, I.; Clark, B.C. Skeletal muscle performance and ageing. *J. Cachexia Sarcopenia Muscle* **2018**, *9*, 3–19. [CrossRef]
18. Landi, F.; Camprubi-Robles, M.; Bear, D.E.; Cederholm, T.; Malafarina, V.; Welch, A.A.; Cruz-Jentoft, A.J. Muscle loss: The new malnutrition challenge in clinical practice. *Clin. Nutr.* **2019**, *38*, 2113–2120. [CrossRef]
19. Ramsey, K.A.; Meskers, C.G.M.; Trappenburg, M.C.; Verlaan, S.; Reijnierse, E.M.; Whittaker, A.C.; Maier, A.B. Malnutrition is associated with dynamic physical performance. *Aging Clin. Exp. Res.* **2020**, *32*, 1085–1092. [CrossRef]
20. Corcoran, C.; Murphy, C.; Culligan, E.P.; Walton, J.; Sleator, R.D. Malnutrition in the elderly. *Sci. Prog.* **2019**, *102*, 171–180. [CrossRef]
21. Volkert, D.; Beck, A.M.; Cederholm, T.; Cereda, E.; Cruz-Jentoft, A.; Goisser, S.; de Groot, L.; Großhauser, F.; Kiesswetter, E.; Norman, K.; et al. Management of Malnutrition in Older Patients—Current Approaches, Evidence and Open Questions. *J. Clin. Med.* **2019**, *8*, 974. [CrossRef] [PubMed]
22. Adly, N.N.; Abd-El-Gawad, W.M.; Abou-Hashem, R.M. Relationship between malnutrition and different fall risk assessment tools in a geriatric in-patient unit. *Aging Clin. Exp. Res.* **2020**, *32*, 1279–1287. [CrossRef] [PubMed]
23. Roy, M.; Gaudreau, P.; Payette, H. A scoping review of anorexia of aging correlates and their relevance to population health interventions. *Appetite* **2016**, *105*, 688–699. [CrossRef] [PubMed]
24. Landi, F.; Lattanzio, F.; Dell'Aquila, G.; Eusebi, P.; Gasperini, B.; Liperoti, R.; Belluigi, A.; Bernabei, R.; Cherubini, A. Prevalence and potentially reversible factors associated with anorexia among older nursing home residents: Results from the ulisse project. *J. Am. Med. Dir. Assoc.* **2013**, *14*, 119–124. [CrossRef]
25. Jadczak, A.D.; Visvanathan, R. Anorexia of Aging—An Updated Short Review. *J. Nutr. Health Aging* **2019**, *23*, 306–309. [CrossRef]

26. Landi, F.; Calvani, R.; Tosato, M.; Martone, A.M.; Ortolani, E.; Savera, G.; Sisto, A.; Marzetti, E. Anorexia of aging: Risk factors, consequences, and potential treatments. *Nutrients* **2016**, *8*, 69. [CrossRef] [PubMed]
27. Volkert, D.; Kiesswetter, E.; Cederholm, T.; Donini, L.M.; Eglseer, D.; Norman, K.; Schneider, S.M.; Ströbele-Benschop, N.; Torbahn, G.; Wirth, R.; et al. Development of a Model on Determinants of Malnutrition in Aged Persons: A MaNuEL Project. *Gerontol. Geriatr. Med.* **2019**, *5*, 233372141985843. [CrossRef]
28. Ter Borg, S.; Verlaan, S.; Hemsworth, J.; Mijnarends, D.M.; Schols, J.M.G.A.; Luiking, Y.C.; De Groot, L.C.P.G.M. Micronutrient intakes and potential inadequacies of community-dwelling older adults: A systematic review. *Br. J. Nutr.* **2015**, *113*, 1195–1206. [CrossRef]
29. Jensen, G.L.; Cederholm, T. The malnutrition overlap syndromes of cachexia and sarcopenia: A malnutrition conundrum. *Am. J. Clin. Nutr.* **2018**, *108*, 1157–1158. [CrossRef]
30. Beaudart, C.; Sanchez-Rodriguez, D.; Locquet, M.; Reginster, J.Y.; Lengelé, L.; Bruyère, O. Malnutrition as a strong predictor of the onset of sarcopenia. *Nutrients* **2019**, *11*, 2883. [CrossRef]
31. Amarya, S.; Singh, K.; Sabharwal, M. Changes during aging and their association with malnutrition. *J. Clin. Gerontol. Geriatr.* **2015**, *6*, 78–84. [CrossRef]
32. Deutz, N.E.P.; Ashurst, I.; Ballesteros, M.D.; Bear, D.E.; Cruz-Jentoft, A.J.; Genton, L.; Landi, F.; Laviano, A.; Norman, K.; Prado, C.M. The Underappreciated Role of Low Muscle Mass in the Management of Malnutrition. *J. Am. Med. Dir. Assoc.* **2019**, *20*, 22–27. [CrossRef] [PubMed]
33. Beaudart, C.; Locquet, M.; Touvier, M.; Reginster, J.Y.; Bruyère, O. Association between dietary nutrient intake and sarcopenia in the SarcoPhAge study. *Aging Clin. Exp. Res.* **2019**, *31*, 815–824. [CrossRef] [PubMed]
34. McLean, R.R.; Mangano, K.M.; Hannan, M.T.; Kiel, D.P.; Sahni, S. Dietary Protein Intake Is Protective Against Loss of Grip Strength Among Older Adults in the Framingham Offspring Cohort. *J. Gerontol. Ser. A Biol. Sci. Med. Sci.* **2016**, *71*, 356–361. [CrossRef]
35. Granic, A.; Mendonça, N.; Sayer, A.A.; Hill, T.R.; Davies, K.; Adamson, A.; Siervo, M.; Mathers, J.C.; Jagger, C. Low protein intake, muscle strength and physical performance in the very old: The Newcastle 85+ Study. *Clin. Nutr.* **2018**, *37*, 2260–2270. [CrossRef]
36. Visser, M.; Deeg, D.J.H.; Lips, P. Low Vitamin D and High Parathyroid Hormone Levels as Determinants of Loss of Muscle Strength and Muscle Mass (Sarcopenia): The Longitudinal Aging Study Amsterdam. *J. Clin. Endocrinol. Metab.* **2003**, *88*, 5766–5772. [CrossRef]
37. Houston, D.K.; Tooze, J.A.; Neiberg, R.H.; Hausman, D.B.; Johnson, M.A.; Cauley, J.A.; Bauer, D.C.; Cawthon, P.M.; Shea, M.K.; Schwartz, G.G.; et al. 25-hydroxyvitamin D status and change in physical performance and strength in older adults. *Am. J. Epidemiol.* **2012**, *176*, 1025–1034. [CrossRef]
38. Fingeret, M.; Vollenweider, P.; Marques-Vidal, P. No association between vitamin C and E supplementation and grip strength over 5 years: The Colaus study. *Eur. J. Nutr.* **2019**, *58*, 609–617. [CrossRef]
39. Granic, A.; Mendonça, N.; Hill, T.R.; Jagger, C.; Stevenson, E.J.; Mathers, J.C.; Sayer, A.A. Nutrition in the very old. *Nutrients* **2018**, *10*, 269. [CrossRef]
40. Giezenaar, C.; Chapman, I.; Luscombe-Marsh, N.; Feinle-Bisset, C.; Horowitz, M.; Soenen, S. Ageing is associated with decreases in appetite and energy intake—A meta-analysis in healthy adults. *Nutrients* **2016**, *8*, 28. [CrossRef]
41. JafariNasabian, P.; Inglis, J.E.; Reilly, W.; Kelly, O.J.; Ilich, J.Z. Aging human body: Changes in bone, muscle and body fat with consequent changes in nutrient intake. *J. Endocrinol.* **2017**, *234*, R37–R51. [CrossRef] [PubMed]
42. Peters, D.M.; Fritz, S.L.; Krotish, D.E. Assessing the reliability and validity of a shorter walk test compared with the 10-Meter Walk Test for measurements of gait speed in healthy, older adults. *J. Geriatr. Phys. Ther.* **2013**, *36*, 24–30. [CrossRef] [PubMed]
43. Schaap, L.A.; Fox, B.; Henwood, T.; Bruyère, O.; Reginster, J.Y.; Beaudart, C.; Buckinx, F.; Roberts, H.; Cooper, C.; Cherubini, A.; et al. Grip strength measurement: Towards a standardized approach in sarcopenia research and practice. *Eur. Geriatr. Med.* **2016**, *7*, 247–255. [CrossRef]
44. Arnault, N. *Table de Composition des Aliments, étude NutriNet-Santé. [Food Composition Table, NutriNet-Santé Study]*; Les éditions INSERM: Paris, France, 2013.
45. Taylor, H.L.; Jacobs, D.R.; Schucker, B.; Knudsen, J.; Leon, A.S.; Debacker, G. A questionnaire for the assessment of leisure time physical activities. *J. Chronic Dis.* **1978**, *31*, 741–755. [CrossRef]

46. Vetrano, D.L.; Landi, F.; Volpato, S.; Corsonello, A.; Meloni, E.; Bernabei, R.; Onder, G. Association of sarcopenia with short- and long-term mortality in older adults admitted to acute care wards: Results from the CRIME study. *J. Gerontol. Ser. A Biol. Sci. Med. Sci.* **2014**, *69*, 1154–1161. [CrossRef]
47. Steffl, M.; Bohannon, R.W.; Petr, M.; Kohlikova, E.; Holmerova, I. Relation between cigarette smoking and sarcopenia: Meta-analysis. *Physiol. Res.* **2015**, *64*, 419–426. [CrossRef]
48. Dallongeville, J.; Maré, N.; Fruchart, J.-C.; Amouyel, P. Community and International Nutrition Cigarette Smoking Is Associated with Unhealthy Patterns of Nutrient Intake: A Meta-analysis. *J. Nutr.* **1998**, *128*, 1450–1457. [CrossRef]
49. Zadak, Z.; Hyspler, R.; Ticha, A.; Vlcek, J. Polypharmacy and malnutrition. *Curr. Opin. Clin. Nutr. Metab. Care* **2013**, *16*, 50–55. [CrossRef]
50. Streicher, M.; van Zwienen-Pot, J.; Bardon, L.; Nagel, G.; Teh, R.; Meisinger, C.; Colombo, M.; Torbahn, G.; Kiesswetter, E.; Flechtner-Mors, M.; et al. Determinants of Incident Malnutrition in Community-Dwelling Older Adults: A MaNuEL Multicohort Meta-Analysis. *J. Am. Geriatr. Soc.* **2018**, *66*, 2335–2343. [CrossRef]
51. Beaudart, C.; Reginster, J.Y.; Petermans, J.; Gillain, S.; Quabron, A.; Locquet, M.; Slomian, J.; Buckinx, F.; Bruyère, O. Quality of life and physical components linked to sarcopenia: The SarcoPhAge study. *Exp. Gerontol.* **2015**, *69*, 103–110. [CrossRef]
52. Thiébaut, A.; Kesse, E.; Com-Nougué, C.; Clavel-Chapelon, F.; Bénichou, J. Ajustement sur l'apport énergétique dans l'évaluation des facteurs de risque alimentaires Adjustment for energy intake in the assessment of dietary risk factors. *Rev. Epidemiol. Sante Publique* **2004**, *52*, 539–557.
53. Conseil Supérieur de la Santé (CSS). *Recommandations Nutritionnelles Pour la Belgique 2016*; CSSAvis n°9285: Bruxelles, Belgium, 2016.
54. Wysokiński, A.; Sobów, T.; Kłoszewska, I.; Kostka, T. Mechanisms of the anorexia of aging—A review. *Age* **2015**, *37*. [CrossRef] [PubMed]
55. Bohannon, R.W. Minimal clinically important difference for grip strength: A systematic review. *Soc. Phys. Ther. Sci.* **2019**, *31*, 75–78. [CrossRef] [PubMed]
56. Beaudart, C.; Rolland, Y.; Cruz-Jentoft, A.J.; Bauer, J.M.; Sieber, C.; Cooper, C.; Al-Daghri, N.; Araujo de Carvalho, I.; Bautmans, I.; Bernabei, R.; et al. Assessment of Muscle Function and Physical Performance in Daily Clinical Practice: A position paper endorsed by the European Society for Clinical and Economic Aspects of Osteoporosis, Osteoarthritis and Musculoskeletal Diseases (ESCEO). *Calcif. Tissue Int.* **2019**, *105*, 1–14. [CrossRef] [PubMed]
57. Robinson, S.; Granic, A.; Sayer, A.A. Nutrition and muscle strength, as the key component of sarcopenia: An overview of current evidence. *Nutrients* **2019**, *11*, 2942. [CrossRef] [PubMed]
58. Úbeda, N.; Achón, M.; Varela-Moreiras, G. Omega 3 fatty acids in the elderly. *Br. J. Nutr.* **2012**, *107*, s131–s151. [CrossRef] [PubMed]
59. Lauretani, F.; Semba, R.D.; Bandinelli, S.; Dayhoff-Brannigan, M.; Giacomini, V.; Corsi, A.M.; Guralnik, J.M.; Ferrucci, L. Low Plasma Carotenoids and Skeletal Muscle Strength Decline Over 6 Years. *J. Gerontol.* **2008**, *63*, 376–383. [CrossRef]
60. Rondanelli, M.; Faliva, M.; Monteferrario, F.; Peroni, G.; Repaci, E.; Allieri, F.; Perna, S. Novel insights on nutrient management of sarcopenia in elderly. *Biomed Res. Int.* **2015**, *2015*. [CrossRef]
61. Dupont, J.; Dedeyne, L.; Dalle, S.; Koppo, K.; Gielen, E. The role of omega-3 in the prevention and treatment of sarcopenia. *Aging Clin. Exp. Res.* **2019**, *31*, 825–836. [CrossRef]
62. Houston, D.K.; Cesari, M.; Ferrucci, L.; Cherubini, A.; Maggio, D.; Bartali, B.; Johnson, M.A.; Schwartz, G.G.; Kritchevsky, S.B. Association Between Vitamin D Status and Physical Performance: The InCHIANTI Study. *J. Gerontol.* **2007**, *62*, 440–446. [CrossRef]
63. Remelli, F.; Vitali, A.; Zurlo, A.; Volpato, S. Vitamin D deficiency and sarcopenia in older persons. *Nutrients* **2019**, *11*, 2861. [CrossRef] [PubMed]
64. Shea, M.K.; Loeser, R.F.; Hsu, F.C.; Booth, S.L.; Nevitt, M.; Simonsick, E.M.; Strotmeyer, E.S.; Vermeer, C.; Kritchevsky, S.B. Vitamin K Status and Lower Extremity Function in Older Adults: The Health Aging and Body Composition Study. *J. Gerontol. Ser. A Biol. Sci. Med. Sci.* **2016**, *71*, 1348–1355. [CrossRef] [PubMed]
65. Azuma, K.; Inoue, S. Multiple modes of vitamin K actions in aging-related musculoskeletal disorders. *Int. J. Mol. Sci.* **2019**, *20*, 2844. [CrossRef] [PubMed]
66. Clausen Torben; Everts Maria Regulation of the Na,K-pump in skeletal muscle. *Int. Soc. Nephrol.* **1989**, *35*, 1–13.

67. McLeod, J.C.; Stokes, T.; Phillips, S.M. Resistance exercise training as a primary countermeasure to age-related chronic disease. *Front. Physiol.* **2019**, *10*. [CrossRef]
68. Deutz, N.E.P.; Bauer, J.M.; Barazzoni, R.; Biolo, G.; Boirie, Y.; Bosy-Westphal, A.; Cederholm, T.; Cruz-Jentoft, A.; Krznariç, Z.; Nair, K.S.; et al. Protein intake and exercise for optimal muscle function with aging: Recommendations from the ESPEN Expert Group. *Clin. Nutr.* **2014**, *33*, 929–936. [CrossRef]
69. Kamo, T.; Ishii, H.; Suzuki, K.; Nishida, Y. The impact of malnutrition on efficacy of resistance training in community-dwelling older adults. *Physiother. Res. Int.* **2019**, *24*. [CrossRef]
70. Nilsson, M.I.; Mikhail, A.; Lan, L.; Carlo, A.D.; Hamilton, B.; Barnard, K.; Hettinga, B.P.; Hatcher, E.; Tarnopolsky, M.G.; Nederveen, J.P.; et al. A five-ingredient nutritional supplement and home-based resistance exercise improve lean mass and strength in free-living elderly. *Nutrients* **2020**, *12*, 2391. [CrossRef]
71. Gropper, S.S.; Tappen, R.M.; Vieira, E.R. Differences In Nutritional And Physical Health Indicators Among Older African Americans, European Americans, And Hispanic Americans. *J. Nutr. Gerontol. Geriatr.* **2019**, *38*, 205–217. [CrossRef]
72. Du, K.; Goates, S.; Arensberg, M.B.; Pereira, S.; Gaillard, T. Prevalence of Sarcopenia and Sarcopenic Obesity Vary with Race/Ethnicity and Advancing Age. *Divers. Equal. Health Care* **2018**, *15*. [CrossRef]
73. Kalonji, E.; Sirot, V.; Noel, L.; Guerin, T.; Margaritis, I.; Leblanc, J.-C. Nutritional Risk Assessment of Eleven Minerals and Trace Elements: Prevalence of Inadequate and Excessive Intakes from the Second French Total Diet Study. *Eur. J. Nutr. Food Saf.* **2015**, *5*, 281–296. [CrossRef]
74. Agence nationale de sécurité sanitaire de l'alimentation, de l'environnement et du travail (ANSES) Avis de l'ANSES, Saisine n°2012-SA-0142; 14 rue Pierre et Marie Curie, 94701 Maisons-Alfort Cedex. 2015. Available online: https://www.anses.fr/fr/system/files/NUT2012sa0142.pdf (accessed on 1 October 2020).
75. Carriquiry, A.L. Assessing the prevalence of nutrient inadequacy. *Public Health Nutr.* **1998**, *2*, 23–33. [CrossRef] [PubMed]

Publisher's Note: MDPI stays neutral with regard to jurisdictional claims in published maps and institutional affiliations.

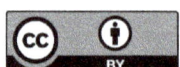

© 2020 by the authors. Licensee MDPI, Basel, Switzerland. This article is an open access article distributed under the terms and conditions of the Creative Commons Attribution (CC BY) license (http://creativecommons.org/licenses/by/4.0/).

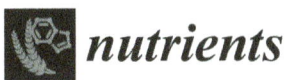

Review

Sodium and Potassium Intake and Cardiovascular Disease in Older People: A Systematic Review

Carla Gonçalves [1,2,3,*] and Sandra Abreu [1,4]

1. CIAFEL—Research Centre in Physical Activity, Health and Leisure, Faculty of Sport, University of Porto, 4099-002 Porto, Portugal; sandramrabreu@gmail.com
2. CITAB, Centre for the Research and Technology of Agro-Environmental and Biological Sciences, 5001-801 Vila Real, Portugal
3. Faculty of Nutrition and Food Sciences, University of Porto, 4099-002 Porto, Portugal
4. Faculty of Psychology, Education and Sports, Lusófona University of Porto, 4000-098 Porto, Portugal
* Correspondence: carlagoncalves.pt@gmail.com; Tel.: +351-22-507-4320

Received: 29 September 2020; Accepted: 4 November 2020; Published: 10 November 2020

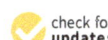

Abstract: This review aims to examine the relationship of sodium and potassium intake and cardiovascular disease (CVD) among older people. Methods: We performed a literature search using PubMed and Web of Science (January 2015 to July 2020) without language restriction. Observational and experimental studies that reported the relationship between sodium, potassium, or sodium-to-potassium ratio with CVD among older adults aged higher than 60 years were included. The authors independently screened all identified studies, extracted information, and assessed the quality of included studies. Risk of bias was assessed using the Risk of Bias Assessment Tool for Nonrandomized Studies (RoBANS) for observational studies and the revised Cochrane risk-of-bias tool (RoB 2 tool) for randomized trials. Results: We included 12 studies (6 prospective cohort studies, 5 cross-sectional studies, and 1 experimental study). Five of the studies reported on sodium-to-potassium ratio ($n = 5$), and the others on potassium and/or sodium intake. Cardiovascular events (e.g., stroke and heart failure) were the most reported outcome ($n = 9$). Of the 12 studies included, five observational studies had low bias risk and the randomized controlled trial was judged as uncertain risk of bias. We found inconsistent results for the effect of the reduction of sodium intake in this population for lower risk of CVD. We found that both the increase of potassium intake and the decrease of sodium-to-potassium ratio were associated with lower risk of hypertension and CVD, particularly stroke. Conclusion: The present review suggests that both higher potassium and lower sodium-to-potassium ratio are associated with lower risk of CVD.

Keywords: cardiovascular disease; hypertension; older people; sodium; potassium

1. Introduction

The world is facing a critical healthcare challenge in rising and potentially unsustainable healthcare costs, mainly due to the increasing prevalence of unhealthy lifestyles, chronic diseases, and a growing ageing population that requires more diversified care and increased societal demands [1,2]. Indeed, the number of older persons (>60 years) in world is expected to double until 2050, when it is projected to reach nearly 2.1 billion of persons; the process of population ageing will be most advanced in Europe and North America [1]. It will be essential for countries to develop and implement policies to face an ageing population with a high burden of chronic conditions, including cardiovascular diseases (CVD). Multi-morbidity will increase the demand to strengthen disease prevention and integrate service delivery around people's needs for health and social care.

On top of health-related age frailty, ageing people have non-communicable chronic diseases such as CVD that are the main contributors to the total burden of disease and mortality in low-, middle- and high-income countries [3,4]. CVD consists of a group of heart and blood vessels disorders that include coronary heart disease (e.g. heart attack), cerebrovascular disease (e.g., stroke), and diseases of the aorta and arteries, including hypertension and peripheral vascular disease [5]. In older persons, CVD imposes a huge burden in terms of mortality, morbidity, disability, functional decline, and healthcare costs [6]. Hypertension is the most powerful preventable risk factor for death and disability from CVD [7] and also for cognitive decline and loss of autonomy later in life [8]. Hypertension prevalence and severity increase with age, and treating healthy subjects aged 75 years and older with moderate to severe hypertension reduces non-fatal strokes, cardiovascular morbidity and mortality, and the incidence of heart failure [9]. The American College of Cardiology/American Heart Association (ACC/AHA) defines for most adults ≥65 years old a blood pressure (BP) goal of <130/80 mmHg [10], and the European Society of Cardiology/European Society of Hypertension (ESC/ESH) recommends for persons between the ages of 65 and 79 years (elderly) and above 80 years (very old) a BP target of <130–139/70–79 mmHg [11].

There is strong scientific evidence that behavioral (such as unhealthy diet) and metabolic (such as hypertension) risk factors play a key role in the etiology of CVD. High dietary intakes of salt and low intake of fruits and vegetables are linked to increase CVD risk [12,13], mainly due to its impact on BP. Both a lower sodium and a higher potassium intake have been associated with lowered BP and a reduction in CVD [14,15], particularly in adults with hypertension. A recent meta-analysis of 32 randomized controlled trials found a U-shaped relationship between potassium supplementation and BP, with stronger lowering effects in participants with hypertension and at higher levels of sodium intake [16]. In this line, the World Health Organization strongly recommends a reduction to <2000 mg/day in sodium intake (5 g/day salt) [17], and an increase in dietary potassium intake of at least 3510 mg/day to reduce BP and the risk of CVD, stroke, and coronary heart disease in adults [18]. Urinary sodium-to-potassium ratio is an alternative indicator of cardiovascular risk, and the proposed ideal ratio of sodium-to-potassium intake (1:1) is achieved when sodium and potassium intake are within WHO recommended values [18]. A recent meta-analysis of prospective and retrospective observational studies reported that higher sodium intake and higher sodium-to-potassium ratio are associated with higher risk of stroke [15]. However, most published systematic reviews and meta-analyses on the relationship between dietary sodium, potassium, and CVD are done among adults regardless of age, ignoring the complexity of older people. Thus, this review aims to examine the relationship of sodium and potassium intake and CVD in older people (>60 years).

2. Materials and Methods

The present systematic review was reported according to the Preferred Reporting Items for Systematic Reviews and Meta-Analyses (PRISMA) statement [19].

2.1. Search Strategy

PubMed and Web of Science were systematically searched from January 2015 up to 10 July 2020, to assess the most recent evidence. The search was performed by one author (CG) using a combination of MeSH terms and keywords related to population, CVD, and dietary sodium and potassium intake, with no restriction on language. The search terms used in PubMed was the following, and then adapted to Web of Science: ("sodium" OR "sodium chloride") AND ("potassium") AND ("cardiovascular disease" OR "coronary heart disease" OR "ischemic heart disease" OR "myocardial infarction" OR "stroke" OR "heart attack" OR "hypertension" OR "high blood pressure") AND ("elderly" OR "older adults" OR aging OR "later life" OR senior OR nonagenarian OR octogenarian OR centenarian). The reference lists of included articles and reviews were also manually reviewed for additional relevant studies.

2.2. Eligibility Criteria and Study Selection

Studies were included in this review if: (1) the study was published in English, French, Portuguese, or Spanish; (2) the study design was cohort, case-cohort, nested case-control, case-control with a follow up of 12 months' length or above, cross-sectional, or intervention studies with randomized groups (the intervention/experimental group and the control group with no intervention/usual sodium or potassium intake), and a minimum intervention duration of 4 weeks; (3) participants' mean or median age were ≥ 60 years old, living in the community or institutionalized (nursing home) (for longitudinal studies mean age were considered at baseline; studies with stratified analyses by age groups were considered if results were available for ages ≥ 60 years); (4) the exposure of interest was sodium, potassium, or both assessed through dietary questionnaires or urinary measurements (for intervention studies the intervention was performed using potassium-containing supplements or through dietary modification only with sodium or potassium as target components); (5) the outcome of interest was CVD (prevalence, incidence, or mortality), hypertension, systolic blood pressure (SBP), or diastolic blood pressure (DBP). We excluded studies performed among participants with kidney disease and studies that not exclusively targeted potassium or sodium intake but multiple health behaviors (e.g., physical activity and diet). If multiple studies were published based on the same sample, we chose to include the study reporting prospective analysis or the study that used the largest sample size (for cross-sectional analyses). The review of titles and abstracts of all identified studies, and full-text assessment were done independently by the authors (CG and SA). Any disagreement was resolved through consensus.

2.3. Data Extraction

Data extraction of eligible studies was done independently by both authors using a standardized form, with any disagreement resolved by consensus. The information extracted comprised: the first author's last name, publication year, country, study design, mean or median age of participants, number of participants/case, sex, exposure identification and assessment method, outcome measure identification, follow-up duration, covariates used in multivariable analysis, and results. For intervention studies, details about the intervention was also extracted.

2.4. Quality Assessment

Both authors independently assessed the risk of bias for observational studies using the Risk of Bias Assessment Tool for Nonrandomized Studies (RoBANS) [20], and the revised Cochrane risk-of-bias tool (RoB 2 tool) for randomized trials [21]. RoBANS evaluated six bias domains: (1) selection of participants; (2) confounding variables; (3) measurement of exposure; (4) outcome assessments; (5) incomplete outcome data; and (6) selective outcome reporting. The risk of bias for each domain was judged as low risk, high risk, or unclear risk. Overall risk of bias was evaluated according to three key domains (the selection of participants, confounding variables, and incomplete outcome data). Then, if one of the three domains was assessed having a risk of bias as low, unclear, or high overall risk was classified according the more frequent classification. If each key domain was assessed differently the overall risk was categorized as unclear.

RoB tool considered the assessment of bias in five domains due to (1) randomization process, (2) deviations from intended interventions, (3) missing outcome data, (4) measurement of the outcome, and (5) selection of the reported results. The possible risk-of-bias judgements in each domain are low risk of bias, some concerns or high risk of bias. Additionally, an overall risk-of-bias judgement was done according to each domain assignment. Therefore high risk of bias was assigned if study it was judged to be at high risk of bias for at least one domain, some concerns if the study it was judged to raise some concerns for at least one domain and low risk if the study it was judged to be at low risk of bias for all domains.

3. Results

The database search resulted in a total of 596 records. Additionally, six papers were identified from the reference list. After the removal of duplicates ($n = 43$), the titles and abstracts of 559 records were screened according to eligibility criteria. Then, from these, the full-text of 92 publication were screened, and 12 papers were included in the present review for data extraction and quality assessment (Figure 1).

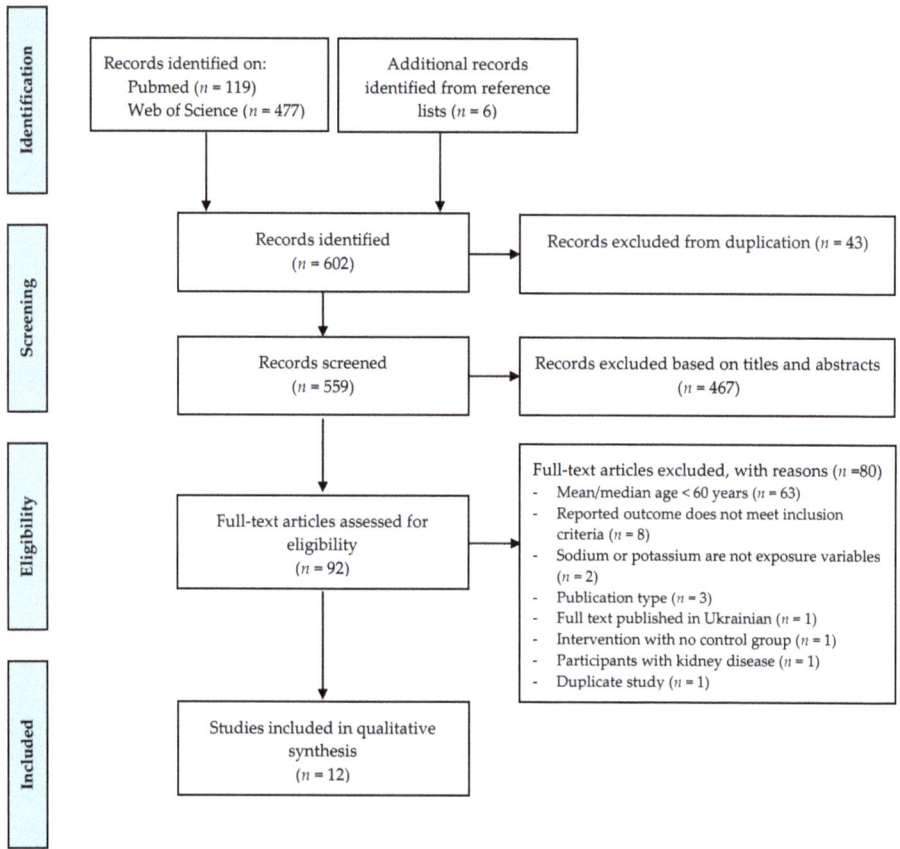

Figure 1. Flowchart of systematic literature search for inclusion in the review of relationship of sodium and potassium intake and cardiovascular disease among older people.

3.1. Characteristics of Studies

Tables 1–3 show the characteristics of the 12 included studies, ordered on publication year, which examined the association between sodium and/or potassium intake and CVD among older people. All included studies were carried out among population from developed countries, including USA ($n = 5$), France ($n = 1$), Italy ($n = 1$), Japan ($n = 1$), Korea ($n = 1$), the Netherlands ($n = 1$), Poland ($n = 1$), and Turkey ($n = 1$). Participants mean age ranged 60 to 79.7 years and all studies were conducted in men and women. Some studies were restricted to population with a specific condition, including type 2 diabetes ($n = 1$) [22], acute stroke ($n = 1$) [23], hypertension ($n = 1$) [24], and pre-hypertension ($n = 1$) [25].

Table 1. Characteristics of included cross-sectional studies in systematic review of dietary sodium, potassium, sodium-to-potassium ratio, and cardiovascular disease.

Author, Year [Reference]	Country	Participants Characteristics	Exposure	Sodium/Potassium Intake Assessment	Outcome Measures	Covariates	Main Findings
Guligowska AR, 2015 [31]	Poland	n = 239 (66 men) mean age = 72.0 ± 9.34 years	Sodium Potassium	24-hour recall questionnaire	Cardiometabolic disease (hypertension, history of ischemic heart disease, chronic HF or MI)	None	No significant differences for dietary sodium and potassium were found between participants with hypertension or disease history and healthy peers, except for sodium intake that was lower in patients with a history of MI (2680 ± 1019 mg vs. 3471 ± 1242 mg, $p = 0.010$) compared to their counterparts.
Dolmatova EV, 2018 [24]	USA	n = 13,033 with self-reported hypertension (6910 men) mean age = 60 ± 14 years	Sodium	24-h recall questionnaire	History of MI, HF, stroke BP	Age	In univariate analysis lower sodium consumption was found among adults with a history of MI, HF, and stroke ($p < 0.001$) but the difference did not remain significant after adjustment for age. Higher SBP and lower DBP were associated with higher sodium in univariate analysis, but the difference was no longer significant after adjustment for age.
Iida, 2019 [32]	Japan	n = 288 (116 men) mean age = 79.7 ± 4.2 years	Salt (NaCl)	Spot urine samples	BP	Age, sex, height, body weight, smoking status, PA, comorbidity (cardiovascular, cerebrovascular, and renal diseases), diabetes mellitus, dyslipidemia, alcohol intake, and medication (antihypertensive agents and diuretics)	A one-unit higher value in estimated salt intake (per g/d) was associated with a higher SBP (adjusted difference: 1.73 mmHg, 95% CI 0.71 to 2.76 mmHg). One SD higher value in estimated salt intake (per g/d) was also associated with a higher SBP (adjusted difference: 4.13 mmHg, 95% CI 1.69 to 6.57 mmHg). A one-unit or SD higher values in estimated salt intake (per g/d) were not associated with higher DPB.
Kyung Kim, 2019 [33]	Korea	n = 217 (94 men) median age = 60 (IQR: 57-63)	Sodium Potassium Sodium to potassium ratio	24-hour urine excretion	24-hour ambulatory BP	Age, gender, BMI, smoking, and use of antihypertensive medications	Nighttime blood pressure linearly increased with 24-h urine sodium (SBP: β = 0.1706, 95% CI 0.0361–0.3052; DBP: β = 0.1440, 95% CI 0.0117–0.2763) and the sodium to potassium ratio (SBP: β = 0.1415, 95% CI 0.0127–0.2703; DBP: β = 0.1441 95% CI 0.0181–0.2700). The 24-h BP was linearly increased with sodium to potassium ratio (SBP: β = 0.1325, 95% CI 0.0031–0.2620; DBP: β = 0.1234 95% CI 0.0025–0.2444). Non-linear associations were found between daytime blood pressure (SBP and DBP), 24-hour SBP and sodium ($p < 0.05$).
Koca TT, 2019 [23]	Turkey	n = 82 (50 patients with stroke (28 men) and 32 controls (13 men)) mean age stroke group = 65.9 ± 14.6 years mean age control group = 60.9 ± 14.1 years	Sodium Potassium Sodium-to-potassium ratio	Spot urine samples	Stroke	None	Urinary sodium to potassium ratio was not significantly different between stroke and control groups. Urinary potassium, sodium, and sodium to potassium ratio excretion was significantly lower in male patients with stroke compared to healthy male ($p < 0.05$ for all).

BP, blood pressure; BMI, body mass index; CI, confidence interval; DBP, diastolic blood pressure; HF, heart failure; MI, myocardial infarction; PA, physical activity; SD, standard deviation; SBP, systolic blood pressure; USA, United States of America; IQR, interquartile range.

Table 2. Characteristics of included longitudinal studies in systematic review of dietary sodium, potassium, sodium-to-potassium ratio, and cardiovascular disease.

Author, Year	Country	Participants Characteristics	Study Design	Follow-Up (Years)	Exposure	Sodium/Potassium Intake Assessment	Outcome Measures	Covariates	Main Findings
Kalogeropoulos AP, 2015 [26]	USA	n = 2642 (1290 men) mean age = 73.6 ± 2.9 years	Prospective cohort	10	Sodium (as continuous variable and categorical variable into 3 groups: <1500 mg/d; 1500–2300 mg/d; >2300 mg/d)	Food frequency questionnaire (at the year 2 visit)	Incident CVD (n_cases = 572) (i.e. coronary heart disease (MI, angina, or coronary revascularization), cerebrovascular disease (stroke, transient ischemic attack, or symptomatic carotid artery disease), peripheral arterial disease) Incident HF (n_cases = 398)	Age, sex, race, baseline hypertensive status, BMI, smoking status, PA, prevalent CVD (for HF events), pulmonary disease, diabetes mellitus, depression, BP, heart rate, electrocardiogram abnormalities, and serum glucose, albumin, creatinine, and cholesterol levels	Ten-year incident CVD, or incident HF, were not associated with sodium intake.
Saulnier PJ, 2017 [22]	France	n = 1439 types 2 diabetes patients (835 men) mean age = 65.3 ± 10.7 years	Prospective cohort	Median = 5.7 (IQR: 3.1–8.8)	Sodium (as continuous variable and categorical variable into tertiles: low, <69 mmol/L; intermediate, 69–103 mmol/L; high, >103 mmol/L) Potassium (as categorical variable into tertiles—not specified)	Spot urinary sample	Cardiovascular death (n_cases = 268)	Age, sex, urinary sodium and potassium, urine to plasma creatine ratio, estimated 24 h sodium excretion, BMI, history of urinary albumin to creatine concentration ratio, N-terminal pro-brain natriuretic peptide	It was found significant relationships between cardiovascular mortality, and sodium and potassium tertiles (Log-rank $p < 0.001$), with patients in the lower tertiles having the highest mortality. For each 1-SD increase of urinary sodium concentration in the adjusted model, cardiovascular mortality was 24% lower (HR: 0.76, 95% CI: 0.66–0.88).
Willey J, 2017 [27]	USA	n = 2496 (902 men) mean age= 68.7 ± 10 years (55% Hispanic)	Prospective cohort	Mean = 12 ± 5	Sodium to potassium ratio	Food frequency questionnaire (at baseline)	Incident stroke (n_cases = 268) Incident ischemic stroke (n_cases = 227)	Age, sex, high-school completion, race ethnicity, total calories, Mediterranean diet score, moderate alcohol use, moderate heavy physical activity, smoking, estimated glomerular filtration rate, body mass index, hypertension, hypercholesterolemia, diabetes mellitus, sodium consumption	In adjusted models, a higher sodium-potassium ratio was associated with increased risk for stroke (HR: 1.6, 95% CI: 1.19–2.14) and ischemic stroke (HR: 1.58, 95% CI: 1.20–2.06). Marginally positive association was observed for potassium intake and stroke among those with <2300 mg sodium/d and an inverse association was observed for potassium intake among those with ≥2300 mg sodium/d.
Lelli D, 2018 [29]	Italy	n = 920 (415 men) mean age = 74.5 ± 6.99 years	Prospective cohort	9	Sodium Potassium (as continuous variables and quartiles)	24-hour urinary excretion	Incident cardiovascular events (n_cases = 169) (i.e. angina pectoris, myocardial infarction, heart failure, and stroke)	Age, sex, education, estimated creatinine clearance, SBP, hypertension, diabetes, BMI, caloric intake/body weight, cigarette smoking, antihypertensive drugs, and diuretics	An association was found between 24-hour sodium excretion and cardiovascular disease (RR 0.95; 95% CI 0.90–1), which did not remain after adjustment for confounders (RR: 0.96, 95% CI: 0.90–1.02).

Table 2. Cont.

Author, Year	Country	Participants Characteristics	Study Design	Follow-Up (Years)	Exposure	Sodium/Potassium Intake Assessment	Outcome Measures	Covariates	Main Findings
Howard G, 2018 [28]	USA	n = 6897 (3125 men; 1807 black participants) mean age = 62 ± 8 years	Prospective cohort	9.4	Sodium to potassium ratio	Food frequency questionnaire (at baseline)	Incident hypertension (n_cases = 836 (298 men) for black and 1679 (837 men) for white participants)	Age, race, and baseline systolic blood pressure for the risk factor of incident hypertension	Among men, the sodium to potassium ratio was associated with incident hypertension (OR: 1.11, 95% CI: 1.01 to 1.20); incidence proportion at 25th percentile, 32.9%, 95% CI: 30.4% to 35.5% and the 75th percentile, 35.8%, 95% CI: 33.5% to 38.2%, absolute risk difference between black and white participants, 2.9%, 95% CI: 0.4% to 5.5%). Among black men, the ratio of sodium to potassium accounted for 12.3% (95% CI: 1.1% to 22.8%) of the excess risk of hypertension. Among women, the sodium to potassium ratio was associated with incident hypertension (OR: 1.13, 95% CI: 1.04 to 1.22; incidence proportion at 25th percentile, 31.1%, 95% CI: 29.1% to 33.5% and the 75th percentile, 34.5%, 95% CI: 32.2% to 36.8%; absolute risk difference between black and white participants, 3.3%, 95% CI: 1.1% to 5.5%). Higher dietary ratio of sodium to potassium accounted for 6.8% (95% CI: 1.6% to 11.9%) of the risk of hypertension among black women.
Averill MM, 2019, USA [36]		n = 6705 (3160 men) mean age= 61.2 ± 10.2	Prospective cohort	11.7 (±2.2)	Sodium to potassium ratio	Spot urine samples (at baseline)	Incident CVD (n_cases = 781) (MI, definite angina, stroke, transient ischemic attack, coronary heart disease death) Incident coronary heart disease (n_cases = 530) (MI and angina) Incident HF (n_cases = 274) Incident peripheral vascular disease (n_cases = 104) Incident stroke (n_cases = 236) SBP	Age, sex, race, diabetes mellitus, smoking (current and former), total cholesterol, high-density lipoprotein cholesterol, treated hypertension, education, SBP, DBP, urine creatinine, hip circumference, BMI, aspirin use, intentional exercise, glomerular filtration rate, dietary energy intake, maximum of common carotid artery intimal medial thickness, and IL-6 (interleukin 6) levels	After adjustment, only sodium-to-potassium ratio >1 was associated with the risk of stroke (HR: 1.47, 95% CI: 1.07–2.00).

BP, blood pressure; BMI, body mass index; CI, confidence interval; CVD, cardiovascular disease; DBP, diastolic blood pressure; HF, heart failure; HR, Hazard ration; MI, myocardial infarction; PA, physical activity; SD, standard deviation; SBP, systolic blood pressure; USA, United States of America; IQR, interquartile range; OR, odds ratio; RR, relative risk.

Table 3. Characteristics of included trials in systematic review of dietary sodium, potassium, sodium-to-potassium ratio, and cardiovascular disease.

Author, Year	Country	Participants Characteristics	Follow-Up	Study Design	Intervention Details	Outcome Measures	Main Findings
Gijsbers L, 2015 [25]	The Netherlands	$n = 36$ untreated (pre)hypertensive (24 men) mean age = 65.8 years	4 weeks	Randomized, double-blind, placebo-controlled crossover	After a 1-week run-in period, subjects were randomly allocated to 3 times in one of the treatments: sodium supplementation (3 g/day, equals 7.6 g/day of salt), potassium supplementation (3 g/day) or placebo.	Fasting office BP 24-h ambulatory BP	During sodium supplementation, office and 24h-ambulatory were significantly increased to ~8 mmHg and ~4 mmHg, respectively. During potassium supplementation, 24-h ambulatory SBP and DBP was significantly reduced by ~4 mmHg and ~2 mmHg, respectively.

BP, blood pressure; DBP, diastolic blood pressure; SBP, systolic blood pressure.

From the 12 included studies, the majority are prospective studies ($n = 6$) [22,26–30] and cross-sectional studies ($n = 5$) [23,24,31–33], and only one was an experimental study [25]. Most of the studies had as exposure variable sodium-to-potassium ratio ($n = 5$) [23,27,28,30,33] and both potassium and sodium intake ($n = 5$) [22,23,25,31,33]. Of the 11 observational studies included, the exposure variable was assessed by self-reported questionnaires ($n = 5$) [24,26–28,31], spot urine ($n = 4$) [22,23,30,32], and 24-h urinary excretion ($n = 2$) [29,33]. Regarding outcome, most of the studies analyzed cardiovascular events ($n = 9$) [22,23,26–31], three BP [25,32], and one both [24,33]. Outcome assessment were derived from medical records [22,26,27,29,31], death certificates [13,22,28], BP monitors [24,25,28,32,33], and self-reported data [24,30]. One study not reported how outcome variable (i.e., stroke) was assessed [23].

3.2. Quality Assessment

For the 12 selected studies, the overall risk of bias was rated high for four studies [23,24,31,32], unclear for three studies [20,25,30] and low for five studies [22,26–29] (Figure 2). The randomized controlled trial included [25] has low risk of bias in the "randomization process errors", "missing outcome data" and "systematic errors in measurement of the outcome" domains of the quality assessment. However, the "deviations from the intended interventions" domain was rated unclear because this is a cross-over trial and does not include a washout period between the treatments as a mean of reducing the carry-over effect. The "selection of the reported result" domain was also rated unclear mainly due to the impossibility to access the baseline differences for all outcome variables in the randomized groups at the start of the cross-over trial. For the 11 observational studies included, the "selection of participants" was judged as low risk of bias, except for four studies due to retrospective data collection and unclear disease diagnosis assessment [31], generation of patients definition by self-report [24], unclear confirmation of excluded patients from control group [32] and insufficient data to prove that case and control group are from a comparable population group [23]. The "confounding variables" domain was only judged as high risk of bias in three studies [23,24,31], mainly due to the fact that major confounding variables (age, gender, body mass index, smoking, alcohol consumption, and race/ethnic group) were not considered. In relation to "incomplete outcome data" domain, two studies was judged unclear risk of bias [20,30], because it is uncertain whether the incomplete outcome data could affect the study outcome or not present data about differences between included and excluded subjects. Finally, the "measurement of exposure" domain was considered as low risk if sodium and/or potassium intake was estimated by 24-hour urinary collection considered the "gold standard" method [20,29], other studies estimates these variables by spot urines, dietary recall or food records and these methods may underestimate sodium consumption and/or do not consider the salt used in food preparations [34–37].

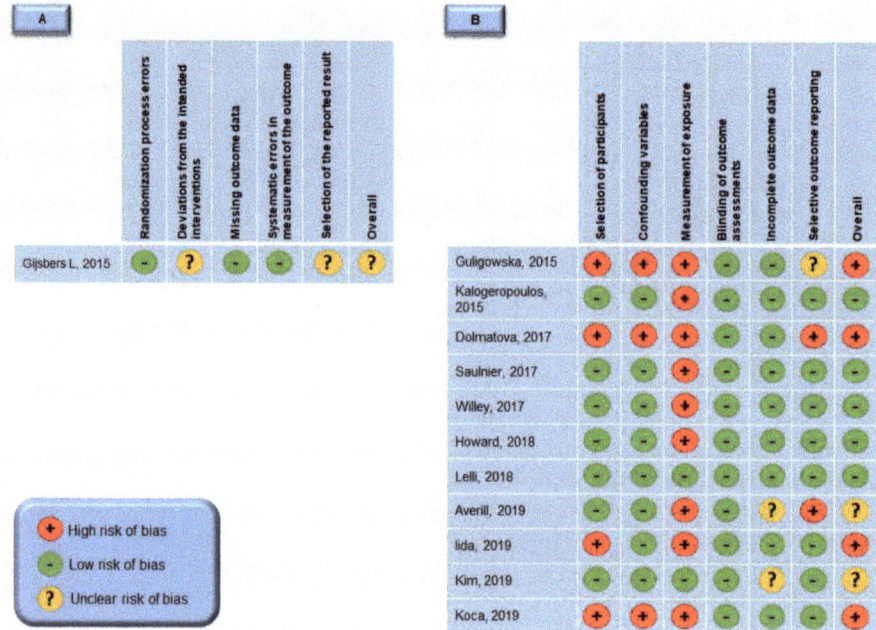

Figure 2. Risk of bias summary: review authors' judgements about each risk of bias item for each included study. (**A**)—randomized controlled trials included; (**B**)—non-randomized studies included.

3.3. Sodium Intake

A total of nine studies analyzed sodium intake, which five are cross-sectional studies [23,24,31–33], three are prospective studies [22,26,29] and one is an experimental study [25]. Kyung Kim et al. [33] evaluated the dose-response association of 24-h urine sodium excretion and 24-h ambulatory blood pressure among community-based participants and found that nighttime BP linearly increased with 24-h urine sodium; however, daytime BP and 24-hour systolic BP (SBP) showed a significant non-linear relationship with sodium excretion. Iida et al. [32] explored the association of salt intake (NaCl) with BP and showed that estimated salt intake (per g/day) (per one-unit mean or standard deviation-SD) was associated with higher SBP, but not with diastolic BP (DBP). In the other hand, in another cross-sectional study [24] in adjusted models no association were found between sodium consumption and cardiovascular events history and higher BP. Furthermore, cross-sectional studies of Guligowska et al. [31] and Koca et al. [23] found that sodium was lower in patients with myocardial infarction and stroke compared to their counterparts, respectively.

From prospective cohort studies, two reported no significant association with cardiovascular events as the result of higher sodium intake [26,29] and one reported increased risk of cardiovascular death as the result of lower urinary sodium concentration [22]. Saulnier et al. [22] evaluated the relationship between spot urine sodium concentration and mortality and cardiovascular death among type 2 diabetes patients and reported that an increase of one SD was associated with a decrease of 22% of cardiovascular death.

Gijsberg et al. [25] conducted a randomized, placebo-controlled crossover study of 36 untreated pre-hypertensive adults who were randomly assigned to three times in one of the following three groups: sodium supplementation (3 g/day, equals 7.6 g/day of salt), potassium supplementation (3 g/day) or placebo. Three times consecutive intervention periods of four weeks, without washout, were conducted for each of these groups. During sodium supplementation, office and 24 h-ambulatory SBP and DPB were significantly increased to ~8 mmHg and ~3 mmHg compared to placebo period, respectively.

3.4. Potassium Intake

Potassium intake was explored in three cross-sectional studies [23,31,33], two prospective studies [22,27] and one experimental study [25]. Among cross-sectional studies, two studies did not find significant results between potassium intake and cardiovascular events [31] or BP [33]. Koca et al. [23] showed that urinary potassium excretion was significantly lower in male patients with stroke compared to healthy counterparts. Willey et al. [27] explored data from the Northern Manhattan Study (NOMAS) and stratified results according to sodium intake. Among those with sodium intake <2300mg/d there was a positive association between potassium intake, total, and ischemic stroke, whereas among those with sodium intake ≥2300 mg/d a marginally inverse association was observed between potassium intake and stroke. Potassium intake was not the main outcome in the other prospective study [22]; however, lower tertiles of urinary potassium concentration was associated with higher cardiovascular mortality. In the experimental study, Gijsberg et al. [25] found during the potassium supplementation that 24-h ambulatory SBP and DBP were significantly reduced by ~4 mmHg and ~2 mmHg, respectively.

3.5. Sodium-to-Potassium Ratio

Most of the studies that explored sodium-to-potassium ratio are prospective studies [27,28,30] and two are cross-sectional studies [20,23]. All of the prospective studies reported increased risk of cardiovascular events as the result of higher sodium-to-potassium ratio. Data from Multi-Ethnic Study of Atherosclerosis (MESA) conducted among 6814 adults from different ethnic groups found in full-adjusted model that a sodium-to-potassium ratio higher than one was associated with the risk of stroke [30]. Likewise, Wiley et al. [27] reported a higher sodium-to-potassium ratio was associated with a greater risk of ischemic and total stroke. Howard et al. [28] conducted a longitudinal cohort study among adults' aged 45 years or older and explored results according to sex and black and white participants. Among men and women, the sodium to potassium ratio was associated with incident hypertension. Additionally, among black men and women the ratio of sodium to potassium accounted for 12.3% and 6.8% of the excess risk of hypertension, respectively. Kyung Kim et al. [33] also found a cross-sectional linear association between nighttime BP and 24-hour BP with sodium-to-potassium ratio. Urinary sodium-to-potassium ratio was not significantly different between stroke and control groups in Koca et al.'s study [23].

4. Discussion

The present review provides summarized evidence on the association between sodium and potassium intake with CVD and hypertension among older people. We identified five non-randomized trials with low bias risk and one randomized controlled trial with uncertain risk of bias that assessed the impact of sodium, potassium, and sodium-to-potassium ratio on CVD. We found inconsistent results that supports the recommendation to reduce sodium intake in this population, however we found strong evidence to support the increase of potassium intake and the decrease of sodium-to-potassium ratio in reducing the risk of hypertension and CVD, particularly stroke.

In the analysis of sodium intake, our findings shown a lack of evidence of an effect of dietary sodium reduction on cardiovascular events and mortality that is in accordance with other authors [38]. Two included studies with low risk of bias shows that dietary sodium intake was not associated with incident of CVD or heart failure [26,29], one study indicate that low sodium intake increased the risk of CVD and mortality [22] and the other related increased BP with increasing sodium intake [25]. This non-linear association between sodium excretion and mortality was already described, suggesting a J-shaped association between sodium intake and cardiovascular events recommending a moderate sodium intake in the general population (3–5 g/d), with targeting the lower end of the moderate range among those with hypertension [39]. Saulnier et al. [22] found that low urinary sodium was associated with an increased risk of CVD and mortality in type 2 diabetes older persons and Lelli et al. [29] found similar association with mortality but not with CVD in frail participants. Diabetes and frailty are two prevalent conditions in older persons, and both have a recognized influence on studied outcomes. The low sodium excretion maybe due to insulin therapy, because the antinatriuretic effect of insulin may contribute to the relationship between insulin resistance and hypertension, the authors also raises the question if kidneys ability to excrete sodium and urine is implicated in the occurrence of fatal cardiovascular diseases [22]. The activation of sympathetic nervous system and the renin–angiotensin–aldosterone system, implicated in the regulation of sodium and volemia, are stimulated in frail persons, which may lead to increased risk for cardiovascular events [29,40]. Another mechanism that could explain the association of the risk of mortality and low sodium intake in frail persons is the lower caloric intake and malnutrition compromising cellular metabolism and several biological processes [41]. Discrepant findings in studies can be also attributable to differences in ranges of sodium intake, study populations and methods of sodium assessments. Some of the included studies uses food frequency questionnaire to estimates sodium intake leading to an underestimation of sodium intake and of an attenuated association between sodium and the outcome [36]. Furthermore, another study used one single spot urine without consideration to the circadian pattern of sodium excretion [42]. Although spot urine and dietary questionnaires may provide useful population sodium estimates, they are poor predictors at individual level [36]. Finally, older adults are inherently at higher risk for CVD and mean sodium intake are lower, mainly due to lower caloric intake; therefore; the effect of high sodium might have been more difficult to ascertain [43]. Although our inconsistent results for the dietary sodium effect on CVD among older people, a large body of evidence showed a favorable effect of low salt consumption on CVD, organ damage, and blood pressure and support the public health recommendation that adult population likely benefit from reducing sodium intake [44–47].

Regarding potassium intake analysis, increase potassium intake seems to be protective to CVD, likewise other meta-analyses verified similar findings [48,49]. Moreover, those persons with high sodium consumption could achieve great benefit with increased intake of potassium-rich foods to lower stroke risk [27,50]. In the other hand, the relationship between dietary potassium and BP seems to be not linear but U-shaped with stronger lowering-BP effect among those with high sodium intake as reported in a recent meta-analysis of randomized clinical trial [15], providing important insight about the combined effect of sodium and potassium intake. The combined association of sodium and potassium was explored as sodium-to-potassium ratio in five of the 12 included studies suggesting an increased risk of CVD and BP with higher sodium-to-potassium ratio. Likewise, it has been suggested that the sodium-to-potassium ratio is more strongly associated with BP than either sodium or potassium alone, being considered a superior metric in the evaluation of BP and incident hypertension [51]. Sodium and potassium are significant regulators of BP. Dependent of pre-exiting electrolyte balance, particularly sodium, reduced potassium intake leads to sodium retention, down regulation of vascular sensitivity to catecholamines, stimulated renin activity and worsening endothelial function [52].

Such as previous systematic reviews of dietary interventions, we observed marked heterogeneity across studies in terms of their population, sample size, methods, and follow-up. Regarding observational studies, few studies included covariates as controlled or well-characterized diet (influences of alcohol, coffee, salt addition in cooking, and DASH scores), dietary supplementation, or physical activity characterization that may influence the association between dietary sodium, potassium, and CVD. Additionally, other potentially important confounders or effect modifiers mediating factors [28] were not taken in consideration such as gender, education level/socioeconomic status, body mass index, waist circumference or stress. Race was also considered only in few studies [26–28,30], all from USA.

Our review has several strengths, including the most up-to-date synthesis of evidence on this topic and focus on older persons. We conducted the review according to guidance from the PRISMA statement. The main limitation of this review is that relevant studies may have been missed since we used only two databases for literature search. However, the PubMed and Web of Science have been used broadly as primary databases in review on nutrition area. Additionally, searching in multiple databases may cover more primary studies than using a single database [53]. Moreover, the inclusion of observational studies do not allow drawing any conclusions related to cause and effect.

Our findings suggests that salt reduction advice in older persons should take in consideration the previous characterization of usual level of consumption, for example by sodium excretion in 24-h urinary samples, in order to recommends reduction to ones that ingest more than 2000 mg/d. This population could benefit with increased potassium-rich foods in daily diet in order to optimize sodium-to-potassium ratio. Frailty, diabetes, ethnicity, and literacy could have an important role in the mediation of these outcomes.

5. Conclusions

The present review suggests that both higher potassium and lower sodium-to-potassium ratio are associated with lower risk of CVD. In contrast, our findings show a lack of evidence of dietary sodium reduction affecting CVD, however, considering the quality of the included studies these results should be interpreted with caution. To strengthen the study of these relationships further rigorous, large long-term, and randomized controlled trials are necessary.

Author Contributions: C.G. and S.A. contributed equally to all steps: conceptualization, methodology, quality analysis, data extraction, and writing the manuscript. All authors have read and agreed to the published version of the manuscript.

Funding: The CIAFEL is supported by FCT/UIDB/00617/2020. The CITAB is supported by FCT/UIDB/04033/2020.

Conflicts of Interest: The authors declare no conflict of interest.

References

1. United Nations. *World Population Ageing 2017: Highlights*; Department of Economic and Social Affairs, P.D.: New York, NY, USA, 2017.
2. Abrignani, M.G.; Aiello, A.; Colivicchi, F.; Lucà, F.; Fattirolli, F.; Gulizia, M.M.; Nardi, F.; Pino, P.G.; Gregorio, G. Cardiovascular prevention in the elderly: Limitations and opportunities. *G. Ital. Cardiol. (Rome)* **2020**, *21*, 619–628. [CrossRef]
3. World Health Organization. *Global Action Plan for the Prevention and Control of Noncommunicable Diseases 2013–2020*; WHO: Geneva, Switzerland, 2013.
4. Wilkins, E.; Wilson, L.; Wickramasinghe, K.; Bhatnagar, P.; Leal, J.; Luengo-Fernandez, R.; Burns, R.; Rayner, M.; Townsend, N. *European Cardiovascular Disease Statistics 2017*; European Heart Network: Brussels, Belgium, 2017.
5. Mendis, S.; Puska, P.; Norrving, B.; World Health Organization. *Global Atlas on Cardiovascular Disease Prevention and Control*; World Health Organization: Geneva, Switzerland, 2011.
6. Yazdanyar, A.; Newman, A.B. The Burden of Cardiovascular Disease in the Elderly: Morbidity, Mortality, and Costs. *Clin. Geriatr. Med.* **2009**, *25*, 563–577. [CrossRef] [PubMed]
7. Damluji, A.A.; Ramireddy, A.; Otalvaro, L.; Forman, D.E. Secondary cardiovascular prevention in older adults: An evidence based review. *J. Geriatr. Cardiol.* **2015**, *12*, 459–464. [CrossRef] [PubMed]
8. Benetos, A.; Petrovic, M.; Strandberg, T. Hypertension Management in Older and Frail Older Patients. *Circ. Res.* **2019**, *124*, 1045–1060. [CrossRef]
9. Schall, P.; Wehling, M. Treatment of arterial hypertension in the very elderly: A meta-analysis of clinical trials. *Arzneimittel-Forschung* **2011**, *61*, 221–228. [CrossRef]
10. Whelton, P.K.; Carey, R.M.; Aronow, W.S.; Casey, D.E.; Collins, K.J.; Himmelfarb, C.D.; DePalma, S.M.; Gidding, S.; Jamerson, K.A.; Jones, D.W. 2017 ACC/AHA/AAPA/ABC/ACPM/AGS/APhA/ASH/ASPC/NMA/PCNA guideline for the prevention, detection, evaluation, and management of high blood pressure in adults: A report of the American College of Cardiology/American Heart Association Task Force on Clinical Practice Guidelines. *J. Am. Coll. Cardiol.* **2018**, *71*, e127–e248.

11. Williams, B.; Mancia, G.; Spiering, W.; Agabiti Rosei, E.; Azizi, M.; Burnier, M.; Clement, D.L.; Coca, A.; de Simone, G.; Dominiczak, A.; et al. 2018 ESC/ESH Guidelines for the management of arterial hypertension: The Task Force for the management of arterial hypertension of the European Society of Cardiology (ESC) and the European Society of Hypertension (ESH). *Eur. Heart J.* **2018**, *39*, 3021–3104. [CrossRef]
12. Aune, D.; Giovannucci, E.; Boffetta, P.; Fadnes, L.T.; Keum, N.; Norat, T.; Greenwood, D.C.; Riboli, E.; Vatten, L.J.; Tonstad, S. Fruit and vegetable intake and the risk of cardiovascular disease, total cancer and all-cause mortality—A systematic review and dose-response meta-analysis of prospective studies. *Int. J. Epidemiol.* **2017**, *46*, 1029–1056. [CrossRef]
13. He, F.J.; MacGregor, G.A. Reducing Population Salt Intake Worldwide: From Evidence to Implementation. *Prog. Cardiovasc. Dis.* **2010**, *52*, 363–382. [CrossRef]
14. O'Donnell, M.; Mente, A.; Rangarajan, S.; McQueen, M.J.; O'Leary, N.; Yin, L.; Liu, X.; Swaminathan, S.; Khatib, R.; Rosengren, A.; et al. Joint association of urinary sodium and potassium excretion with cardiovascular events and mortality: Prospective cohort study. *BMJ* **2019**, *364*, l772. [CrossRef]
15. Jayedi, A.; Ghomashi, F.; Zargar, M.S.; Shab-Bidar, S. Dietary sodium, sodium-to-potassium ratio, and risk of stroke: A systematic review and nonlinear dose-response meta-analysis. *Clin. Nutr.* **2019**, *38*, 1092–1100. [CrossRef] [PubMed]
16. Filippini, T.; Naska, A.; Kasdagli, M.; Torres, D.; Lopes, C.; Carvalho, C.; Moreira, P.; Malavolti, M.; Orsini, N.; Whelton, P.K.; et al. Potassium Intake and Blood Pressure: A Dose-Response Meta-Analysis of Randomized Controlled Trials. *J. Am. Hear. Assoc.* **2020**, *9*, e015719. [CrossRef] [PubMed]
17. World Health Organization. *Guideline: Sodium Intake for Adults and Children*; World Health Organization: Geneva, Switzerland, 2012.
18. World Health Organization. *Guideline: Potassium Intake for Adults and Children*; World Health Organization: Geneva, Switzerland, 2012.
19. Moher, D.; Liberati, A.; Tetzlaff, J.; Altman, D.G.; Group, P. Preferred reporting items for systematic reviews and meta-analyses: The PRISMA statement. *PLoS Med.* **2009**, *6*, e1000097. [CrossRef] [PubMed]
20. Kim, S.Y.; Park, J.E.; Lee, Y.J.; Seo, H.J.; Sheen, S.S.; Hahn, S.; Jang, B.H.; Son, H.J. Testing a tool for assessing the risk of bias for nonrandomized studies showed moderate reliability and promising validity. *J. Clin. Epidemiol.* **2013**, *66*, 408–414. [CrossRef] [PubMed]
21. Sterne, J.A.C.; Savović, J.; Page, M.J.; Elbers, R.G.; Blencowe, N.S.; Boutron, I.; Cates, C.J.; Cheng, H.-Y.; Corbett, M.S.; Eldridge, S.M.; et al. RoB 2: A revised tool for assessing risk of bias in randomised trials. *BMJ* **2019**, *366*, l4898. [CrossRef] [PubMed]
22. Saulnier, P.-J.; Gand, E.; Ragot, S.; Bankir, L.; Piguel, X.; Fumeron, F.; Rigalleau, V.; Halimi, J.-M.; Marechaud, R.; Roussel, R.; et al. Urinary Sodium Concentration Is an Independent Predictor of All-Cause and Cardiovascular Mortality in a Type 2 Diabetes Cohort Population. *J. Diabetes Res.* **2017**, *2017*, 1–10. [CrossRef] [PubMed]
23. Koca, T.T.; Tugan, C.B.; Seyithanoglu, M.; Koçyiğit, B.F. The Clinical Importance of the Plasma Atherogenic Index, Other Lipid Indexes, and Urinary Sodium and Potassium Excretion in Patients with Stroke. *Eurasian J. Med.* **2019**, *51*, 171–175. [CrossRef] [PubMed]
24. Dolmatova, E.V.; Moazzami, K.; Bansilal, S. Dietary sodium intake among US adults with hypertension, 1999–2012. *J. Hypertens.* **2018**, *36*, 237–242. [CrossRef]
25. Gijsbers, L.; Dower, J.I.; Mensink, M.; Siebelink, E.; Bakker, S.J.L.; Geleijnse, J.M. Effects of sodium and potassium supplementation on blood pressure and arterial stiffness: A fully controlled dietary intervention study. *J. Hum. Hypertens.* **2015**, *29*, 592–598. [CrossRef]
26. Kalogeropoulos, A.P.; Georgiopoulou, V.V.; Murphy, R.A.; Newman, A.B.; Bauer, D.C.; Harris, T.B.; Yang, Z.; Applegate, W.B.; Kritchevsky, S.B. Dietary sodium content, mortality, and risk for cardiovascular events in older adults: The Health, Aging, and Body Composition (Health ABC) Study. *JAMA Intern. Med.* **2015**, *175*, 410–419. [CrossRef]
27. Willey, J.; Gardener, H.; Cespedes, S.; Cheung, Y.K.; Sacco, R.L.; Elkind, M.S. Dietary Sodium to Potassium Ratio and Risk of Stroke in a Multiethnic Urban Population: The Northern Manhattan Study. *Stroke* **2017**, *48*, 2979–2983. [CrossRef]
28. Howard, G.; Cushman, M.; Moy, C.S.; Oparil, S.; Muntner, P.; Lackland, D.T.; Manly, J.J.; Flaherty, M.L.; Judd, S.E.; Wadley, V.G.; et al. Association of Clinical and Social Factors With Excess Hypertension Risk in Black Compared With White US Adults. *JAMA* **2018**, *320*, 1338–1348. [CrossRef]

29. Lelli, D.; Antonelli-Incalzi, R.; Bandinelli, S.; Ferrucci, L.; Pedone, C. Association between Sodium Excretion and Cardiovascular Disease and Mortality in the Elderly: A Cohort Study. *J. Am. Med. Dir. Assoc.* **2018**, *19*, 229–234. [CrossRef]
30. Averill, M.M.; Young, R.L.; Frazier-Wood, A.C.; Kurlak, E.O.; Kramer, H.; Steffen, L.M.; McClelland, R.L.; Delaney, J.A.; Drewnowski, A. Spot Urine Sodium-to-Potassium Ratio Is a Predictor of Stroke. *Stroke* **2019**, *50*, 321–327. [CrossRef] [PubMed]
31. Guligowska, A.; Pigłowska, M.; Śmigielski, J.; Kostka, T. Inappropriate pattern of nutrient consumption and coexistent cardiometabolic disorders in elderly people from Poland. *Pol. Arch. Intern. Med.* **2015**, *125*, 521–531. [CrossRef] [PubMed]
32. Iida, H.; Kurita, N.; Takahashi, S.; Sasaki, S.; Nishiwaki, H.; Omae, K.; Yajima, N.; Fukuma, S.; Hasegawa, T.; Fukuhara, S.; et al. Salt intake and body weight correlate with higher blood pressure in the very elderly population: The Sukagawa study. *J. Clin. Hypertens* **2019**, *21*, 942–949. [CrossRef] [PubMed]
33. Kim, M.K.; Kwon, M.; Rhee, M.-Y.; Kim, K.-I.; Nah, D.-Y.; Kim, S.-W.; Gu, N.; Sung, K.-C.; Hong, K.-S.; Cho, E.-J.; et al. Dose–response association of 24-hour urine sodium and sodium to potassium ratio with nighttime blood pressure at older ages. *Eur. J. Prev. Cardiol.* **2019**, *26*, 952–960. [CrossRef]
34. Mattes, R.D.; Donnelly, D. Relative contributions of dietary sodium sources. *J. Am. Coll. Nutr.* **1991**, *10*, 383–393. [CrossRef]
35. Gonçalves, C.; Abreu, S.; Padrão, P.; Pinho, O.; Graça, P.; Breda, J.J.; Santos, R.; Moreira, P. Sodium and potassium urinary excretion and dietary intake: A cross-sectional analysis in adolescents. *Food Nutr. Res.* **2016**, *60*, 29442. [CrossRef]
36. McLean, R.M. Measuring Population Sodium Intake: A Review of Methods. *Nutrients* **2014**, *6*, 4651–4662. [CrossRef]
37. He, F.J.; Campbell, N.R.C.; Ma, Y.; MacGregor, G.A.; Cogswell, M.E.; Cook, N.R. Errors in estimating usual sodium intake by the Kawasaki formula alter its relationship with mortality: Implications for public health. *Int. J. Epidemiol.* **2018**, *47*, 1784–1795. [CrossRef] [PubMed]
38. Taylor, R.S.; Ashton, K.E.; Moxham, T.; Hooper, L.; Ebrahim, S. Reduced dietary salt for the prevention of cardiovascular disease. *Cochrane Database Syst. Rev.* **2011**, Cd009217. [CrossRef]
39. O'Donnell, M.; Mente, A.; Yusuf, S. Sodium Intake and Cardiovascular Health. *Circ. Res.* **2015**, *116*, 1046–1057. [CrossRef] [PubMed]
40. Verma, S.; Gupta, M.; Holmes, D.T.; Xu, L.; Teoh, H.; Gupta, S.; Yusuf, S.; Lonn, E.M. Plasma renin activity predicts cardiovascular mortality in the Heart Outcomes Prevention Evaluation (HOPE) study. *Eur. Hear. J.* **2011**, *32*, 2135–2142. [CrossRef]
41. McCullough, P.A.; Fallahzadeh, M.K.; Hegazi, R.M. Nutritional Deficiencies and Sarcopenia in Heart Failure: A Therapeutic Opportunity to Reduce Hospitalization and Death. *Rev. Cardiovasc. Med.* **2016**, *17* (Suppl. 1), S30–S39.
42. Johnston, J.G.; Pollock, D.M. Circadian regulation of renal function. *Free. Radic. Biol. Med.* **2018**, *119*, 93–107. [CrossRef]
43. Moreira, P.; Sousa, A.S.; Guerra, R.S.; Santos, A.; Borges, N.; Afonso, C.; Amaral, T.F.; Padrão, P. Sodium and potassium urinary excretion and their ratio in the elderly: Results from the Nutrition UP 65 study. *Food Nutr. Res.* **2018**, *62*. [CrossRef]
44. Aburto, N.J.; Ziolkovska, A.; Hooper, L.; Elliott, P.; Cappuccio, F.P.; Meerpohl, J.J. Effect of lower sodium intake on health: Systematic review and meta-analyses. *BMJ* **2013**, *346*, f1326. [CrossRef]
45. D'Elia, L.; La Fata, E.; Giaquinto, A.; Strazzullo, P.; Galletti, F. Effect of dietary salt restriction on central blood pressure: A systematic review and meta-analysis of the intervention studies. *J. Clin. Hypertens.* **2020**, *22*, 814–825. [CrossRef]
46. D'Elia, L.; Galletti, F.; La Fata, E.; Sabino, P.; Strazzullo, P. Effect of dietary sodium restriction on arterial stiffness: Systematic review and meta-analysis of the randomized controlled trials. *J. Hypertens.* **2018**, *36*, 734–743. [CrossRef] [PubMed]
47. Strazzullo, P.; D'Elia, L.; Kandala, N.-B.; Cappuccio, F.P. Salt intake, stroke, and cardiovascular disease: Meta-analysis of prospective studies. *BMJ* **2009**, *339*, b4567. [CrossRef] [PubMed]
48. D'Elia, L.; Iannotta, C.; Sabino, P.; Ippolito, R. Potassium-rich diet and risk of stroke: Updated meta-analysis. *Nutr. Metab. Cardiovasc. Dis.* **2014**, *24*, 585–587. [CrossRef] [PubMed]
49. D'Elia, L.; Barba, G.; Cappuccio, F.P.; Strazzullo, P. Potassium intake, stroke, and cardiovascular disease a meta-analysis of prospective studies. *J. Am. Coll. Cardiol.* **2011**, *57*, 1210–1219. [CrossRef] [PubMed]

50. Du, S.; Batis, C.; Wang, H.; Zhang, B.; Zhang, J.; Popkin, B.M. Understanding the patterns and trends of sodium intake, potassium intake, and sodium to potassium ratio and their effect on hypertension in China. *Am. J. Clin. Nutr.* **2013**, *99*, 334–343. [CrossRef]
51. Perez, V.; Chang, E.T. Sodium-to-potassium ratio and blood pressure, hypertension, and related factors. *Adv. Nutr.* **2014**, *5*, 712–741. [CrossRef]
52. Kanbay, M.; Bayram, Y.; Solak, Y.; Sanders, P.W. Dietary potassium: A key mediator of the cardiovascular response to dietary sodium chloride. *J. Am. Soc. Hypertens.* **2013**, *7*, 395–400. [CrossRef]
53. Vassar, M.; Yerokhin, V.; Sinnett, P.M.; Weiher, M.; Muckelrath, H.; Carr, B.; Varney, L.; Cook, G. Database selection in systematic reviews: An insight through clinical neurology. *Heal. Inf. Libr. J.* **2017**, *34*, 156–164. [CrossRef]

Publisher's Note: MDPI stays neutral with regard to jurisdictional claims in published maps and institutional affiliations.

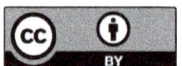

© 2020 by the authors. Licensee MDPI, Basel, Switzerland. This article is an open access article distributed under the terms and conditions of the Creative Commons Attribution (CC BY) license (http://creativecommons.org/licenses/by/4.0/).

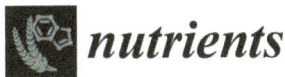

Review

Age-Related Changes and Sex-Related Differences in Brain Iron Metabolism

Tanja Grubić Kezele [1,2,*,†] and Božena Ćurko-Cofek [1,†]

1. Department of Physiology and Immunology, Faculty of Medicine, University of Rijeka, Braće Branchetta 20, 51000 Rijeka, Croatia; bozena.curko.cofek@medri.uniri.hr
2. Clinical Department for Clinical Microbiology, Clinical Hospital Center Rijeka, Krešimirova 42, 51000 Rijeka, Croatia
* Correspondence: tanja.grubic@medri.uniri.hr; Tel.: +385-917-550-647
† These authors contributed equally to this work.

Received: 7 August 2020; Accepted: 25 August 2020; Published: 27 August 2020

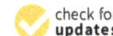

Abstract: Iron is an essential element that participates in numerous cellular processes. Any disruption of iron homeostasis leads to either iron deficiency or iron overload, which can be detrimental for humans' health, especially in elderly. Each of these changes contributes to the faster development of many neurological disorders or stimulates progression of already present diseases. Age-related cellular and molecular alterations in iron metabolism can also lead to iron dyshomeostasis and deposition. Iron deposits can contribute to the development of inflammation, abnormal protein aggregation, and degeneration in the central nervous system (CNS), leading to the progressive decline in cognitive processes, contributing to pathophysiology of stroke and dysfunctions of body metabolism. Besides, since iron plays an important role in both neuroprotection and neurodegeneration, dietary iron homeostasis should be considered with caution. Recently, there has been increased interest in sex-related differences in iron metabolism and iron homeostasis. These differences have not yet been fully elucidated. In this review we will discuss the latest discoveries in iron metabolism, age-related changes, along with the sex differences in iron content in serum and brain, within the healthy aging population and in neurological disorders such as multiple sclerosis, Parkinson's disease, Alzheimer's disease, and stroke.

Keywords: aging; Alzheimer's disease; iron metabolism; multiple sclerosis; Parkinson's disease; sex differences; stroke

1. Introduction

Iron is an essential micronutrient because of its importance in the process of erythropoiesis, oxidative metabolism, and cellular immune responses [1]. Healthy adults contain 4–5 g of iron, which is mostly (65%) found in red blood cell hemoglobin (Hb), and 30–35% is stored in the liver in the form of ferritin. Only 1–2% is in the form of iron-sulfur clusters or heme in the enzymes and multiprotein complexes [2]. Despite its essential role in the human body [3], there are no effective means of excreting iron [4]. Thus, a critical point in iron homeostasis is the regulation of the absorption of dietary iron from the duodenum. The body absorbs 1–2 mg of dietary iron a day, and this intake must be balanced with losses in the form of sloughed intestinal mucosal cells, menstruation, and other blood losses [5]. Maintaining the balance is very important because free iron is able to generate free radicals through Fenton reaction, and it is highly toxic [6,7]. Therefore, organisms have developed sophisticated pathways to import, chaperone, sequester, and export iron in order to maintain an appropriate iron balance [8]. Any disruption of iron homeostasis leads to either iron deficiency (ID) or iron overload (IO) [9].

The pathophysiological consequences of ID are impairments in cognitive development, cardiovascular diseases, endothelial disorders, and other health complications [10], especially in elderly. A chronic low-grade inflammation present in the elderly leads to less efficient absorption through hepcidin regulation and subsequent increase in ferritin concentrations. ID becomes more of a problem because of age-related changes in Hb and sex hormones, effects of medication prescribed for age-related diseases, and metabolic changes associated with inflammatory states [11].

IO leads to adverse manifestations in different tissues (brain, heart, liver, adipose, muscle, pancreas) and it is implicated in the pathogenesis of several metabolic (e.g., type 2 diabetes, non-alcoholic steatohepatitis, atherosclerosis, stroke, etc.) [12] and neurodegenerative diseases (e.g., Alzheimer's disease (AD), Parkinson's disease (PD), multiple sclerosis (MS), etc.) [13], which could be found more often in elderly.

Although physiological iron requirements do not differ between adult and elderly men, and post-menopausal and elderly women, there is growing evidence that iron metabolism is affected by the aging process [11]. Age-related cellular and molecular alterations in iron metabolism can lead to iron dyshomeostasis and deposition [14]. Iron deposits can contribute to the development of inflammation, abnormal protein aggregation and degeneration, especially in the central nervous system (CNS), leading to the progressive decline in cognitive processes [13], and contributing to pathophysiology of stroke [15].

An increased number of recent experimental and clinical discoveries about the sex-related differences in iron metabolism present in certain neurological disorders [16–22] is raising attention, and pointing to the need for future research exploring possible underlying mechanisms, which could be responsible for the sex differences in the susceptibility to these diseases.

Whereas environmental factors are involved in most of the cases of neurodegenerative diseases, it is important to take into consideration the role of nutrition in both neuroprotection and neurodegeneration. Furthermore, there is sufficient evidence regarding ID having adverse health effects to justify correcting it through diet or iron therapy. At the same time, it is important to ensure that the risk of high body iron stores is not increased as this may have detrimental effects on the brain and cause neurodegeneration and other neurological disorders [23,24]. Therefore, the aim of this review is to provide an up-to-date discussion in iron metabolism, age-related changes, along with the sex differences in iron content in serum and brain, within the healthy aging population and in neurological disorders such as MS, PD, AD, and stroke.

2. Systemic Iron Metabolism

In the last 15 years, many new iron genes, proteins and pathways have been discovered thanks to the application of genetic screens and transgenic technology in biomedical research. They brought a new light in the understanding of iron absorption, trafficking, utilization, and regulation [25].

2.1. Iron Absorption

All iron enters the body from the diet. Normal diet should contain 13–18 mg of iron per day but only 1–2 mg is absorbed [26]. Absorption of dietary iron mainly occurs at the apical surface of the mature duodenal enterocytes [27]. Low pH of duodenum favors solubility of iron while further down the intestine the formation of insoluble ferric complexes probably reduces bioavailability [26]. It is well known that vitamin C enhances iron uptake in the duodenum but it is also important at cellular level since it enables efficient uptake of iron from transferrin, which is the only source of iron for erythropoiesis [28].

Dietary iron can be in heme (10%) and non-heme (ionic, 90%) forms and they absorb via different mechanisms [26]. Dietary non-heme iron primarily exists in an oxidized (Fe^{3+}) ferric form that is not bioavailable, and therefore must be reduced to the ferrous (Fe^{2+}) form before the transport across the intestinal epithelium [29,30]. The reduction of iron from the ferric to the ferrous state occurs at the enterocyte brush border by a duodenal cytochrome b (DCYTB), an iron-regulated ferric reductase enzyme [27,29].

Ferrous iron is then transported across the apical plasma membrane of the enterocyte by divalent metal transporter-1 (DMT1) [31,32]. Inside the enterocyte, iron may be stored as ferritin and excreted in the faeces when the senescent enterocyte is sloughed. The other possibility is the transfer of iron out of the enterocyte across the basolateral membrane to the plasma by the basolateral iron exporter ferroportin-1 (FPN1) [33,34]. FPN1 is a 12 transmembrane domain protein (also known as SLC40A1, IREG1, or MTP1) [35]. It transports ferrous iron, which must be oxidized by a multi-copper oxidase protein called hephaestin (HEPH) to ferric iron [30,36], which binds to plasma transferrin (Tf) [37,38].

The research supports the existence of transferrin-independent routes of iron uptake. DMT1 was thought to be responsible for non-transferrin-bound iron (NTBI) uptake by liver cells, but iron loading of DMT1-deficient mouse hepatocytes indicates that there is at least one alternative transferrin-independent uptake pathway [39]. The main candidate for this alternative pathway is a zinc transporter Zrt–Irt-like protein 14 (ZIP14, SLC39A14). It is considered as the second major carrier involved in NTBI uptake by hepatocytes [40].

Heme iron is absorbed into enterocytes by a heme carrier protein 1 (HCP1). It is a membrane protein in the proximal intestine, where heme absorption is the greatest [41,42]. Once internalized in the enterocytes, the most dietary heme iron is released as ferrous iron by heme oxygenase (HO) and enters a common pathway with dietary non-heme iron before it leaves the enterocytes [1]. It remains unclear whether some heme traverses the cells intact and leaves the enterocytes through the action of the heme exporters breast cancer resistance protein/ATP-binding cassette subfamily G member 2 (BCRP/ABCG2) and feline leukemia virus C receptor (FLVCR) [41].

2.2. Iron Transport and Distribution

Except for the duodenal enterocytes, the sources of iron in the plasma are iron-recycling reticuloendothelial macrophages [43]. When iron enters the circulation, it binds to Tf and is transported to sites of use and storage [44]. Human Tf is a 76-kDa glycoprotein mainly produced in the liver. One Tf molecule can carry two ferric ions. Serum Tf can be in the non-iron bind (apo-Tf), monoferric, or diferric (holo-Tf) forms [45,46].

The interaction between Fe^{3+} and Tf is dependent on pH. Fe^{3+} efficiently binds to Tf at pH 7.4 and dissociates from Tf at acidic pH [46]. Iron enters cells that require iron through a transferrin receptor 1 (TfR1)-mediated mechanism [47]. Holo-Tf has a much higher affinity for TfR than monoferric-Tf. Therefore, holo-Tf binds to TfR1 on the cell surface and the whole complex is internalized by clathrin-mediated endocytosis forming clathrin-coated endosomes (siderosomes) [44]. In the acidic endosomal milieu, Fe^{3+} dissociates from Tf and is converted to Fe^{2+} by metalloreductases [48]. Fe^{2+} is transported into the cytosol by DMT1 while Tf/TfR1 complex is transported to the cell surface and both elements are reused in another cycle of cellular iron uptake [46]. TfR1 is expressed in all tissues [49] and its expression is regulated by the cellular iron status at both the transcriptional and post-transcriptional levels. In the presence of hypoxia or ID, the expression of hypoxia-inducible factors (HIF-1α and HIF-2α) increases, and these proteins bind to the hypoxia response element (HRE) in the promoter of transferrin receptor (TFRC) gene, thereby promoting TFRC transcription [50]. At the post-transcriptional level, the iron regulatory protein (IRP)/iron responsive element (IRE) system plays an important role [51]. Under intracellular iron-deficient conditions, intracellular iron sensors IRP1 and IRP2 bind to IREs to stabilize the TFRC mRNA and enhance the expression of TfR1 protein. In the case of iron excess, IRPs lose their interactions with IREs. IRP1 becomes an aconitase through conformational changes [52] and IRP2 is degraded after ubiquitination [53,54], resulting in destabilization and degradation of TFRC mRNA.

Transferrin receptor 2 (TfR2) mRNA is highly expressed in the liver and to a lesser extent in spleen, lung, muscle, prostate and peripheral blood mononuclear cells [46,55]. It binds to holo-Tf with 20-fold lower affinity than TfR1 [56]. Since TfR2 lacks an IRE, it is not regulated in response to the plasma iron level. Instead, TfR2 expression is reciprocally regulated by Tf saturation, and consequently upregulated in IO [5]. It was also suggested that TfR2 could be involved in the uptake of NTBI [57].

2.3. Iron Storage and Recycling

The liver is the main storage site for excess iron [49]. The uptake of Tf-bound iron from plasma to liver cells is through the TfR1 and TfR2. Since free intracellular iron is toxic, most of the iron in the cells is stored in ferritin [58]. The poly(rC)-binding proteins act as intracellular iron chaperones and deliver iron to ferritin and several enzymes [59].

Ferritin is the main form of iron storage and can be found in all tissues, but mostly in the liver, spleen, and in bone marrow. It has the capacity to sequester up to 4500 atoms of non-heme iron in its spherical structure [60]. This spherical structure consists of 24 subunits of heavy (H) and light (L) ferritin in different ratios, depending on the tissue [61]. Within the ferritin, iron is stored in the ferric form [62]. Ferritin shows enzymatic properties by converting ferric to ferrous iron as iron is sequestered in the ferritin mineral core [63]. When high concentrations of iron-laden ferritin accumulate within the cell, the ferritin molecules aggregate, and fuse with lysosomes. This process leads to the degradation of ferritin, and the resulting mixture of Fe^{3+} cores and peptides is known as hemosiderin [64]. Iron can be efficiently mobilized from both ferritin and hemosiderin when it is required elsewhere in the body.

Another important feature of ferritin is that small amounts are secreted from the cell, and this amount strongly correlates with the concentration of intracellular iron. This association makes serum ferritin concentrations an accurate indicator of body iron stores [65].

Mitochondrial ferritin is also an iron-storage protein. Its amino acid sequence shares high homology with H-chain ferritin, indicating similar functions [66,67]. It has been shown that mitochondrial ferritin expression is limited to tissues with high metabolic activity and oxygen consumption, such as brain, testis, and heart [68].

A significant part of iron (600 mg) is deposited in tissue macrophages [69], which respond to systemic iron requirements by the interaction of hepcidin and FPN1 [70,71]. Iron storage at the macrophages is safe and does not lead to oxidative damage [72]. The amount of iron required for daily production of red blood cells (20–30 mg) is provided mostly by iron recycling by macrophages [1,73]. Splenic and hepatic macrophages phagocytize and degrade senescent and damaged erythrocytes to recover iron, mainly to produce Hb in new erythrocytes but also for other carriers and enzymes requiring iron [69]. In the phagocytic vesicles, heme is metabolized by HO and iron is exported to the cytoplasm by a protein similar to DMT1 [1].

Erythropoietin reduces iron retention in macrophages by decreasing DMT1 and increasing FPN1 expression [72]. Macrophages obtain a certain amount of iron from plasma through the action of DMT1 and TfR1, and from apoptotic cells and bacteria [44].

2.4. Regulation of Systemic Iron Homeostasis

All the processes involved in maintaining iron homeostasis are regulated at the different levels, mainly by the interaction and cooperation of three systems [74]. The first system consists of hormone hepcidin and iron export protein FPN1. They act on systemic level and regulate serum iron levels [75]. The post-transcriptional regulation of iron genes involved in intracellular iron homeostasis is mediated by the interaction of IRPs and IRE while HIF2 α mediates transcriptional regulation of iron homeostasis [76].

Hepcidin is a key regulator of iron level. Variations in body iron demand are communicated to the liver which, in turn, modulates the expression of hepcidin [77], encoded by the hepcidin antimicrobial peptide gene (HAMP) [78]. Hepcidin is primarily produced by liver sinusoidal endothelial cells in response to iron levels [75,79], and in the small quantity by macrophages [80] and adipocytes [81]. Different physiological and pathological conditions such as increased erythropoiesis, hypoxia, anemia, IO, endocrine, metabolic, and inflammatory processes affect hepcidin synthesis in hepatocytes [63,82].

Hepcidin is upregulated in response to iron loading and inflammation and decreases in response to ID and hypoxia [83,84].

Hepcidin transcription is regulated by bone morphogenic protein 6 (BMP6) [85], which acts on hepatocytes through BMP receptor (BMPR) [86]. BMPR creates a supercomplex with hemojuvelin (HJV), matriptase 2 (MT2) and neogenin [87].

Activated BMPR induces phosphorylation of s-mothers against decapentaplegic (SMAD) molecules, which then cause an increase in hepcidin expression through activation of HAMP gene [38]. Tumor necrosis factor (TNF), pathogens, and interleukin-6 (IL-6) stimulate hepcidin synthesis via signal transducer and activator of transcription 3 (STAT-3) activation [77,88]. Hepcidin expression in macrophages is regulated mainly through toll-like receptor 4 (TLR4) associated with adaptor proteins [89].

Iron sensing is dependent on an interaction of Tf, TfR1 and TfR2, aided by the hemochromatosis protein (HFE). HFE has an extracellular transferrin receptor-binding region and forms a stable complex with TfR1 [90]. When HFE binds to TfR1, HFE changes the conformation of the Tf-Fe binding site, decreasing the affinity of TfR1 for Tf and iron entry into cells [49,84,91].

Hepcidin expression decreases the iron absorption from the duodenal enterocytes, iron release from macrophages and its transport across the placenta [92,93]. The iron exporter required for iron egress from enterocytes, macrophages, as well as all other iron exporting cells including placental syncytiotrophoblasts and hepatocytes, is FPN1. It is not only the effector of cellular iron export, but also the receptor for hepcidin, its primary regulator [94]. Hepcidin binds to FPN1 present on the cell surface and induces the phosphorylation of amino acids located on an intracellular loop of FPN1, triggering the internalization of the hepcidin-FPN1 complex, leading to the ubiquitination of FPN1 and lysosomal degradation of both proteins [65].

In the inflammatory conditions, upregulation of hepcidin is mainly through IL-6 [93,95], which induces STAT-3 activation and its binding to the hepcidin promoter [96]. The increased hepcidin synthesis causes iron sequestration in macrophages and decreases iron availability in tissues, limiting the growth of microbes [70] and causing the characteristic hypoferremia and eventually anemia of inflammation [93,95].

3. Brain Iron Metabolism

The brain is a very metabolically active organ and accounts for about 20% of the body's total energy consumption. These high-energy needs must be supported with an adequate supply of iron [97]. Therefore, iron is the most abundant metal in the brain [14]. It has an essential role as a co-factor for many physiological processes in the CNS, including oxidative metabolism, myelination, and the biosynthesis of neurotransmitters [98]. To ensure the normal course of these processes, brain iron levels are tightly regulated [99].

The entry of iron from the blood into the brain is controlled by the blood–brain barrier (BBB) [100] and to a lesser extent by the blood–cerebrospinal fluid barrier (BCSFB) [101]. The role of the BBB is to prevent the brain from neurotoxic plasma components and pathogens [102]. At the same time, it controls chemical composition of the neuronal milieu by regulating the transport of molecules required for normal neuronal functioning [103]. The BBB is formed by a monolayer of tightly sealed microvascular endothelial cells extending along the vascular tree [104] and expressing low paracellular and transcellular permeability [105]. Those endothelial cells are surrounded by basal lamina and astrocytic perivascular end-feet, forming the neurovascular unit [106]. Tf-bound iron cannot cross the BBB directly and the mechanism of iron transcellular entry into the brain is not entirely clear [107]. According to the recent models [108,109], there are two possible iron transport pathways: transferrin-bound iron (Tf-Fe) and NTBI [107] (Figure 1).

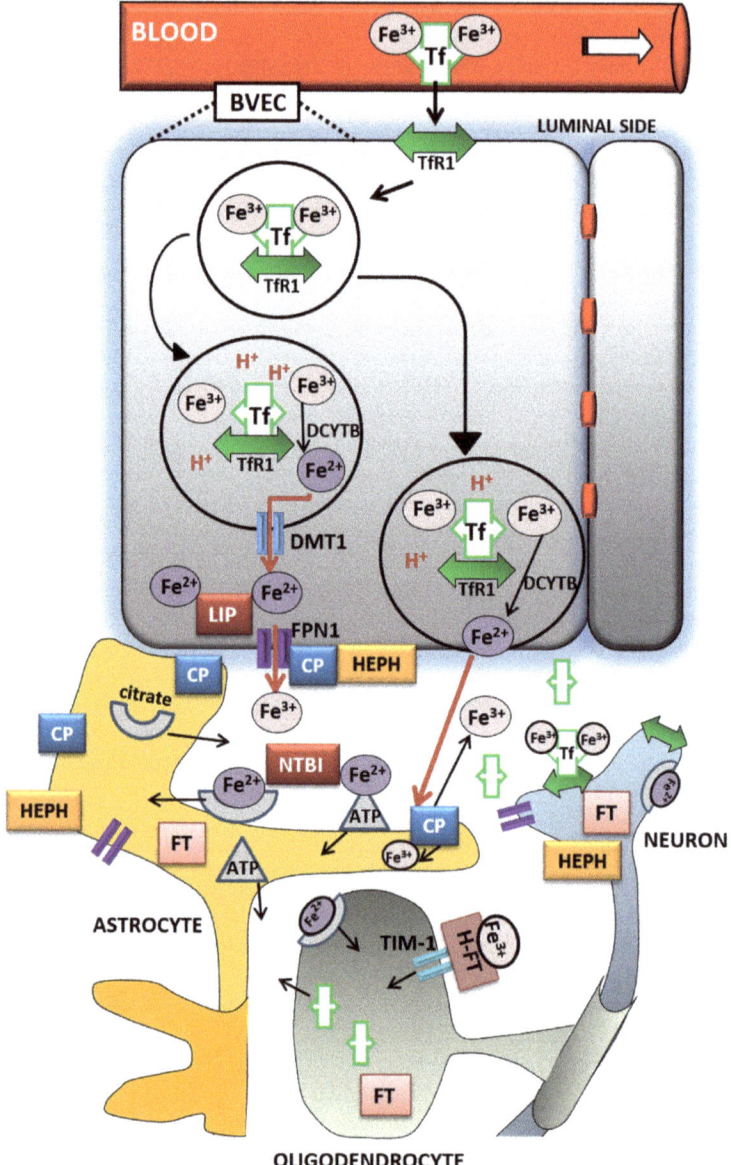

Figure 1. Iron transport inside the brain. A scheme of proposed transferrin-bound and non-transferrin bound iron transport pathways in the brain. *Abbreviations*: BVEC—blood vascular endothelial cell, Tf—transferrin, TfR1—transferrin receptor 1, Fe^{3+}—ferric iron, Fe^{2+}—ferrous iron, DCYTB—duodenal cytochrome b, DMT1—divalent metal transporter-1, FPN1—ferroportin-1, LIP—labile iron pool, CP—ceruloplasmin, HEPH—hephaestin, NTBI—non-transferrin-bound iron, FT—ferritin, H-FT—H-ferritin, TIM-1—T-cell immunoglobulin and mucin domain.

The Tf/TfR1 pathway is considered to be the major route for iron transport across the luminal membrane of the capillary endothelium [107]. According to the widely established transcytosis mechanism, Tf binds to TfR at the luminal side of the brain capillaries [32]. The complex traverses the cell in the endocytosis vesicle, where the acid environment facilitates the release of ferric iron from Tf and its reduction to ferrous iron by endosomal reductase [110], possibly DCYTB or six-transmembrane epithelial antigen of the prostate-2 (STEAP2) [111]. The next steps in this pathway are still not completely clear. One possibility is that ferrous iron is transported from the endosome to the cytosol by the DMT1 [112] and joins the intracellular labile iron pool (LIP) [113] (Figure 1). It could be further utilized for metabolic purposes by the endothelial cells, stored in endothelial cell ferritin [114] or imported into mitochondria via mitoferrins and TfR2 [115]. It could be also released into the extracellular fluid by action of export protein FPN1 [108], and reoxidized to Fe^{3+} by ferroxidases HEPH and ceruloplasmin (CP) [100]. Studies have confirmed that capillary endothelium of the BBB, neurons, and astrocytes, has the ability to express FPN1 and HEPH [116,117]. The alternative mechanism that has been proposed is that the endosome containing Tf-TfR1 complex goes all the way to the abluminal side and releases iron between the endothelial cells and astrocyte end-foot processes [99]. The released ferrous iron is then oxidized to ferric iron by the ferroxidase activity of CP or HEPH expressed on the end-foot processes [112]. Oxidized iron binds to apo-Tf circulating within the brain [113] (Figure 1). The main source of Tf in the brain interstitium is its diffusion from the ventricles and a certain amount is synthesized in oligodendrocytes [118]. Because of the low concentrations of Tf in the cerebrospinal fluid (CSF), iron saturation of CSF Tf is almost 100%, while serum Tf is saturated by about 30% [99]. Consequently, under conditions of IO, CSF Tf has much lower buffering capacity [119], NTBI levels may be quite high [120], and the vulnerability of neuronal cells to iron toxicity increases [119].

Iron may also enter the brain through epithelial cells of the choroid plexus, which form the BCSFB [121]. The choroid plexus consists of fenestrated capillaries so the holo-Tf can cross them and reach the choroidal epithelium [122]. Further, the iron is released the same way as from the BBB endothelial cells by means of DMT1, FPN1 and ferroxidases [14]. When iron enters the CSF, there is no diffusional barrier between CSF and interstitial fluid. Iron binds to Tf in CSF and supplies CNS cells expressing TfR1 [123].

Different cell types in the brain acquire iron by distinct pathways. Neurons express high levels of TfR1. Therefore, Tf is the main source of iron for neurons [112], although neurons can also uptake NTBI from interstitial fluid [124]. Unlike them, oligodendrocytes and astrocytes do not express TfR1 and their main source of iron is NTBI [110]. Namely, ferrous iron in the brain interstitium can also bind to ATP or citrate released from astrocytes and it is transported to oligodendrocytes and astrocytes as NTBI [99] (Figure 1).

Oligodendrocytes acquire NTBI via the T-cell immunoglobulin and mucin domain (Tim-1). It is a ferritin receptor exclusively expressed in oligodendrocytes that binds H-ferritin [125]. Astrocytes express ferri-reductase on their plasma membranes to reduce ferric to ferrous iron and facilitate iron uptake [126] (Figure 1). Once iron enters the brain cells, the iron pool is tightly regulated. It has to provide enough iron for cellular functions and prevent the development of oxidative stress [110]. Ferritin has an important role in iron sequestration and free iron level reduction [127], whereas neuromelanin captures large amounts of iron in certain neurons for longer-term storage [128]. Namely, the pigment neuromelanin acts as a scavenger binding redox-active metal ion such as iron. The expression of ferritin varies in different cell types according to their functional requirements for iron. Neurons contain the least, and microglia contain the most amount of cytosolic ferritin [129] but in the hypoxic conditions ferritin synthesis increases in cortical neurons and decreases in glial cells [130]. Ferritin degradation by the autophagy-lysosome system [131] initiates iron release, mainly through FPN1 [132]. Since hepcidin regulates the expression of FPN1, it modulates cellular iron level as well [13]. Recent studies revealed that hepcidin can be produced by the brain endothelium [108] or systemically derived by passing the BBB [133], and it is widely distributed in the brain [134,135]. Hence, hepcidin may be involved in the regulation of iron availability and circulation in the brain [108]. Cellular iron levels are also modulated at the post-transcriptional level by binding to the IREs of mRNA of IRPs [13].

When some of these cellular and molecular mechanisms of iron regulation are disrupted, the brain iron homeostasis is disturbed as well. If there is either too much or too little iron in the brain, numerous neurologic disorders can occur [14]. Excessive brain iron accumulation is found in MS, PD and AD, amyotrophic lateral sclerosis (ALS), neurodegeneration with brain iron accumulation, and Huntington's disease [114]. ID is associated with significant cognitive, performance and brain structural deficits [136].

4. Age-Related Iron Dyshomeostasis

Many iron homeostatic mechanisms appear to be affected during physiological aging (Figure 2). Therefore, older age is associated with increased risk of ID, elevated body iron stores and increased brain iron levels [23].

Iron deficiency is the most common nutrient deficiency worldwide [137]. The causes underlying ID, i.e., ID anemia are diverse and include: inadequate oral iron intake resulting from poor diets, excessive milk intake or vegetarian diets, inadequate iron absorption as a result of celiac disease and others, or excessive iron loss, mainly because of the blood loss or as a result of parasitic infection [137]. Inadequate iron supply leads to cerebral hypoxia [138], insufficient neurotransmitter synthesis [13], poor myelin integrity [139,140], and consequently to poor cognition, cognitive decline, and dementia [141].

Body iron levels may be elevated in older adults due to consumption of highly bioavailable forms of iron, such as supplemental iron and red meat, or enhancers of nonheme-iron absorption like vitamin C [142]. Studies have shown that high body iron stores were associated with increased risk of coronary heart disease [143], type 2 diabetes [144], and cognitive impairment and dementia [145].

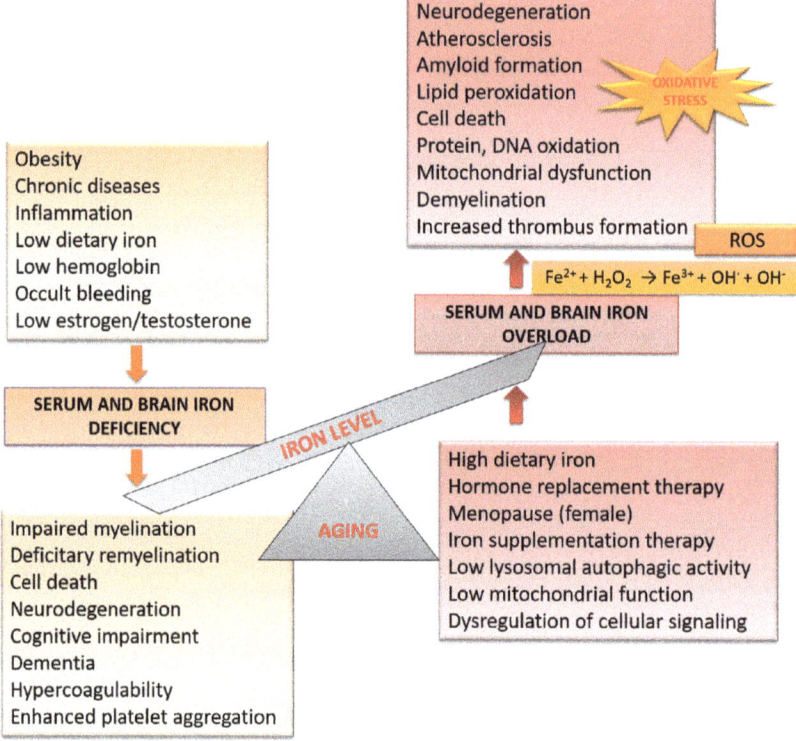

Figure 2. Age-related changes in iron level and consequent brain disorders.

Brain iron accumulation is considered as a hallmark of aging [146] and it is associated with the progressive imbalance between antioxidant defenses and intracellular generation of reactive oxygen species (ROS) [147]. This may explain the increased susceptibility of the aged brain to disease and the reason why aging is the major risk factor in neurodegenerative diseases [14].

Post-mortem analyses showed a positive correlation between iron deposition and age as well as the different iron contents in different brain regions [148]. Iron staining in older individuals (60–90 years of age) showed a larger content of iron in the microglia and astrocytes of the cortex, hippocampus, cerebellum, basal ganglia, and amygdala [149,150].

Increase in iron concentration, in the form of H- and L-ferritin, occurs in the *substantia nigra* [114] with many extraneuronal iron deposits in individuals over 80 years of age, especially in oligodendrocytes. Neuronal deposits in the *substantia nigra* are found in the neurons that do not contain neuromelanin [151]. Modern non-invasive methods, such as magnetic resonance imaging (MRI), revealed an age-related increase in the non-heme iron concentration in the *nucleus caudatus, putamen* and *globus pallidus* [152,153].

The mechanism of increase in iron concentration in certain brain regions is not completely clear. One of the proposed mechanisms is altered vascularization. It is observed during aging and in neurodegenerative diseases [154]. Region-specific increase of total iron could be probably triggered by inflammation [155], increased BBB permeability [156], redistribution of iron within the brain, and changes in the iron homeostasis [13]. The increase in iron concentration inside the CNS cells might directly damage these cells or affect the cellular environment, making it more susceptible to toxins and activation of pathogenic processes [151]. Besides, during brain aging, iron is partially converted from its stable and soluble form (ferritin) into hemosiderin and other oxyhydroxides that contain iron at higher reactivity [157], inducing the neuronal vulnerability to oxidative stress [158]. An additional feature of brain aging that contributes to the development of oxidative stress is an increase in the levels of monoamine oxidase (MAO). This enzyme catalyzes the oxidative deamination of neurotransmitters, in which hydrogen peroxide (H_2O_2) and aldehydes as highly toxic by-products are subsequently generated [159]. Since those by-products are inductors of lipid peroxidation, it is assumed that activation of MAO is associated with age-related disturbances of the homeostasis and generation of free radicals in the nervous tissue [160].

5. Sex-Related Differences in Iron Homeostasis during Healthy Aging and in Neurological Disorders

Increasing experimental and clinical evidence concerning iron metabolism support the idea that healthy aging processes, as well as neurological disorders, differ between women and men, suggesting the existence of different underlying mechanisms involved in the iron homeostasis and the pathogenesis of diseases (Figure 3) [16–22,161]. Age and sex are important co-factors to consider when establishing the differences between the pathological neurodegeneration from healthy aging.

As for healthy aging, a sex-specific negative association was found between dietary iron intake and cellular aging markers. Iron intake showed deleterious effects on the peripheral blood leukocyte telomere length in women and on the number of mitochondrial DNA copies in men [162].

These effects of iron imbalance on genomic stability and cellular aging markers must be considered during dietary iron intake and iron supplementation [162]. In addition, brain iron concentration differs between older men and women, showing that women have lower total subcortical brain iron levels after expected menopause onset [17]. These findings indicate that age-related changes in estrogen levels may be a mediating factor of such associations.

However, the overall data that involve sex-related differences in iron dyshomeostasis and concomitant brain disorders are still limited and mainly concentrated on estrogen functions. Thus, we are far away from the actual understanding of what underlies these differences in iron metabolism during aging processes and therefore need further assessment.

FEMALE	AGING	MALE
MULTIPLE SCLEROSIS		
• earlier onset of disease • ↑ serum ferritin • ↓ serum Fe (↓ shift from serum to brain) • ↓ Fe accumulation in CNS • ↓ estrogen (↑ inflammation, ↓Fe)		• worse clinical course, ↓ serum ferritin, ↑ oxidative stress reaction to Fe • ↑ serum Fe (↑ shift from serum to brain) • ↑ Fe accumulation in CNS • ↓ vitamin D (↑ hepcidin, ↓Fe) • ↓ testosterone (↑ inflammation, ↓Fe)
PARKINSON'S DISEASE		
• ↑ mitochondrial respiratory activity (brain) • ↑ neuromelanin (*substantia nigra*) • ↓ estrogen (↑ Fe-induced autophagy) • ↓ estrogen (↓Fe, ↓ FPN1, ↑ DMT1 in neurons, ↓ FPN1, ↓ DMT1 in astrocytes, ↑ inflammation) • ↓ serum Fe (↓ shift from serum to brain)		• ↓ mitochondrial respiratory activity in brain • ↑ *striatum* susceptibility to Fe accumulation • Fe deficiency anemia • ↓ testosterone (↑ inflammation, ↓Fe) • ↑ serum Fe (↑ shift from serum to brain)
ALZHEIMER'S DISEASE		
• ↑ regulatory control between Fe and glutamate metabolism • Fe deficiency anemia (↓ cognition) • ↓ estrogen (↑ Fe-induced lipid peroxidation, ↑ amiloid, ↑ inflammation, ↓Fe) • ↓ serum Fe (↓ shift from serum to brain)		• ↑ Fe accumulation in brain • ↑ carriers for HFE H63D/TfC2 • Fe deficiency anemia (↓ cognition) • ↓ testosterone (↑ amiloid, ↑ inflammation, ↓ Fe) • ↑ serum Fe (↑ shift from serum to brain)
STROKE		
• ↑ serum ferritin level • Fe deficiency anemia • ↑Fe • ↓ estrogen (↑ inflammation, ↓Fe)		• ↓ serum ferritin level • Fe deficiency anemia • ↑Fe • ↓ testosterone (↑ inflammation, ↓Fe)

Figure 3. The summary of features that involve iron impact on increased susceptibility to certain neurological disorders or increased progression of already present disorders in males and females during aging. The summary includes data from the references in this review. *Abbreviations*: CNS—central nervous system, Fe—ferrum, FPN1—ferroportin-1, DMT1—divalent metal transporter-1, HFE H63D—hemochromatosis H63D, TfC2—transferrin C2.

5.1. Iron and Multiple Sclerosis

Investigations in animal model of MS, experimental autoimmune encephalomyelitis (EAE), showed worsening of clinical course in iron overloaded animals, which had an iron accumulation in CNS (brain and spinal cord) [16]. Although female IO rats developed symptoms earlier, male IO rats showed more severe clinical course and higher mortality rate, indicating the existence of sex-dependent mechanisms [163]. During the acute phase of EAE, female IO rats sequestered more iron in the liver and produced more ferritin than male EAE rats. Male rats, however, reacted on IO by higher production of oxidative stress markers, malondialdehyde and 4-hydroxynonenal, in the neural tissues and showed greater signs of plaque formation and gliosis in the spinal cord [16]. The data point to sexual dimorphism in mechanisms that regulate peripheral and brain iron homeostasis and imply that men and women during MS might be differentially vulnerable to exogenous IO.

In patients with MS, iron content is elevated in deep grey matter structures and in the vicinity of lesions and reduced in the white matter [164]. Iron content is low in remyelinated plaques [164], suggesting that dynamic shuttling of iron continues through the MS disease process. This reveals that the iron dysregulation associated with MS is, in fact, a redistribution of iron between different areas of the brain [165]. Furthermore, quantitative MRI technique, i.e., quantitative susceptibility mapping suggests that altered deep grey matter iron is associated with the evolution of MS and on disability accrual, independent of tissue atrophy [166]. Excess iron enhances the generation of ROS, leading to myelin and neuron loss followed by demyelination and neurodegeneration [140].

Contrary to the belief that iron is harmful and invariably causes oxidative damage, it may paradoxically represent the key component of the entire antioxidant protection system of the oligodendrocyte. Namely, oligodendrocytes need iron for the extremely high energy requirements of producing and maintaining the complex myelin sheath [167], indicating that ID could seriously compromise the viability of these cells. Iron is also an important element for the maturation of oligodendrocyte progenitor cells (OPCs) into oligodendrocytes [168,169]. During remyelination, the OPCs are recruited to the MS lesions and differentiated into mature oligodendrocytes, which can further remyelinate the damaged axons. Considering the requirement for iron-containing enzymes in all these processes, iron levels in oligodendrocytes have an important influence on remyelination and neuronal repair. In the situation of reduced iron availability and iron-deficient oligodendrocytes, whether through global ID [170], impaired iron trafficking [171] or its export from astrocytes [11,172], it leads to reduced OPCs proliferation, disturbances in oligodendrocyte differentiation and following remyelination. Furthermore, OPCs are very sensitive to oxidation and the depletion of antioxidants such as glutathione, even more than mature oligodendrocytes [140]. This implies that these cells need antioxidant protection during patient relapses when there is an increased concentration of inflammatory mediators and ROS. Namely, iron is required for the production of ATP, which is essential for the synthesis of NADPH. NADPH is the reducing power of the cell [173] needed for the synthesis of lipids such as cholesterol, which are produced by oligodendrocytes for their membranes [173,174]. Heme cofactors in cytochrome P450 enzymes catalyze the essential hydroxylation reactions in the synthesis of cholesterol.

Furthermore, the hydroxylations that produce active vitamin D ($1,25(OH)_2 D_3$) from cholesterol are carried out by a cytochrome P450 enzyme called CYP27B1 [175]. Oligodendrocytes express vitamin D_3 receptors and respond to $1,25(OH)_2 D_3$ [176]. Thus, the relevant cytochrome P450 enzyme with a heme group is synthesized only in the presence of sufficient iron. It is already well known that sufficient vitamin D is protective against MS [177] and is associated with improved clinical and MRI outcomes [178]. In addition, Vitamin D has been shown to decrease hepcidin, which inversely regulates serum iron level, and the optimal function of hepcidin may be predicated upon the adequate presence of vitamin D in the blood [179].

Recent data showed that elderly males suffer from a serious vitamin D deficiency compared to elderly females. Nevertheless, old age is an independent risk factor for vitamin D deficiency, so together with ID could worsen the MS progression [180]. A possible reason could be the connection of ID with the age-related changes associated with chronic inflammatory states [11].

The link between ID and obesity may also be of relevance in MS, since obesity may be a risk factor for MS [181]. Obesity is often present in elderly people, and ID in obese has been ascribed to chronic, low-grade inflammation [182]. There is sufficient evidence linking ID, even moderate one, with adverse health effects to justify the use of iron therapy. Therapy should be performed with caution to prevent the risk of high body iron stores and its detrimental effects on the brain [23].

Females exhibit lower levels of serum iron [183] and lower levels of brain iron compared to men from midlife to old age [184]. Pre-menstrual blood loss reduces serum iron levels in women and may contribute to sex differences in brain iron accumulation [185]. Namely, histological data suggest that lower serum iron levels may influence brain iron levels since anemia was found to reduce brain iron in people postmortem [186]. Men have shown higher iron concentrations in the cortical white matter and subcortical nuclei according to MRI images [183,185,187]. Changing of the sex steroids levels in post-menopause [188] may influence sex-related variations of brain iron levels as well [17]. However, a lack of sex-related differences in brain iron levels have also been reported [153].

On the other hand, although elderly patients with late onset of MS (LOMS) represent a growing minority of all patients with the diagnosis of MS, the LOMS (aged >65 years) has a worse prognosis, which is still subject to debate [189]. However, it could be associated with the facts that brain iron levels increase with age in healthy individuals [190] and that serum iron level is lowering at the same time [23]. Namely, it can be hypothesized that a shift of iron from the blood compartment to the brain compartment occurred due to iron dysregulation because of aging and leading to iron deposition due to excess iron in the brain. If the iron does play a role in the etiology of MS, it could be possible that some patients may need supplementation, and others' attenuation of iron intake depending on their genetic background, making the individualized treatment approach for subgroups of MS.

Another reason for taking into consideration the iron supplementation is the fact that MS patients eat a more limited diet, with a lower average of 31 nutrients, including zinc, thiamin, and iron, when compared with healthy controls. In a study by Armon-Omer et al., 2019 blood tests showed that MS patients had significantly lower iron levels, with the lowest measures in the severe MS group [191]. In conclusion, it is possible that inadequate iron levels (both low and high) may be harmful in MS. Iron excess might increase free radicals, which may elevate oxidative stress, while iron reduction could decrease immune system function and cause an energy deficit due to loss of mitochondrial membrane potential [11]. In addition, Armon-Omer and coworkers found lower dietary copper intake in the MS group, which is an essential cofactor for many oxidative enzymes and is necessary for iron absorption and transfer [191].

Some studies suggest that ID may play a role in MS disease progression as MS patients display clinical improvement upon iron supplementation. However, other studies indicate improved disease outcome in iron-limited MS patients [11]. These contradictory results may be due to differences in nutritional, biochemical and sex-related factors between subjects, requiring further investigation.

5.2. Iron and Stroke

Both iron deficiency and excess have been associated with stroke risk. Previous studies have found that both increase the risk of venous thromboembolism and carotid atherosclerosis [192]. Higher iron status is protective against some forms of the atherosclerotic disease but increases the risk of thrombosis related to stasis and is associated with increased stroke risk, in particular, cardioembolic stroke [15]. Further investigation is required to determine the precise mechanism of these effects. As previously reported, iron is a prooxidant cofactor associated with increased production of ROS. In the animal model, a moderate IO markedly accelerated thrombus formation, impaired vasoreactivity, and enhanced the production of ROS and systemic markers of oxidative stress [193]. Furthermore, the administration of ROS scavenger completely abrogates the iron load-induced thrombus formation, thus confirming that the iron accelerates thrombosis through a prooxidant mechanism [194].

Over the last few years, the association of ID and thrombophilia has also been increasingly studied. Various kinds of thrombotic diseases including central retinal vein occlusion, cerebral venous sinus thrombosis and carotid artery thrombus were observed to be associated with an ID. In addition, numbers of cases of embolic and ischemic stroke have been reported to be associated with the ID [195].

An increased plasma Tf level is often seen in patients suffering from ID anemia [196]. Beside the role of binding and transporting the plasma iron, Tf is also an important clotting regulator and an adjuster in the maintenance of coagulation balance, which modifies the coagulation cascade. In atherosclerosis, abnormally upregulated Tf interact with and potentiate thrombin/FXIIa and blocks antithrombin's inactivation effect on coagulation proteases by binding to antithrombin, thus inducing hypercoagulability [197]. Furthermore, elevated Tf found in plasma or CSF of patients with ischemic stroke, ID anemia and venous thromboembolism interacts with clotting factors, suggesting that elevated Tf causes thromboembolic diseases [195]. Another consequence of ID that would be highly relevant to stroke pathogenesis is enhanced platelet aggregation. The platelet aggregation is enhanced as a response to serotonin (5 hydroxytryptophan, 5HT) in ID patients [198,199] because ID impairs the activity of the iron-containing platelet monoamine oxidase that metabolizes 5HT [200].

Gender plays an important role in the incidence of stroke. The overall incidence of stroke in men is estimated to be 33% higher than in women throughout most of the adulthood [201]. Findings from the prospective study in men from Kaluza et al., 2013 indicate that a high heme iron intake, particularly in normal-weight individuals, may increase the risk of stroke [202].

The epidemiology of stroke changes as women age and coincide with the loss of estrogen after menopause [18]. Furthermore, elderly women have more severe strokes, poorer recovery, and greater long-term disability [203], compared with men of the same age.

Estrogen is an immunomodulatory and neuroprotective agent with a suppressive action on inflammation [204]. It is known that postmenopausal women have higher levels of circulating TNF-α [205], which is involved in many neurodegenerative diseases [206].

Research evidence showed that TNF is beneficial in injury repair, but high levels of TNF can be neurotoxic [207]. Physiological levels of estrogen appear to attenuate TNF expression [208] while estrogen deficiency (as in postmenopausal period) represents a loss of this attenuation with a subsequent increase in TNF expression [18]. An increase of inflammatory agents in postmenopausal period could be associated with the higher hepcidin production and subsequent decrease in iron absorption, which could be an additional potential risk factor for ischemic stroke in women [205,209].

On the other hand, in the study from Miller [210], hormone replacement therapy was associated with lower iron stores in post-reproductive women in the absence of uterine blood loss, indicating potential homeostatic hormonal control of the iron status. Namely, higher serum iron in post-menopause has traditionally been attributed to reduced menstrual bleeding and lack of iron loss that women experience with menopause, in addition to estrogen deficiency [210]. With findings from studies on the levels of ferritin and sex hormones, it can be concluded that as women age, their serum levels of estrogen decrease, while serum ferritin levels increase [211]. This is probably due to an increase in the iron regulatory hormone hepcidin since elevated levels of estrogen usually reduce hepcidin synthesis [209], which regulates ferritin. Before the onset of menopause hepcidin levels in women are nearly 50% lower than in males of corresponding ages. After the menopause, hepcidin levels tend to be similar in both sexes [212,213] or slightly increased in men [214]. These results demonstrate a negative correlation between ferritin and estrogen levels during the menopausal transition period [215]. On the other hand, a synchronized pattern of changes in ferritin and testosterone levels was observed in men. Namely, as the men age, ferritin levels decrease gradually following »andropause« [216]. These results indicate that iron accumulation was a common process in aging women (but without the IO), which may account for the observed differences between genders in the incidence of the aging disorder, including the stroke [217].

Among older men with low testosterone levels, testosterone treatment can increase the serum iron levels and correct ID anemia [218]. Also, data are showing significant overlap between the testosterone administration and IO [219].

Furthermore, as the body is unable to eliminate excess iron, a negative feedback mechanism that allows iron to inhibit testosterone production to maintain body iron homeostasis is proposed [219]. The body iron stores can be regulated by testosterone, and vice versa, the testosterone may be reciprocally regulated by iron. Crosstalk between testosterone and iron has significant implications in testosterone deficiency and therapy. Additionally, the regulation of testosterone by iron may indicate a significant role of iron in the development of the hypogonadotropic hypogonadism in aging and chronic disease in men [219–221]. In a study from Jeppesen et al., 1996 both total and free testosterone were significantly inversely associated with stroke severity, and total testosterone was significantly inversely associated with infarct size [222]. Furthermore, a study from Zeller et al., 2018 suggested that low testosterone levels are associated with increased risk of future ischemic stroke in men [19]. The possible explanation lies in an increased level of hepcidin, which is inversely regulated by testosterone [223] and leads to ID anemia with greater susceptibility to stroke.

These data also suggest another mechanism regarding stroke pathogenesis, which includes initially increased serum iron level that negatively regulates testosterone level in men and promotes susceptibility to stroke. However, low testosterone level is probably not an independent risk factor for stroke, especially in older men. Low testosterone level is more likely to be found in overweight or obese, which is significantly associated with cardiovascular risk factors, such as diabetes, high blood pressure and high cholesterol. Namely, adipose tissue is able to control several functions of the testis through its products secreted in the bloodstream (e.g., leptin, adipocytokines), which have a negative impact on Leydig cell's function and testosterone secretion [224].

On the other hand, testosterone exerts a significant inhibitory effect on adipose tissue formation and the expression of various adipocytokines, such as leptin, TNF-α, IL-6, and IL-1, whereas a low testosterone level correlates with increased expression of markers of inflammation [225]. Furthermore, low chronic inflammation due to the excess adipose tissue upregulates hepcidin, which lowers the iron serum levels and its absorption [163,226], so eventually serum iron levels will decrease and subsequently lead to ID, present at the same time with the low testosterone level.

5.3. Iron and Parkinson's Disease

Dopaminergic neurons in the *substantia nigra* are highly vulnerable to stress conditions, compared to other neuronal types. Different factors seem to contribute to oxidative stress in PD, including IO, neuroinflammation and aging [14,206,227].

Several researches have documented an increase in total iron concentration in the *substantia nigra* in the most severe cases of PD, but no changes were found in milder cases [228,229]. Increased iron concentrations in the *substantia nigra* might result from mutations in genes important for iron transport and binding [230] or from peripheral iron influx through a damaged and discontinued BBB via the Permeability-glycoprotein [165]. Furthermore, the ability of the lysosome to participate in autophagy becomes slower with age, resulting in an increase of non-protein »garbage« within the cells, especially in age-related diseases like PD [227].

Accumulated iron increases protein aggregation via enhanced generation of ROS and oxidative stress [231]. As already mentioned, iron accumulation in the *substantia nigra* in PD patients was confirmed, but the studies on alteration of iron levels in blood and CFS reported inconsistent results. Blood levels of iron did not differ significantly between PD patients and the controls, but CSF iron levels tended to be lower in PD patients compared to the controls [232].

Increasing experimental and clinical evidence supports the idea that PD differs between women and men [21]. Although males exhibit greater susceptibility, most studies concentrate on the neuroprotective effects of estrogens in females. It was shown that men and women experience the disease differently, suggesting different mechanisms involved in the pathogenesis of the disease [21].

Although the sexual dimorphism in brain mitochondria has been proven [20], there are few recent studies that have dealt with other possible causes of sex-related differences. A recent neuromelanin imaging study found a larger neuromelanin-rich volume in the women *substantia nigra* compared with men older than 47 years, suggesting that this difference may be the underlying cause of the high male-to-female ratio of the PD prevalence [233]. Furthermore, experimental and epidemiological evidence suggest that estrogens play a regulatory role in brain iron metabolism [223,234]. The striatum of male mice showed greater susceptibility to iron accumulation than female [235]. A study conducted on humans showed that at the same serum iron concentrations, women had a lower probability of having PD [236]. Recently, several different pathways related to estrogen effects on iron metabolism in both sexes were found. GPER1 (G Protein-Coupled Estrogen Receptor 1) mediates the suppressive effects of estrogen on IO-induced autophagy in males, while estrogen receptor suppresses induced lipid peroxidation in females [237]. Furthermore, the results from the study of Xu and coworkers, showed that estrogen regulates differently the iron metabolism in astrocytes and neurons, i.e., increases the expression of iron exporter FPN1 and iron importer DMT1 by inducing HIF-1α in astrocytes, whereas decreased expression of IRP-1 may account for the decreased DMT1 and increased FPN1 expression in neurons [238].

Nutrition plays an important role in both neuroprotection and neurodegeneration, although there are many conflicting results. A recent epidemiological study found that intake of meat was inversely associated with PD risk in women [239]. Usually, the higher incidence of mortality, cardiovascular diseases, and diabetes is associated with higher meat consumption [240,241]. Furthermore, a positive correlation between red meat consumption and PD may be explained by the heme content that increases intracellular iron concentrations and subsequent ROS production, contributing to iron deposits and cell damage. In this context, iron intake from dietary nutrients may be related to a higher risk for PD [242]. However, blood donations, which can decrease systemic iron stores, do not lower the risk of PD [243]. On the other hand, conflicting results from Miyake et al., 2011 study showed that higher intake of iron could be associated with neuroprotection in PD [244].

In contrast to higher iron level content in the body, certain authors disagree about the implication of ID on the pathogenesis of PD [165]. ID anemia and low Hb have also been associated with PD i.e., with increased risk and disease severity [245]. Furthermore, it has been documented that PD patients exhibit lower ferritin, TIBC, and serum iron levels [245]. A positive correlation between anemia and PD was found in a recent large study of 86,334 newly diagnosed anemic patients. The study suggested that de novo anemic patients may develop PD 4 or more years after the initial diagnosis of anemia [246] and a higher risk for PD was independent of iron supplementation [247].

On the other hand, the meta-analysis from Mariani et al., 2013 showed that there is no difference in iron between PD patients and healthy controls [248].

Possible reasons for these discrepancies may be that the total amount and the serum iron in patients with PD did not change, but the distribution of iron changed [249], i.e., iron aggregated in the *substantia nigra*. Besides, this heterogeneity can manifest as highly variable iron metabolism due to sex-specific differences [250], which could lead to inconsistent results. However, epidemiological studies have not identified any sex-specific factors in the risk of developing PD among anemic patients.

We must take into account that besides the dysregulated iron metabolism, the presence of anemia in PD could also be an indicator of poor absorption of other nutrients [251].

5.4. Iron and Alzheimer's Disease

Alzheimer's disease is the most common cause of dementia characterized by short term memory loss and a progressive decline in cognitive and motor functions [165]. In neurodegenerative diseases including AD, where age is the major risk factor, iron dyshomeostasis coincides with neuroinflammation, abnormal protein aggregation, neurodegeneration, and neurobehavioral deficits. Disruption of iron homeostasis in the brain, both deficiency and overload, can affect neurophysiological mechanisms, cognition, and social behavior, which eventually contributes to the development of a diverse set of neuro-pathologies. Using MRI, it was found that the iron content in the brains of AD patients was significantly increased [252].

Whether the iron accumulation present in neurodegenerative diseases is a primary event or a secondary effect of the disease is unclear. However, it is for sure that aging is the major risk factor for age-related iron accumulation and neurodegeneration [13]. Iron seems to promote both deposition of amyloid-β protein and oxidative stress, which is associated with the plaques [7,253]. In contrast, some argued that, by binding iron, Aβ-protein might protect the surrounding neurons from oxidative stress [254].

Decreased antioxidant defenses and mitochondrial dysfunction present in elderly can allow the release of excessive iron [255]. This can cause pathological IO, resulting in cellular damage that is considered to be a contributing factor in neurodegenerative diseases more prevalent with aging, such as AD [165]. The results from recent studies showed that elevated ferritin in CSF was associated with poor cognitive function and probably can be used as a biomarker to measure the progression of mild cognitive impairment and early AD [256,257].

Brain iron increases with age and is abnormally elevated early in the disease [258]. Higher brain iron levels were associated with male gender and the presence of allelic variants in genes encoding for iron metabolism proteins (hemochromatosis H63D (HFE H63D) and transferrin C2 (TfC2)). This genotype effect was not observed in women, who had lower iron content in the brain than men [22,258]. The results showed worse verbal-memory performance associated with higher hippocampal iron deposition in men but not in women, independent of gene status. Furthermore, independent of gender, worse verbal working memory performance was associated with higher basal ganglia iron in the non-carrier for HFE H63D/TfC2 gene variant but not in the carrier. These results suggest that in healthy older individuals, increased deposits of iron in vulnerable gray matter regions may negatively impact memory functions and could represent a risk factor for faster cognitive decline [22].

Furthermore, it was shown in many in vivo and in vitro studies that iron metabolism is integrally involved in the regulation of glutamate metabolism and vice versa. The results from Burger et al., 2020, showed association between iron metabolism and glutamate concentration in female, suggesting stronger regulatory control between iron and glutamate metabolism than in men [259].

Aging is associated with a gradual decline in sex hormone levels in men and women, together with a deterioration in general health, mood, and cognitive abilities [260,261]. Sex hormones are also protective in keeping amyloid down, while depleted estrogen and testosterone levels result in a massive rise in this toxic protein in the brain [260,262].

Estrogens are considered as potent neuroprotectants and the best-studied in vitro and in vivo class of drugs for potential use in the prevention of AD [260]. In cell-free systems, estrogens inhibit iron-induced lipid peroxidation [263,264]. However, this effect was not found with testosterone [264].

In elderly, anemia or abnormal Hb concentrations are associated with higher morbidity and mortality, and with an increased risk for dementia and rapid cognitive decline [265].

The studies in elderly populations have confirmed that anemia and lower serum Hb were associated with a twofold increased risk for developing AD over approximately 3 years [266,267]. The findings from Carlson, et al. 2008 suggest a role of neonatal ID in dysregulation of genes that may set the stage for long-term AD and that this may occur through a histone modification mechanism [268].

It is important to have in mind that iron supplementation improves attention and concentration irrespective of baseline iron status [269]. However, as said before, excess of iron mediates the oxidative stress and causes neuronal disorders and neurodegeneration. In addition, it is thought that imbalance in iron homeostasis is a precursor to AD as well, thus it is strongly suggested that older people should be careful with diets excessive in iron.

6. Conclusions

Older age is associated with increased risk of ID, elevated body iron stores and increased brain iron levels [23]. Inadequate iron supply, which often accompanies aging, leads to cerebral hypoxia [138], insufficient neurotransmitter synthesis [13], impaired myelination [139], and consequently to poorer cognition, cognitive decline, and dementia [141]. On the other hand, brain iron accumulation is considered as a hallmark of aging [146] and it is associated with the progressive imbalance between antioxidant defenses and intracellular generation of ROS [147]. This increases susceptibility of aged brain to diseases and thus makes aging a major risk factor for neurodegenerative diseases development [14]. Therefore, it would be very important for the future research to determine the exact cellular and molecular mechanisms related to perturbations in iron metabolism in the aging brain to distinguish between physiological and pathological aging and find possible therapeutic targets for neurodegenerative diseases.

To counteract the ID during aging, one should certainly consider iron supplements recommended by a physician to correct the anemic state.

However, it should be noted how this supplementation may not be warranted for healthy elderly people consuming a balanced diet. In contrary, it could be detrimental for those who are homozygous or heterozygous for the HFE mutations, since recent studies showed that even moderate increases in body iron may increase the risk for body disorders including neurological ones [270], or cause irreparable damage to the brain neurons [137,271]. Because of that, older people should be careful consuming a high-iron content diet as well.

The major unknown is still the sex-related differences in iron metabolism that come with aging. Increasing experimental and clinical evidence support the idea that neurological disorders differ between women and men, suggesting the existence of different underlying mechanisms involved in their pathogenesis [16–22]. However, we are still far away from the actual understanding of what underlies these differences. We need a better understanding of the underlying mechanisms of how sex hormones can influence the iron metabolism and further, the development of neurological disorders. New insights into aging processes, which include the impact of sex hormones on iron metabolism as well, could enlighten the understanding of these differences during aging.

Author Contributions: Both authors contributed equally to the conception of the review, to the interpretation of data, and to the writing of the manuscript. All authors have read and agreed to the published version of the manuscript.

Funding: This work has been funded by the University of Rijeka (grant number: uniri-biomed-18-41).

Conflicts of Interest: The authors declare no conflict of interest.

References

1. Munoz, M.; Villar, I.; Garcia-Erce, J.A. An Update on Iron Physiology. *World J. Gastroenterol.* **2009**, *15*, 4617–4626. [CrossRef] [PubMed]
2. Darshan, D.; Frazer, D.M.; Anderson, G.J. Molecular Basis of Iron-Loading Disorders. *Expert Rev. Mol. Med.* **2010**, *12*, e36. [CrossRef] [PubMed]
3. Sheftel, A.; Stehling, O.; Lill, R. Iron-Sulfur Proteins in Health and Disease. *Trends Endocrinol. Metab.* **2010**, *21*, 302–313. [CrossRef] [PubMed]
4. Chen, C.; Paw, B.H. Cellular and Mitochondrial Iron Homeostasis in Vertebrates. *Biochim. Biophys. Acta* **2012**, *1823*, 1459–1467. [CrossRef]
5. Siah, C.W.; Ombiga, J.; Adams, L.A.; Trinder, D.; Olynyk, J.K. Normal Iron Metabolism and the Pathophysiology of Iron Overload Disorders. *Clin. Biochem. Rev.* **2006**, *27*, 5–16.
6. Gammella, E.; Recalcati, S.; Cairo, G. Dual Role of ROS as Signal and Stress Agents: Iron Tips the Balance in Favor of Toxic Effects. *Oxid. Med. Cell. Longev.* **2016**, *2016*, 8629024. [CrossRef]
7. Zhao, Z. Iron and Oxidizing Species in Oxidative Stress and Alzheimer's Disease. *Aging Med.* **2019**, *2*, 82–87. [CrossRef]
8. Hentze, M.W.; Muckenthaler, M.U.; Galy, B.; Camaschella, C. Two to Tango: Regulation of Mammalian Iron Metabolism. *Cell* **2010**, *142*, 24–38. [CrossRef]
9. Ye, H.; Rouault, T.A. Human Iron-Sulfur Cluster Assembly, Cellular Iron Homeostasis, and Disease. *Biochemistry* **2010**, *49*, 4945–4956. [CrossRef]
10. Musallam, K.M.; Taher, A.T. Iron Deficiency Beyond Erythropoiesis: Should We Be Concerned? *Curr. Med. Res. Opin.* **2018**, *34*, 81–93. [CrossRef]
11. Van Rensburg, S.J.; Kotze, M.J.; van Toorn, R. The Conundrum of Iron in Multiple Sclerosis—Time for an Individualised Approach. *Metab. Brain Dis.* **2012**, *27*, 239–253. [CrossRef] [PubMed]
12. Fernandez-Real, J.M.; Manco, M. Effects of Iron Overload on Chronic Metabolic Diseases. *Lancet Diabetes Endocrinol.* **2014**, *2*, 513–526. [CrossRef]
13. Ward, R.J.; Zucca, F.A.; Duyn, J.H.; Crichton, R.R.; Zecca, L. The Role of Iron in Brain Ageing and Neurodegenerative Disorders. *Lancet Neurol.* **2014**, *13*, 1045–1060. [CrossRef]
14. Ashraf, A.; Clark, M.; So, P.-W. The Aging of Iron Man. *Front. Aging Neurosci.* **2018**, *10*, 65. [CrossRef] [PubMed]
15. Gill, D.; Monori, G.; Tzoulaki, I.; Dehghan, A. Iron Status and Risk of Stroke. A Mendelian Randomization Study. *Stroke* **2018**, *49*, 2815–2821. [CrossRef]

16. Ćurko-Cofek, B.; Grubić Kezele, T.; Marinić, J.; Tota, M.; Starčević Čizmarević, N.; Milin, Č.; Ristić, S.; Radošević-Stašić, B.; Barac-Latas, V. Chronic Iron Overload Induces Gender-Dependent Changes in Iron Homeostasis, Lipid Peroxidation and Clinical Course of Experimental Autoimmune Encephalomyelitis. *Neurotoxicology* **2016**, *27*, 1–12. [CrossRef]
17. Persson, N.; Wu, J.; Zhang, Q.; Liu, T.; Shen, J.; Bao, R.; Ni, M.; Liu, T.; Wang, Y.; Spincemaille, P. Age and Sex Related Differences in Subcortical Brain Iron Concentrations Among Healthy Adults. *Neuroimage* **2015**, *122*, 385–398. [CrossRef]
18. Koellhoffer, E.C.; McCullough, L.D. The Effects of Estrogen in Ischemic Stroke. *Transl. Stroke Res.* **2013**, *4*, 390–401. [CrossRef]
19. Zeller, T.; Schnabel, R.B.; Appelbaum, S.; Ojeda, F.; Berisha, F.; Schulte-Steinberg, B.; Brueckmann, B.E.; Kuulasmaa, K.; Jousilahti, P.; Blankenberg, S.; et al. Low Testosterone Levels Are Predictive for Incident Atrial Fibrillation and Ischaemic Stroke in Men, but Protective in Women—Results from the FINRISK Study. *Eur. J. Prev. Cardiol.* **2018**, *25*, 1133–1139. [CrossRef]
20. Khalifa, A.R.M.; Abdel-Rahman, E.A.; Mahmoud, A.M.; Ali, M.H.; Noureldin, M.; Saber, S.H.; Mohsen, M.; Ali, S.S. Sex-Specific Differences in Mitochondria Biogenesis, Morphology, Respiratory Function, and ROS Homeostasis in Young Mouse Heart and Brain. *Physiol. Rep.* **2017**, *5*, e13125. [CrossRef]
21. Jurado-Coronel, J.C.; Cabezas, R.; Rodríguez, M.F.A.; Echeverria, V.; García-Segura, L.M.; Barreto, G.E. Sex Differences in Parkinson's Disease: Features on Clinical Symptoms, Treatment Outcome, Sexual Hormones and Genetics. *Front. Neuroendocrinol.* **2018**, *50*, 18–30. [CrossRef] [PubMed]
22. Bartzokis, G.; Lu, P.H.; Tingus, K.; Peters, D.G.; Amar, C.P.; Tishler, T.A.; Finn, J.P.; Villablanca, P.; Altshuler, L.L.; Mintz, J. Gender and Iron Genes may Modify Associations Between Brain Iron and Memory in Healthy Aging. *Neuropsychopharmacology* **2011**, *36*, 1375–1384. [CrossRef] [PubMed]
23. Fairweather-Tait, S.J.; Wawer, A.A.; Gillings, R.; Jennings, A.; Myint, P.K. Iron Status in the Elderly. *Mech. Ageing Dev.* **2014**, *136*, 22–28. [CrossRef] [PubMed]
24. Belaidi, A.A.; Bush, A.I. Iron Neurochemistry in Alzheimer's Disease and Parkinson's Disease: Targets for Therapeutics. *J. Neurochem.* **2016**, *139*, 179–197. [CrossRef]
25. Camaschella, C.; Nai, A.; Silvestri, L. Iron Metabolism and Iron Disorders Revisited in the Hepcidin Era. *Haematologica* **2020**, *105*, 260–272. [CrossRef]
26. Miret, S.; Simpson, R.J.; McKie, A.T. Physiology and Molecular Biology of Dietary Iron Absorption. *Annu. Rev. Nutr.* **2003**, *23*, 283–301. [CrossRef]
27. Fuqua, B.K.; Vulpe, C.D.; Anderson, G.J. Intestinal Iron Absorption. *J. Trace Elem. Med. Biol.* **2012**, *26*, 115–119. [CrossRef]
28. Lane, D.J.R.; Richardson, D.R. The Active Role of Vitamin C in Mammalian Iron Metabolism: Much More than just Enhanced Iron Absorption! *Free Radic. Biol. Med.* **2014**, *75*, 69–83. [CrossRef]
29. McKie, A.T.; Barrow, D.; Latunde-Dada, G.O.; Rolfs, A.; Sager, G.; Mudaly, M.; Richardson, C.; Barlow, D.; Bomford, A.; Peters, T.J.; et al. An Iron-Regulated Ferric Reductase Associated with the Absorption of Dietary Iron. *Science* **2001**, *291*, 1755–1759. [CrossRef]
30. Ems, T.; St Lucia, K.; Huecker, M.R. Biochemistry, Iron Absorption. In: StatPearls [Internet]. (Updated 30 April 2020). Available online: http://www.ncbi.nlm.nih.gov/books/NBK448204/ (accessed on 15 May 2020).
31. Fleming, R.E.; Bacon, B.R. Orchestration of Iron Homeostasis. *N. Engl. J. Med.* **2005**, *352*, 1741–1744. [CrossRef]
32. Duck, K.A.; Connor, J.R. Iron Uptake and Transport Across Physiological Barriers. *Biometals* **2016**, *29*, 573–591. [CrossRef] [PubMed]
33. Abboud, S.; Haile, D.J. A Novel Mammalian Iron-Regulated Protein Involved in Intracellular Iron Metabolism. *J. Biol. Chem.* **2000**, *275*, 19906–19912. [CrossRef]
34. Bogdan, A.R.; Miyazawa, M.; Hashimoto, K.; Tsuji, Y. Regulators of Iron Homeostasis: New Players in Metabolism, Cell Death, and Disease. *Trends Biochem. Sci.* **2016**, *41*, 274–286. [CrossRef] [PubMed]
35. Donovan, A.; Lima, C.A.; Pinkus, J.L.; Pinkus, G.S.; Zon, L.I.; Robine, S.; Andrews, N.C. The Iron Exporter Ferroportin/Slc40a1 Is Essential for Iron Homeostasis. *Cell Metab.* **2005**, *1*, 191–200. [CrossRef] [PubMed]
36. De Domenico, I.; Ward, D.M.; Bonaccorsi di Patti, M.C.; Jeong, S.Y.; David, S.; Musci, G.; Kaplan, J. Ferroxidase Activity Is Required for the Stability of Cell Surface Ferroportin in Cells Expressing GPI-ceruloplasmin. *EMBO J.* **2007**, *26*, 2823–2831. [CrossRef]

37. Vulpe, C.D.; Kuo, Y.M.; Murphy, T.L.; Cowley, L.; Askwith, C.; Libina, N.; Gitschier, J.; Anderson, G.J. Hephaestin, a Ceruloplasmin Homologue Implicated in Intestinal Iron Transport, Is Defective in the SLA Mouse. *Nat. Genet.* **1999**, *21*, 195–199. [CrossRef]
38. Coffey, R.; Ganz, T. Iron Homeostasis: An Anthropocentric Perspective. *J. Biol. Chem.* **2017**, *292*, 12727–12734. [CrossRef]
39. Gunshin, H.; Fujiwara, Y.; Custodio, A.O.; Direnzo, C.; Robine, S.; Andrews, N.C. Slc11a2 Is Required for Intestinal Iron Absorption and Erythropoiesis but Dispensable in Placenta and Liver. *J. Clin. Investig.* **2005**, *115*, 1258–1266. [CrossRef]
40. Liuzzi, J.P.; Aydemir, F.; Nam, H.; Knutson, M.D.; Cousins, R.J. Zip14 (Slc39a14) Mediates Non-Transferrin-Bound Iron Uptake into Cells. *Proc. Natl. Acad. Sci. USA* **2006**, *103*, 13612–13617. [CrossRef]
41. Krishnamurthy, P.; Xie, T.; Schuetz, J.D. The Role of Transporters in Cellular Heme and Porphyrin Homeostasis. *Pharmacol. Ther.* **2007**, *114*, 345–358. [CrossRef]
42. Le Blanc, S.; Garrick, M.D.; Arredondo, M. Heme Carrier Protein 1 Transports Heme and Is Involved in Heme-Fe Metabolism. *Am. J. Physiol. Cell Physiol.* **2012**, *302*, C1780–C1785. [CrossRef] [PubMed]
43. Muckenthaler, M.U.; Rivella, S.; Hentze, M.W.; Galy, B. A Red Carpet for Iron Metabolism. *Cell* **2017**, *168*, 344–361. [CrossRef] [PubMed]
44. Crichton, R.R.; Danielsson, B.G.; Geisser, P. *Iron Therapy with Special Emphasis on Intravenous Administration*, 4th ed.; Crichton, R.R., Danielsson, B.G., Geisser, P., Eds.; UNI-MED Verlag AG: Bremen, Germany, 2008; pp. 14–24.
45. Peyrin-Biroulet, L.; Williet, N.; Cacoub, P. Guidelines on the Diagnosis and Treatment of Iron Deficiency Across Indications: A Systematic Review. *Am. J. Clin. Nutr.* **2015**, *102*, 1585–1594. [CrossRef] [PubMed]
46. Kawabata, H. Transferrin and Transferrin Receptors Update. *Free Radic. Biol. Med.* **2019**, *133*, 46–54. [CrossRef]
47. Lambert, L.A.; Mitchell, S.L. Molecular Evolution of the Transferrin Receptor/Glu-tamate Carboxypeptidase II Family. *J. Mol. Evol.* **2007**, *64*, 113–128. [CrossRef] [PubMed]
48. Ohgami, R.S.; Campagna, D.R.; Greer, E.L.; Antiochos, B.; McDonald, A.; Chen, J.; Sharp, J.J.; Fujiwara, Y.; Barker, J.E.; Fleming, M.D. Identification of a Ferrireductase Required for Efficien Ttransferrin-Dependent Iron Uptake in Erythroid Cells. *Nat. Genet.* **2005**, *37*, 1264–1269. [CrossRef]
49. Rishi, G.; Subramaniam, V.N. The Liver in Regulation of Iron Homeostasis. *Am. J. Physiol. Gastrointest. Liver Physiol.* **2017**, *313*, G157–G165. [CrossRef]
50. Xu, M.M.; Wang, J.; Xie, J.X. Regulation of Iron Metabolism by Hypoxia-Inducible Factors. *Sheng Li Xue Bao* **2017**, *69*, 598–610.
51. Rouault, T.A. The Role of Iron Regulatory Proteins in Mammalian Iron Homeostasis and Disease. *Nat. Chem. Biol.* **2006**, *2*, 406–414. [CrossRef]
52. Yikilmaz, E.; Rouault, T.A.; Schuck, P. Self-Association and Ligand-Induced Conformational Changes of Iron Regulatory Proteins 1 and 2. *Biochemistry* **2005**, *44*, 8470–8478. [CrossRef]
53. Iwai, K.; Drake, S.K.; Wehr, N.B.; Weissman, A.M.; LaVaute, T.; Minato, N.; Klausner, R.D.; Levine, R.L.; Rouault, T.A. Iron-Dependent Oxidation, Ubiquitination, and Degradation of Iron Regulatory Protein 2: Implications for Degradation of Oxidized Proteins. *Proc. Natl. Acad. Sci. USA* **1998**, *95*, 4924–4928. [CrossRef] [PubMed]
54. Vashisht, A.A.; Zumbrennen, K.B.; Huang, X.; Powers, D.N.; Durazo, A.; Sun, D.; Bhaskaran, N.; Persson, A.; Uhlen, M.; Sangfelt, O.; et al. Control of Iron Homeostasis by an Iron-Regulated Ubiquitin Ligase. *Science* **2009**, *326*, 718–721. [CrossRef] [PubMed]
55. Worthen, C.A.; Enns, C.A. The Role of Hepatic Transferrin Receptor 2 in the Regulation of Iron Homeostasis in the Body. *Front. Pharmacol.* **2014**, *5*, 34. [CrossRef] [PubMed]
56. West, A.P.; Bennett, M.J.; Sellers, V.M.; Andrews, N.C.; Enns, C.A.; Bjorkman, P.J. Comparison of the Interactions of Transferrin Receptor And transferrin Receptor 2 with Transferrin and the Hereditary Hemochromatosis Protein HFE. *J. Biol. Chem.* **2000**, *275*, 38135–38138. [CrossRef] [PubMed]
57. Graham, R.M.; Reutens, G.M.; Herbison, C.E.; Delima, R.D.; Chua, A.C.; Olynyk, J.K.; Trinder, D. Transferrin Receptor 2 Mediates Uptake of Transferrin-Bound and Non-Transferrin-Bound Iron. *J. Hepatol.* **2008**, *48*, 327–334. [CrossRef]
58. Anderson, E.R.; Shah, Y.M. Iron Homeostasis in the Liver. *Compr. Physiol.* **2013**, *3*, 315–330. [CrossRef]

59. Leidgens, S.; Bullough, K.Z.; Shi, H.; Li, F.; Shakoury-Elizeh, M.; Yabe, T.; Subramanian, P.; Hsu, E.; Natarajan, N.; Nandal, A.; et al. Each Member of the Poly-r(C)-binding Protein 1 (PCBP) Family Exhibits Iron Chaperone Activity toward Ferritin. *J. Biol. Chem.* **2013**, *288*, 17791–17802. [CrossRef]
60. Bondi, A.; Valentino, P.; Daraio, F.; Porporato, P.; Gramaglia, E.; Canturan, S.; Gottardi, E.; Camaschella, C.; Roetto, A. Hepatic Expression of Hemochromatosis Genes in Two Mouse Strains After Phleotomy and Iron Overload. *Haematologica* **2005**, *90*, 1161–1167.
61. Theil, E.C. Ferritin Protein Nanocages-The Story. *Nanotechnol. Percept.* **2012**, *8*, 7–16. [CrossRef]
62. Torti, F.M.; Torti, S.V. Regulation of Ferritin Genes and Protein. *Blood* **2002**, *99*, 3505–3516. [CrossRef]
63. Waldvogel-Abramowski, S.; Waeber, G.; Gassner, C.; Buser, A.; Frey, B.M.; Favrat, B.; Tissot, J.-D. Physiology of Iron Metabolism. *Transfus. Med. Hemother.* **2014**, *41*, 213–221. [CrossRef] [PubMed]
64. Theil, E.C. Ferritin: The Protein Nanocage and Iron Biomineral in Health and in Disease. *Inorg. Chem.* **2013**, *52*, 12223–12233. [CrossRef] [PubMed]
65. Anderson, G.J.; Frazer, D.M. Current Understanding of Iron Homeostasis. *Am. J. Clin. Nutr.* **2017**, *106*, 1559S–1566S. [CrossRef] [PubMed]
66. Langlois d'Estaintot, B.; Santambrogio, P.; Granier, T.; Gallois, B.; Chevalier, J.M.; Precigoux, G.; Levi, S.; Arosio, P. Crystal Structure and Biochemical Properties of the Human Mitochondrial Ferritin and its Mutant Ser144Ala. *J. Mol. Biol.* **2004**, *340*, 277–293. [CrossRef]
67. Ward, D.M.; Cloonan, S.M. Mitochondrial Iron in Human Health and Disease. *Annu. Rev. Physiol.* **2019**, *81*, 453–482. [CrossRef]
68. Finazzi, D.; Arosio, P. Biology of Ferritin in Mammals: An Update on Iron Storage, Oxidative Damage and Neurodegeneration. *Arch. Toxicol.* **2014**, *88*, 1787–1802. [CrossRef]
69. Hentze, M.W.; Muckenthaler, M.U.; Andrews, N.C. Balancing Acts: Molecular Control of Mammalian Iron. *Cell* **2004**, *117*, 285–297. [CrossRef]
70. Ganz, T. Macrophages and Systemic Iron Homeostasis. *J. Innate Immun.* **2012**, *4*, 446–453. [CrossRef]
71. Sukhbaatar, N.; Weichhart, T. Iron Regulation: Macrophages in Control. *Pharmaceuticals* **2018**, *11*, 137. [CrossRef]
72. Kong, W.N.; Zhao, S.E.; Duan, X.L.; Yang, Z.; Qian, Z.M.; Chang, Y.Z. Decreased DMT1 and Increased Ferroportin 1 Expression Is the Mechanisms of Reduced Iron Retention in Macrophages by Erythropoietin in Rats. *J. Cell. Biochem.* **2008**, *104*, 629–641. [CrossRef]
73. Singh, A.K. Erythropoiesis: The Roles of Erythropoietin and Iron. In *Textbook of Nephro-Endocrinology*, 2nd ed.; Singh, A.K., Williams, G.H., Eds.; Academic Press: Bucharest, Romania, 2017; Volume 13, pp. 207–215.
74. Zhang, D.L.; Ghosh, M.C.; Rouault, T.A. The Physiological Functions of Iron Regulatory Proteins in Iron Homeostasis—An Update. *Front. Pharmacol.* **2014**, *5*, 124. [CrossRef] [PubMed]
75. Ganz, T.; Nemeth, E. Hepcidin and Iron Homeostasis. *Biochim. Biophys. Acta* **2012**, *1823*, 1434–1443. [CrossRef] [PubMed]
76. Shah, Y.M.; Matsubara, T.; Ito, S.; Yim, S.H.; Gonzales, E.J. Intestinal Hypoxia-Inducible Transcription Factors are Essential for Iron Absorption Following Iron Deficiency. *Cell Metab.* **2009**, *9*, 152–164. [CrossRef] [PubMed]
77. Agarwal, A.K.; Yee, J. Hepcidin. *Adv. Chronic Kidney Dis.* **2019**, *26*, 298–305. [CrossRef]
78. Rochette, R.; Gudjoncik, A.; Guenancia, C.; Zeller, M.; Cottin, Y.; Vergely, C. The Iron-Regulator Hormone Hepcidin: A Possible Therapeutic Target? *Pharmacol. Ther.* **2015**, *146*, 35–52. [CrossRef]
79. Canali, S.; Zumbrennen-Bullough, K.B.; Core, A.B.; Wang, C.-Y.; Nairz, M.; Bouley, R.; Swirski, F.K.; Babitt, J.L. Endothelial Cells Produce Bone Morphogenetic Protein 6 Required for Iron Homeostasis in Mice. *Blood* **2017**, *129*, 405–414. [CrossRef]
80. Liu, X.B.; Nguyen, N.B.; Marquess, K.D.; Yang, F.; Haile, D.J. Regulation of Hepcidin and Ferroportin Expression by Lipopolysaccharide in Splenic Macrophages. *Blood Cells Mol. Dis.* **2005**, *35*, 47–56. [CrossRef]
81. Bekri, S.; Gual, P.; Anty, R.; Luciani, N.; Dahman, M.; Ramesh, B.; Iannelli, A.; Staccini-Myx, A.; Casanova, D.; Amor, I.B.; et al. Increased Adipose Tissue Expression of Hepcidin in Severe Obesity Is Independent from Diabetes and NASH. *Gastroenterology* **2006**, *131*, 788–796. [CrossRef]
82. Darshan, D.; Anderson, G.J. Interacting Signals in the Control of Hepcidin Expression. *BioMetals* **2009**, *22*, 77–87. [CrossRef]

83. Nicolas, G.; Chauvet, C.; Viatte, L.; Danan, J.L.; Bigard, X.; Devaux, I.; Beaumont, C.; Kahn, A.; Vaulont, S. The Gene Encoding the Iron Regulatory Peptide Hepcidin Is Regulated by Anemia, Hypoxia, and Inflammation. *J. Clin. Investig.* **2002**, *110*, 1037–1044. [CrossRef]
84. Rishi, G.; Wallace, D.F.; Subramaniam, V.N. Hepcidin: Regulation of the Master Iron Regulator. *Biosci. Rep.* **2015**, *35*, e00192. [CrossRef] [PubMed]
85. Babitt, J.L.; Huang, F.W.; Wrighting, D.M.; Xia, Y.; Sidis, Y.; Samad, T.A.; Campagna, J.A.; Chung, R.T.; Schneyer, A.L.; Woolf, C.J.; et al. Bone Morphogenetic Protein Signaling by Hemojuvelin Regulates Hepcidin Expression. *Nat. Genet.* **2006**, *38*, 531–539. [CrossRef] [PubMed]
86. Galaris, D.; Barbouti, A.; Pantopoulos, K. Iron Homeostasisand Oxidative Stress: An Intimate Relationship. *Biochim. Biophys. Acta Mol. Cell Res.* **2019**, *1866*, 118535. [CrossRef] [PubMed]
87. Zhao, N.; Maxson, J.E.; Zhang, R.H.; Wahedi, M.; Enns, C.A.; Zhang, A.-S. Neogenin Facilitates the Induction of Hepcidin Expression by Hemojuvelin in the Liver. *J. Biol. Chem.* **2016**, *291*, 12322–12335. [CrossRef]
88. Wu, H.; Yung, L.M.; Cheng, W.H.; Yu, P.B.; Babitt, J.L.; Lin, H.Y.; Xia, Y. Hepcidin Regulation by BMP Signaling in Macrophages Is Lipopolysaccharide Dependent. *PLoS ONE* **2012**, *7*, e44622. [CrossRef]
89. Tangudu, N.K.; Vujić Spasić, M. Heme Activates Macrophage Hepcidin Expression via Toll like Receptor 4 and Extracellular Signal-Regulated Kinases Signaling Pathway. *Clin. Pharmacol. Biopharm.* **2017**, *6*, 166. [CrossRef]
90. Barton, J.C.; Edwards, C.Q.; Acton, R.T. HFE Gene: Structure, Function, Mutations, and Associated Iron Abnormalities. *Gene* **2015**, *574*, 179–192. [CrossRef]
91. Lebron, J.A.; Bennett, M.J.; Vaughn, D.E.; Chirino, A.J.; Snow, P.M.; Mintier, G.A.; Feder, J.N.; Bjorkman, P.J. Crystal Structure of the Hemochromatosis Protein HFE and Characterization of its Interaction with Transferrin Receptor. *Cell* **1998**, *93*, 111–123. [CrossRef]
92. Camaschella, C.; Silvestri, L. New and Old Players in the Hepcidin Pathway. *Haematologica* **2008**, *93*, 1441–1444. [CrossRef]
93. Pagani, A.; Nai, A.; Silvestri, L.; Camaschella, C. Hepcidin and Anemia: A Tight Relationship. *Front. Physiol.* **2019**, *10*, 1294. [CrossRef]
94. Nemeth, E.; Tuttle, M.S.; Powelson, J.; Vaughn, M.B.; Donovan, A.; McVey Ward, D.; Ganz, T.; Kaplan, J. Hepcidin Regulates Cellular Iron Efflux by Binding to Ferroportin and Inducing Its Internalization. *Science* **2004**, *306*, 2090–2093. [CrossRef] [PubMed]
95. Nemeth, E.; Rivera, S.; Gabayan, V.; Keller, C.; Taudorf, S.; Pedersen, B.K.; Ganz, T. IL-6 Mediates Hypoferremia of Inflammation by Inducing the Synthesis of the Iron Regulatory Hormone Hepcidin. *J. Clin. Investig.* **2004**, *113*, 1271–1276. [CrossRef]
96. Verga Falzacappa, M.V.; Vujic Spasic, M.; Kessler, R.; Stolte, J.; Hentze, M.W.; Muckenthaler, M.U. STAT3 Mediates Hepatic Hepcidin Expression and Its Inflammatory Stimulation. *Blood* **2007**, *109*, 353–358. [CrossRef] [PubMed]
97. Magistretti, P.J.; Allaman, I. A Cellular Perspective on Brain Energy Metabolism and Functional Imaging. *Neuron* **2015**, *86*, 883–901. [CrossRef] [PubMed]
98. Salvador, G.A. Iron in Neuronal Function and Dysfunction. *Biofactors* **2010**, *36*, 103–110. [CrossRef]
99. Moos, T.; Nielsen, T.R.; Skjørringe, T.; Morgan, E.H. Iron Trafficking Inside the Brain. *J. Neurochem.* **2007**, *103*, 1730–1740. [CrossRef]
100. McCarthy, R.C.; Kosman, D.J. Iron Transport Across the Blood-Brain Barrier: Development, Neurovascular Regulation and Cerebral Amyloid Angiopathy. *Cell. Mol. Life Sci.* **2015**, *72*, 709–727. [CrossRef]
101. Moos, T.; Morgan, E.H. Transferrin and Transferrin Receptor Function in Brain Barrier Systems. *Cell. Mol. Neurobiol.* **2000**, *20*, 77–95. [CrossRef]
102. Montagne, A.; Zhao, Z.; Zlokovic, B.V. Alzheimer's Disease: A Matter of Blood-Brain Barrier Dysfunction? *J. Exp. Med.* **2017**, *214*, 3151–3169. [CrossRef]
103. Zhao, Z.; Nelson, A.R.; Betsholtz, C.; Zlokovic, B.V. Establishment and Dysfunction of the Blood-Brain Barrier. *Cell* **2015**, *163*, 1064–1078. [CrossRef]
104. Sweeney, M.D.; Zhao, Z.; Montagne, A.; Nelson, A.R.; Zlokovic, B.V. Blood-Brain Barrier: From Physiology to Disease and Back. *Physiol. Rev.* **2019**, *99*, 21–78. [CrossRef] [PubMed]
105. Zlokovic, B.V. Neurovascular Pathways to Neurodegeneration in Alzheimer's Disease and Other Disorders. *Nat. Rev. Neurosci.* **2011**, *12*, 723–738. [CrossRef] [PubMed]

106. Iadecola, C. The Neurovascular Unit Coming of Age: A Journey Through Neurovascular Coupling in Health and Disease. *Neuron* **2017**, *96*, 17–42. [CrossRef] [PubMed]
107. Ke, Y.; Qian, Z.M. Brain Iron Metabolism: Neurobiology and Neurochemistry. *Prog. Neurobiol.* **2007**, *83*, 149–173. [CrossRef] [PubMed]
108. Simpson, I.A.; Ponnuru, P.; Klinger, M.E.; Myers, R.L.; Devraj, K.; Coe, C.L.; Lubach, G.R.; Carruthers, A.; Connor, J.R. A Novel Model for Brain Iron Uptake: Introducing the Concept of Regulation. *J. Cereb. Blood Flow Metab.* **2015**, *35*, 48–57. [CrossRef]
109. Khan, A.I.; Liu, J.; Dutta, P. Iron Transport Kinetics Through Blood-Brain Barrier Endothelial Cells. *Biochim. Biophys. Acta* **2018**, *1862*, 1168–1179. [CrossRef]
110. Rouault, T.A.; Cooperman, S. Brain Iron Metabolism. *Semin. Pediatr. Neurol.* **2006**, *13*, 142–148. [CrossRef]
111. De Domenico, I.; McVey Ward, D.; Kaplan, J. Regulation of Iron Acquisition and Storage: Consequences for Iron-Linked Disorders. *Nat. Rev. Mol. Cell Biol.* **2008**, *9*, 72–81. [CrossRef]
112. Benarroch, E.E. Brain Iron Homeostasis and Neurodegenerative Disease. *Neurology* **2009**, *72*, 1436–1440. [CrossRef]
113. Burkhart, A.; Skjørringe, T.; Johnsen, K.B.; Siupka, P.; Thomsen, L.B.; Nielsen, M.S.; Thomsen, L.L.; Moos, T. Expression of Iron-Related Proteins at the Neurovascular Unit Supports Reduction and Reoxidation of Iron for Transport Through the Blood-Brain Barrier. *Mol. Neurobiol.* **2016**, *53*, 7237–7253. [CrossRef]
114. Zecca, L.; Stroppolo, A.; Gatti, A.; Tampellini, D.; Toscani, M.; Gallorini, M.; Giaveri, G.; Arosio, P.; Santambrogio, P.; Fariello, R.G.; et al. The Role of Iron and Copper Molecules in the Neuronal Vulnerability of Locus Coeruleus and Substantia Nigra during Aging. *Proc. Natl. Acad. Sci. USA* **2004**, *101*, 9843–9848. [CrossRef] [PubMed]
115. Horowitz, M.P.; Greenamyre, J.T. Mitochondrial Iron Metabolism and Its Role in Neurodegeneration. *J. Alzheimers Dis.* **2010**, *20*, S551–S568. [CrossRef] [PubMed]
116. Wu, L.J.; Leenders, A.G.; Cooperman, S.; Meyron-Holtz, E.; Smith, S.; Land, W.; Tsai, R.Y.; Berger, U.V.; Sheng, Z.H.; Rouault, T.A. Expression of the Iron Transporter Ferroportin in Synaptic Vesicles and the Blood–Brain Barrier. *Brain Res.* **2004**, *1001*, 108–117. [CrossRef] [PubMed]
117. Qian, Z.M.; Chang, Y.Z.; Du, J.R.; Ho, K.P.; Zhu, L.; Xu, Y.J.; Li, L.Z.; Wang, C.Y.; Wang, Q.; Ge, X.H.; et al. Development and Iron-Dependent Expression of Hephaestin in Different Brain Regions of Rats. *J. Cell. Biochem.* **2007**, *102*, 1225–1233. [CrossRef] [PubMed]
118. De Arriba Zerpa, G.A.; Saleh, M.C.; Fernandez, P.M.; Guillou, F.; Espinosa de los Monteros, A.; De Vellis, J.; Zakin, M.M.; Baron, B. Alternative Splicing Prevents Transferrin Secretion During Differentiation of a Human Oligodendrocyte Cell Line. *J. Neurosci. Res.* **2000**, *61*, 388–395. [CrossRef]
119. Singh, N.; Haldar, S.; Tripathi, A.K.; Horback, K.; Wong, J.; Sharma, D.; Beserra, A.; Suda, S.; Anbalagan, C.; Dev, S.; et al. Brain Iron Homeostasis: From Molecular Mechanisms to Clinical Significance and Therapeutic Opportunities. *Antioxid. Redox Signal.* **2014**, *20*, 1324–1363. [CrossRef]
120. Nnah, I.C.; Wessling-Resnick, M. Brain Iron Homeostasis: A Focus on Microglial Iron. *Pharmaceuticals* **2018**, *11*, 129. [CrossRef]
121. Rouault, T.A.; Zhang, D.L.; Jeong, S.Y. Brain Iron Homeostasis, the Choroid Plexus, and Localization of Iron Transport Proteins. *Metab. Brain Dis.* **2009**, *24*, 673–684. [CrossRef]
122. Brown, P.D.; Davies, S.L.; Speake, T.; Millar, I.D. Molecular Mechanisms of Cerebrospinal Fluid Production. *Neuroscience* **2004**, *129*, 957–970. [CrossRef]
123. Leitner, D.F.; Connor, J.R. Functional Roles of Transferrin in the Brain. *Biochim. Biophys. Acta* **2012**, *1820*, 393–402. [CrossRef]
124. Burdo, J.R.; Menzies, S.L.; Simpson, I.A.; Garrick, L.M.; Garrick, M.D.; Dolan, K.G.; Haile, D.J.; Beard, J.L.; Connor, J.R. Distribution of Divalent Metal Transporter 1 and Metal Transport Protein 1 in the Normal and Belgrade Rat. *J. Neurosci. Res.* **2001**, *66*, 1198–1207. [CrossRef] [PubMed]
125. Han, J.; Seaman, W.E.; Di, X.; Wang, W.; Willingham, M.; Torti, F.M.; Torti, S.V. Iron Uptake Mediated by Binding of H-ferritin to the Tim-2 Receptor in Mouse Cells. *PLoS ONE* **2011**, *6*, e23800. [CrossRef] [PubMed]
126. Bishop, G.M.; Scheiber, I.F.; Dringen, R.; Robinson, S.R. Synergistic Accumulation of Iron and Zinc by Cultured Astrocytes. *J. Neural Transm.* **2010**, *117*, 809–817. [CrossRef] [PubMed]
127. Vidal, R.; Miravalle, L.; Gao, X.; Barbeito, A.G.; Baraibar, M.A.; Hekmatyar, S.K.; Widel, M.; Bansal, N.; Delisle, M.B.; Ghetti, B. Expression of a Mutant Form of the Ferritin Light Chain Gene Induces Neurodegeneration and Iron Overload in Transgenic Mice. *J. Neurosci.* **2008**, *28*, 60–67. [CrossRef]

128. Zucca, F.A.; Segura-Aguilar, J.; Ferrari, E.; Muñoz, P.; Paris, I.; Sulzer, D.; Sarna, T.; Casella, L.; Zecca, L. Interactions of Iron, Dopamine and Neuromelanin Pathways in Brain Aging and Parkinson's Disease. *Prog. Neurobiol.* **2017**, *155*, 96–119. [CrossRef]
129. MacKenzie, E.L.; Iwasaki, K.; Tsuji, Y. Intracellular Iron Transport and Storage: From Molecular Mechanisms to Health Implications. *Antioxid. Redox Signal.* **2008**, *10*, 997–1030. [CrossRef]
130. Irace, C.; Scorziello, A.; Maffettone, C.; Pignataro, G.; Matrone, C.; Adornetto, A.; Santamaria, R.; Annunziato, L.; Colonna, A. Divergent Modulation of Iron Regulatory Proteins and Ferritin Biosynthesis by Hypoxia/Reoxygenation in Neurons and Glial Cells. *J. Neurochem.* **2005**, *95*, 1321–1331. [CrossRef]
131. Asano, T.; Komatsu, M.; Yamaguchi, Y.; Ishikawa-Iwai, F.; Mizushima, N.; Iwai, K. Distinct Mechanisms of Ferritin Delivery to Lysosomes in Iron-Depleted and Iron-Replete Cells. *Mol. Cell. Biol.* **2011**, *31*, 2040–2052. [CrossRef]
132. Biasiotto, G.; Di Lorenzo, D.; Archetti, S.; Zanella, I. Iron and Neurodegeneration: Is Ferritinophagy the Link? *Mol. Neurobiol.* **2016**, *53*, 5542–5574. [CrossRef]
133. Vela, D. The Dual Role of Hepcidin in Brain Iron Load and Inflammation. *Front. Neurosci.* **2018**, *12*, 740. [CrossRef]
134. Zechel, S.; Huber-Wittmer, K.; Von Bohlen und Halbach, O. Distribution of the Iron-Regulating Protein Hepcidin in the Murine Central Nervous System. *J. Neurol. Res.* **2006**, *84*, 790–800. [CrossRef] [PubMed]
135. Wang, Q.; Du, F.; Qian, Z.M.; Ge, X.H.; Zhu, L.; Yung, W.H.; Yang, L.; Ke, Y. Lipopolysaccharide Induces a Significant Increase in Expression of Iron Regulatory Hormone Hepcidin in the Cortex and Substantia Nigra in Rat Brain. *Endocrinology* **2008**, *149*, 3920–3925. [CrossRef] [PubMed]
136. Beard, J.L.; Connor, J.R. Iron Status and Neural Functioning. *Annu. Rev. Nutr.* **2003**, *23*, 41–58. [CrossRef] [PubMed]
137. Ferreira, A.; Neves, P.; Gozzelino, R. Multilevel Impacts of Iron in the Brain: The Cross Talk between Neurophysiological Mechanisms, Cognition, and Social Behavior. *Pharmaceuticals* **2019**, *12*, 126. [CrossRef] [PubMed]
138. Petranovic, D.; Batinac, T.; Petranovic, D.; Ruzic, A.; Ruzic, T. Iron Deficiency Anaemia Influences Cognitive Functions. *Med. Hypotheses* **2008**, *70*, 70–72. [CrossRef]
139. Bourre, J.M. Effects of Nutrients (in Food) on the Structure and Function of the Nervous System: Update on Dietary Requirements for Brain. Part 1: Micronutrients. *J. Nutr. Health Aging* **2006**, *10*, 377–385.
140. Kuhn, S.; Gritti, L.; Crooks, D.; Dombrowski, Y. Oligodendrocytes in Development, Myelin Generation and Beyond. *Cells* **2019**, *8*, 1424. [CrossRef]
141. Andro, M.; Le Squere, P.; Estivin, S.; Gentric, A. Anaemia and Cognitive Performances in the Elderly: A Systematic Review. *Eur. J. Neurol.* **2013**, *20*, 1234–1240. [CrossRef]
142. Fleming, D.J.; Tucker, K.L.; Jacques, P.F.; Dallal, G.E.; Wilson, P.W.; Wood, R.J. Dietary Factors Associated with the Risk of High Iron Stores in the Elderly Framingham Heart Study Cohort. *Am. J. Clin. Nutr.* **2002**, *76*, 1375–1384. [CrossRef]
143. Hunnicutt, J.; He, K.; Xun, P. Dietary Iron Intake and Body Iron Stores Are Associated with Risk of Coronary Heart Disease in a Meta-Analysis of Prospective Cohort Studies. *J. Nutr.* **2013**, *144*, 359–366. [CrossRef]
144. Bao, W.; Rong, Y.; Rong, S.; Liu, L. Dietary Iron Intake, Body Iron Stores, and the Risk of Type 2 Diabetes: A Systematic Review and Meta-Analysis. *BMC Med.* **2012**, *10*, 119. [CrossRef] [PubMed]
145. Penke, L.; Valdés Hernández, M.C.; Maniega, S.M.; Gow, A.J.; Murray, C.; Starr, J.M.; Bastin, M.E.; Deary, I.J.; Wardlaw, J.M. Brain Iron Deposits Are Associated with General Cognitive Ability and Cognitive Aging. *Neurobiol. Aging* **2012**, *33*, 510–517.e512. [CrossRef] [PubMed]
146. Hosking, D.E.; Ayton, S.; Beckett, N.; Booth, A.; Peters, R. More Evidence Is Needed. Iron, Incident Cognitive Decline and Dementia: A Systematic Review. *Ther. Adv. Chronic. Dis.* **2018**, *9*, 241–256. [CrossRef] [PubMed]
147. Poon, H.F.; Calabrese, V.; Calvani, M.; Butterfield, D.A. Proteomics Analyses of Specific Protein Oxidation and Protein Expression in Aged Rat Brain and its Modulation by L-Acetylcarnitine: Insights into the Mechanisms of Action of this Proposed Therapeutic Agent for CNS Disorders Associated with Oxidative Stress. *Antioxid. Redox Signal.* **2006**, *8*, 381–394. [CrossRef] [PubMed]
148. Lu, L.-N.; Qian, Z.-M.; Wu, K.-C.; Yung, W.-H.; Ke, Y. Expression of Iron Transporters and Pathological Hallmarks of Parkinson's and Alzheimer's Diseases in the Brain of Young, Adult, and Aged Rats. *Mol. Neurobiol.* **2016**, *54*, 5213–5224. [CrossRef] [PubMed]

149. Connor, J.R.; Menzies, S.L.; St Martin, S.M.; Mufson, E.J. Cellular Distribution of Transferrin, Ferritin and Iron in Normal and Aged Human Brains. *J. Neurosci. Res.* **1990**, *27*, 595–611. [CrossRef] [PubMed]
150. Hare, D.J.; Gerlach, M.; Riederer, P. Considerations for Measuring Iron in Post-Mortem Tissue of Parkinson's Disease Patients. *J. Neural Transm.* **2012**, *119*, 1515–1521. [CrossRef]
151. Zecca, L.; Youdim, M.B.; Riederer, P.; Connor, J.R.; Crichton, R.R. Iron, Brain Ageing and Neurodegenerative Disorders. *Nat. Rev. Neurosci.* **2004**, *5*, 863–873. [CrossRef]
152. Yan, S.-Q.; Sun, J.-Z.; Yan, Y.-Q.; Wang, H.; Lou, M. Evaluation of Brain Iron Content Based on Magnetic Resonance Imaging (MRI): Comparison among Phase Value, R2* and Magnitude Signal Intensity. *PLoS ONE* **2012**, *7*, e31748. [CrossRef]
153. Xu, X.; Wang, Q.; Zhang, M. Age, Gender, and Hemispheric Differences in Iron Deposition in the Human Brain: An in Vivo MRI Study. *Neuroimage* **2008**, *40*, 35–42. [CrossRef]
154. Iadecola, C. Neurovascular Regulation in the Normal Brain and in Alzheimer's Disease. *Nat. Rev. Neurosci.* **2004**, *5*, 347–360. [CrossRef] [PubMed]
155. Conde, J.R.; Streit, W.J. Microglia in the Aging Brain. *J. Neuropathol. Exp. Neurol.* **2006**, *65*, 199–203. [CrossRef] [PubMed]
156. Farrall, A.J.; Wardlaw, J.M. Blood-Brain Barrier: Ageing and Microvascular Disease–Systematic Review and Meta-Analysis. *Neurobiol. Aging* **2009**, *30*, 337–352. [CrossRef] [PubMed]
157. Crichton, R.R. *Inorganic Biochemistry of Iron Metabolism: From Molecular Mechanisms to Clinical Consequences*, 2nd ed.; John Wiley & Sons: Chichester, UK, 2001; pp. 1–21.
158. Weinreb, O.; Amit, T.; Youdim, M.B.H. Targeting Dysregulation of Brain Iron Homeostasis in Ageing. *Nutr. Aging* **2012**, *1*, 27–39. [CrossRef]
159. Kumar, M.J.; Andersen, J.K. Perspectives on MAO-B in Aging and Neurological Disease: Where Do We Go from Here? *Mol. Neurobiol.* **2004**, *30*, 77–89. [CrossRef]
160. Shemyakov, S.E. Monoamine Oxidase Activity, Lipid Peroxidation, and Morphological Changes in Human Hypothalamus During Aging. *Bull. Exp. Biol. Med.* **2001**, *131*, 586–588. [CrossRef]
161. Carrasquilla, G.D.; Frumento, P.; Berglund, A.; Borgfeldt, C.; Bottai, M.; Chiavenna, C.; Eliasson, M.; Engström, G.; Hallmans, G.; Jansson, J.H.; et al. Postmenopausal hormone therapy and risk of stroke: A pooled analysis of data from population-based cohort studies. *PLoS Med.* **2017**, *14*, e1002445. [CrossRef]
162. Yu, J.; Liu, H.; He, S.; Li, P.; Ma, C.; Ma, M.; Liu, Y.; Lv, L.; Ping, F.; Zhang, H.; et al. Sex-Specific Negative Association between Iron Intake and Cellular Aging Markers: Mediation Models Involving TNFα. *Oxid. Med. Cell. Longev.* **2019**, *2019*, 4935237. [CrossRef]
163. Ćurko-Cofek, B.; Grubić Kezele, T.; Barac-Latas, V. Hepcidin and Metallothioneins as Molecular Base for Sex-Dependent Differences in Clinical Course of Experimental Autoimmune Encephalomyelitis in Chronic Iron Overload. *Med. Hypotheses* **2017**, *107*, 51–54. [CrossRef]
164. Hametner, S.; Wimmer, I.; Haider, L.; Pfeifenbring, S.; Brück, W.; Lassmann, H. Iron and Neurodegeneration in the Multiple Sclerosis Brain. *Ann. Neurol.* **2013**, *74*, 848–861. [CrossRef]
165. Grubić Kezele, T. Iron. In *Trace Elements and Minerals in Health and Longevity*, 1st ed.; Malavolta, M., Mocchegiani, E., Eds.; Springer Nature: Cham, Switzerland, 2018; Volume 8, pp. 1–34.
166. Zivadinov, R.; Tavazzi, E.; Bergsland, N.; Hagemeier, J.; Lin, F.; Dwyer, M.G.; Carl, E.; Kolb, C.; Hojnacki, D.; Ramasamy, D.; et al. Brain Iron at Quantitative MRI Is Associated with Disability in Multiple Sclerosis. *Radiology* **2018**, *289*, 487–496. [CrossRef] [PubMed]
167. Rosko, L.; Smith, V.N.; Yamazaki, R.; Huang, J.K. Oligodendrocyte Bioenergetics in Health and Disease. *Neuroscientist* **2019**, *5*, 334–343. [CrossRef] [PubMed]
168. Morath, D.J.; Mayer-Pröschel, M. Iron Modulates the Differentiation of a Distinct Population of Glial Precursor Cells into Oligodendrocytes. *Dev. Biol.* **2001**, *237*, 232–243. [CrossRef] [PubMed]
169. Morath, D.J.; Mayer-Pröschel, M. Iron Deficiency During Embryogenesis and Consequences for Oligodendrocyte Generation in Vivo. *Dev. Neurosci.* **2002**, *24*, 197–207. [CrossRef] [PubMed]
170. Schonberg, D.L.; McTigue, D.M. Iron is Essential for Oligodendrocyte Genesis following Intraspinal Macrophage Activation. *Exp. Neurol.* **2009**, *218*, 64–74. [CrossRef] [PubMed]
171. Grishchuk, Y.; Peña, K.A.; Coblentz, J.; King, V.E.; Humphrey, M.D.; Wang, S.L.; Kiselyov, K.I.; Slaugenhaupt, S.A. Impaired Myelination and Reduced Brain Ferric Iron in the Mouse Model of Mucolipidosis IV. *Dis. Model Mech.* **2015**, *8*, 1591–1601. [CrossRef]

172. Schulz, K.; Kroner, A.; David, S. Iron Efflux from Astrocytes Plays a Role in Remyelination. *Soc. Neurosci.* **2012**, *32*, 4841–4847. [CrossRef]
173. Todorich, B.; Pasquini, J.M.; Garcia, C.I.; Paez, P.M.; Connor, J.R. Oligodendrocytes and Myelination: The Role of Iron. *Glia* **2009**, *57*, 467–478. [CrossRef]
174. Morell, P.; Jurevics, H. Origin of Cholesterol in Myelin. *Neurochem. Res.* **1996**, *21*, 463–470. [CrossRef]
175. Jones, G.; Prosser, D.E.; Kaufmann, M. Cytochrome P450-mediated Metabolism of Vitamin D. *J. Lipid Res.* **2014**, *55*, 13–31. [CrossRef]
176. Fuente, A.G.F.; Errea, O.; Van Wijngaarden, P.; Gonzalez, G.A.; Kerninon, C.; Jarjour, A.A.; Lewis, H.J.; Jones, C.A.; Nait-Oumesmar, B.; Zhao, C. Vitamin D Receptor–Retinoid X Receptor Heterodimer Signaling Regulates Oligodendrocyte Progenitor Cell Differentiation. *J. Cell Biol.* **2015**, *211*, 975–985. [CrossRef] [PubMed]
177. Sintzel, M.B.; Rametta, M.; Reder, A.T. Vitamin D and Multiple Sclerosis: A Comprehensive Review. *Neurol. Ther.* **2018**, *7*, 59–85. [CrossRef] [PubMed]
178. Abbatemarco, J.R.; Fox, R.J.; Li, H.; Ontaneda, D. Vitamin D and MRI Measures in Progressive Multiple Sclerosis. *Mult. Scler. Relat. Disord.* **2019**, *35*, 276–282. [CrossRef] [PubMed]
179. Bacchetta, J.; Zaritsky, J.J.; Sea, J.L.; Chun, R.F.; Lisse, T.S.; Zavala, K.; Nayak, A.; Wesseling-Perry, K.; Westerman, M.; Hollis, B.W.; et al. Suppression of Iron-regulatory Hepcidin by Vitamin D. *J. Am. Soc. Nephrol.* **2014**, *25*, 564–572. [CrossRef] [PubMed]
180. Kweder, H.; Eidi, H. Vitamin D Deficiency in Elderly: Risk Factors and Drugs Impact on Vitamin D Status. *Avicenna J. Med.* **2018**, *8*, 139–146. [CrossRef]
181. Munger, K.L.; Chitnis, T.; Ascherio, A. Body Size and Risk of MS in Two Cohorts of US Women. *Neurology* **2009**, *73*, 1543–1550. [CrossRef]
182. Gianfrancesco, M.A.; Barcellos, L.F. Obesity and Multiple Sclerosis Susceptibility: A Review. *J. Neurol. Neuromed.* **2016**, *1*, 1–5. [CrossRef]
183. Low, M.S.Y.; Speedy, J.; Styles, C.E.; De-Regil, L.M.; Pasricha, S.R. Daily iron supplementation for improving anaemia, iron status and health in menstruating women. *Cochrane Database Syst. Rev.* **2016**, *4*, CD009747. [CrossRef]
184. Ramos, P.; Santos, A.; Pinto, N.R.; Mendes, R.; Magalhães, T.; Agostinho Almeida, A. Iron Levels in the Human Brain: A Post-Mortem Study of Anatomical Region Differences and Age-Related Changes. *J. Trace Elem. Med. Biol.* **2014**, *28*, 13–17. [CrossRef]
185. Tishler, T.A.; Raven, E.P.; Lu, P.H.; Altshuler, L.L.; Bartzokis, G. Pre-menopausal Hysterectomy Is Associated with Increased Brain Ferritin Iron. *Neurobiol. Aging* **2012**, *33*, 1950–1958. [CrossRef]
186. Hallgren, B.; Sourander, P. The Effect of Age on the Non-Haemin Iron in the Human Brain. *J. Neurochem.* **1958**, *3*, 41–51. [CrossRef] [PubMed]
187. Hagemeier, J.; Weinstock-Guttman, B.; Heininen-Brown, M.; Poloni, G.U.; Bergsland, N.; Schirda, C.; Magnano, C.R.; Kennedy, C.; Carl, E.; Dwyer, M.G.; et al. Gray Matter SWI-filtered Phase and Atrophy Are Linked to Disability in MS. *Front. Biosci.* **2013**, *5*, 525–532. [CrossRef] [PubMed]
188. Schmidt, P.J.; Rubinow, D.R. Sex Hormones and Mood in the Perimenopause. *Ann. N. Y. Acad. Sci.* **2009**, *1179*, 70–85. [CrossRef] [PubMed]
189. Awad, A.; Stüve, O. Multiple Sclerosis in the Elderly Patient. *Drugs Aging* **2010**, *27*, 283–294. [CrossRef]
190. Bartzokis, G.; Mintz, J.; Sultzer, D.; Marx, P.; Herzberg, J.S.; Phelan, C.K.; Marder, S.R. In Vivo MR Evaluation of Age-Related Increases in Brain Iron. *Am. J. Neuroradiol.* **1994**, *15*, 1129–1138.
191. Armon-Omer, A.; Waldman, C.; Simaan, N.; Neuman, H.; Tamir, S.; Shahien, R. New Insights on the Nutrition Status and Antioxidant Capacity in Multiple Sclerosis Patients. *Nutrients* **2019**, *11*, 427. [CrossRef]
192. Gill, D.; Brewer, C.F.; Monori, G.; Trégouët, D.A.; Franceschini, N.; Giambartolomei, C.; Tzoulaki, I.; Dehghan, A. Effects of Genetically Determined Iron Status on Risk of Venous Thromboembolism and Carotid Atherosclerotic Disease: A Mendelian Randomization Study. *J. Am. Heart Assoc.* **2019**, *8*, e012994. [CrossRef]
193. Menon, R.G.; Khan, B.V.; Rajagopalan, S.; Fay, W.P. Chronic Iron Administration Increases Vascular Oxidative Stress and Accelerates Arterial Thrombosis. *Circulation* **2003**, *107*, 2601–2606.
194. Franchini, M.; Targher, G.; Montagnana, M.; Lippi, G. Iron and Thrombosis. *Ann. Hematol.* **2008**, *87*, 167–173. [CrossRef]

195. Tang, X.; Fang, M.; Cheng, R.; Zhang, Z.; Wang, Y.; Shen, C.; Han, Y.; Lu, Q.; Du, Y.; Liu, Y.; et al. Iron-Deficiency and Estrogen Are Associated with Ischemic Stroke by Up-Regulating Transferrin to Induce Hypercoagulability. *Circ. Res.* **2020**, *127*, 651–663. [CrossRef]
196. Ogun, A.S.; Adeyinka, A. Biochemistry, Transferrin. In *StatPearls [Internet]*; StatPearls Publishing: St. Petersburg, FL, USA, 2019. Available online: https://www.ncbi.nlm.nih.gov/books/NBK532928/ (accessed on 30 May 2020).
197. Tang, X.; Zhang, Z.; Fang, M.; Han, Y.; Wang, G.; Wang, S.; Xue, M.; Li, Y.; Zhang, L.; Wu, J.; et al. Transferrin Plays a Central Role in Coagulation Balance by Interacting with Clotting Factors. *Cell Res.* **2020**, *30*, 119–132. [CrossRef] [PubMed]
198. Woods, H.F.; Youdim, M.B.H.; Boullin, D.; Callender, S. Monoamine Metabolism and Platelet Function in Iron-Deficiency Anaemia. In *Ciba Foundation Symposium 51-Iron Metabolism*; John Wiley & Sons, Ltd.: Chichester, UK, 1977; Volume 51, pp. 227–248.
199. Jackson, S. The Growing Complexity of Platelet Aggregation. *Blood* **2007**, *109*, 5087–5095. [CrossRef] [PubMed]
200. Shovlin, C.L.; Chamali, B.; Santhirapala, V.; Livesey, J.A.; Angus, G.; Manning, R.; Laffan, M.A.; Meek, J.; Tighe, H.C.; Jackson, J.E. Ischaemic Strokes in Patients with Pulmonary Arteriovenous Malformations and Hereditary Hemorrhagic Telangiectasia: Associations With Iron Deficiency and Platelets. *PLoS ONE* **2014**, *9*, e88812. [CrossRef] [PubMed]
201. Appelros, P.; Stegmayr, B.; Terent, A. Sex Differences in Stroke Epidemiology: A Systematic Review. *Stroke* **2009**, *40*, 1082–1090. [CrossRef] [PubMed]
202. Kaluza, J.; Wolk, A.; Larsson, S.C. Heme Iron Intake and Risk of Stroke: A Prospective Study of Men. *Stroke* **2013**, *44*, 334–339. [CrossRef]
203. Fukuda, M.; Kanda, T.; Kamide, N.; Akutsu, T.; Sakai, F. Gender Differences in Long-term Functional Outcome after First-ever Ischemic Stroke. *Intern. Med.* **2009**, *48*, 967–973. [CrossRef]
204. Petrone, A.B.; Simpkins, J.W.; Barr, T.L. 17β-Estradiol and Inflammation: Implications for Ischemic Stroke. *Aging Dis.* **2014**, *5*, 340–345. [CrossRef]
205. Malutan, A.M.; Dan, M.; Nicolae, C.; Carmen, M. Proinflammatory and Anti-Inflammatory Cytokine Changes Related to Menopause. *Prz. Menopauzalny* **2014**, *13*, 162–168. [CrossRef]
206. Montgomery, S.L.; Bowers, W.J. Tumor Necrosis Factor-alpha and the Roles it Plays in Homeostatic and Degenerative Processes within the Central Nervous System. *J. Neuroimmune Pharmacol.* **2012**, *7*, 42–59. [CrossRef]
207. Doll, D.N.; Rellick, S.L.; Barr, T.L.; Ren, X.; Simpkins, J.W. Rapid Mitochondrial Dysfunction Mediates TNF-Alpha-Induced Neurotoxicity. *J. Neurochem.* **2015**, *132*, 443–451. [CrossRef]
208. Liao, S.L.; Chen, W.Y.; Chen, C.J. Estrogen Attenuates Tumor Necrosis Factor-Alpha Expression to Provide Ischemic Neuroprotection in Female Rats. *Neurosci. Lett.* **2002**, *330*, 159–162. [CrossRef]
209. Vela, D. Hepcidin, an Emerging and Important Player in Brain Iron Homeostasis. *J. Transl. Med.* **2018**, *16*, 25. [CrossRef] [PubMed]
210. Miller, E.M. Hormone Replacement Therapy Affects Iron Status More than Endometrial Bleeding in Older US Women: A Role for Estrogen in Iron Homeostasis? *Maturitas* **2016**, *88*, 46–51. [CrossRef]
211. Zacharski, L.R.; Ornstein, D.L.; Woloshin, S.; Schwartz, L.M. Association of Age, Sex, and Race with Body Iron Stores in Adults: Analysis of NHANES III Data. *Am. Heart J.* **2000**, *140*, 98–104. [CrossRef] [PubMed]
212. Bajbouj, K.; Shafarin, J.; Allam, H.; Madkour, M.; Awadallah, S.; El-Serafy, A.; Sandeep, D.; Hamad, M. Elevated Levels of Estrogen Suppress Hepcidin Synthesis and Enhance Serum Iron Availability in Premenopausal Women. *Exp. Clin. Endocrinol. Diabetes* **2018**, *126*, 453–459. [CrossRef]
213. Busti, F.; Campostrini, N.; Martinelli, N.; Girelli, D. Iron Deficiency in the Elderly Population, Revisited in the Hepcidin era. *Front. Pharmacol.* **2014**, *5*, 83. [CrossRef]
214. Ilkovska, B.; Kotevska, B.; Trifunov, G.; Kanazirev, B. Serum Hepcidin Reference Range, Gender Differences, Menopausal Dependence and Biochemical Correlates in Healthy Subjects. *J. IMAB Annu. Proc. Sci. Pap.* **2016**, *22*, 1127–1131. [CrossRef]
215. Jian, J.; Pelle, E.; Huang, X. Iron and Menopause: Does Increased Iron Affect the Health of Postmenopausal Women? *Antioxid. Redox Signal.* **2009**, *11*, 2939–2943. [CrossRef]
216. Huang, X.; Xu, Y.; Partridge, N.C. Dancing with Sex Hormones, Could Iron Contribute to the Gender Difference in Osteoporosis? *Bone* **2013**, *55*, 458–460. [CrossRef]

217. Chen, B.; Li, G.F.; Shen, Y.; Huang, X.I.; Xu, Y.J. Reducing Iron Accumulation: A Potential Approach for the Prevention and Treatment of Postmenopausal Osteoporosis. *Exp. Ther. Med.* **2015**, *10*, 7–11. [CrossRef]
218. Roy, C.N.; Snyder, P.J.; Stephens-Shields, A.J.; Artz, A.S.; Bhasin, S.; Cohen, H.J.; Farrar, J.T.; Gill, T.M.; Zeldow, B.; Cella, D.; et al. Association of Testosterone Levels with Anemia in Older Men: A Controlled Clinical Trial. *JAMA Intern. Med.* **2017**, *177*, 480–490. [CrossRef]
219. Gabrielsen, J.S. Iron and Testosterone: Interplay and Clinical Implications. *Curr. Sex. Health Rep.* **2017**, *9*, 5–11. [CrossRef]
220. Grubić Kezele, T. Androgen-driven COVID-19 Infectio—Is Testosterone an Enemy or a Friend? *Horm. Mol. Biol. Clin. Investig.* **2020**, *41*. [CrossRef]
221. Grubić Kezele, T. Cryptozoospermia after Treatment with Clomiphene Citrate Following Long-Term Use of Intramuscular Testosterone Undecanoate Depot Injection (Nebido®). *Horm. Mol. Biol. Clin. Investig.* **2019**, *39*. [CrossRef] [PubMed]
222. Jeppesen, L.L.; Jørgensen, H.S.; Nakayama, H.; Raaschou, H.O.; Olsen, T.S.; Winther, K. Decreased Serum Testosterone in Men with Acute Ischemic Stroke. *Arterioscler. Thromb. Vasc. Biol.* **1996**, *16*, 749–754. [CrossRef] [PubMed]
223. Sangkhae, V.; Nemeth, E. Regulation of the Iron Homeostatic Hormone Hepcidin. *Adv. Nutr.* **2017**, *8*, 126–136. [CrossRef]
224. Mammi, C.; Calanchini, M.; Antelmi, A.; Cinti, F.; Rosano, G.M.C.; Lenzi, A.; Caprio, M.; Fabbri, A. Androgens and Adipose Tissue in Males: A Complex and Reciprocal Interplay. *Int. J. Endocrinol.* **2012**, *2012*, 789653. [CrossRef]
225. Bianchi, V.E. The Anti-Inflammatory Effects of Testosterone. *J. Endocr. Soc.* **2019**, *3*, 91–107. [CrossRef]
226. Dhindsa, S.; Ghanim, H.; Batra, M.; Kuhadiya, N.D.; Abuaysheh, S.; Green, K.; Antoine Makdissi, A.; Chaudhuri, A.; Dandona, P. Effect of Testosterone on Hepcidin, Ferroportin, Ferritin and Iron Binding Capacity in Patients with Hypogonadotropic Hypogonadism and Type 2 Diabetes. *Clin. Endocrinol.* **2016**, *85*, 772–780. [CrossRef]
227. Peng, W.; Minakaki, G.; Nguyen, M.; Krainc, D. Preserving Lysosomal Function in the Aging Brain: Insights from Neurodegeneration. *Neurotherapeutics* **2019**, *16*, 611–634. [CrossRef]
228. Liu, Z.; Shen, H.; Lian, T.; Mao, L.; Tang, S.; Sun, L.; Huang, X.; Guo, P.; Cao, C.; Yu, S.; et al. Iron Deposition in Substantia Nigra: Abnormal Iron Metabolism, Neuroinflammatory Mechanism and Clinical Relevance. *Sci. Rep.* **2017**, *7*, 14973. [CrossRef] [PubMed]
229. Ghassaban, K.; He, N.; Sethi, S.K.; Huang, P.; Chen, S.; Yan, F.; Haacke, E.M. Regional High Iron in the Substantia Nigra Differentiates Parkinson's Disease Patients From Healthy Controls. *Front. Aging Neurosci.* **2019**, *11*, 106. [CrossRef] [PubMed]
230. Li, K.; Ge, Y.L.; Gu, C.C.; Zhang, J.R.; Jin, H.; Li, J.; Cheng, X.Y.; Yang, Y.P.; Wang, F.; Zhang, Y.C.; et al. Substantia Nigra Echogenicity is Associated with Serum Ferritin, Gender and Iron-Related Genes in Parkinson's Disease. *Sci. Rep.* **2020**, *10*, 8660. [CrossRef] [PubMed]
231. Joppe, K.; Roser, A.E.R.; Maass, F.; Lingor, P. The Contribution of Iron to Protein Aggregation Disorders in the Central Nervous System. *Front. Neurosci.* **2019**, *13*, 15. [CrossRef] [PubMed]
232. Shen, X.; Yang, H.; Zhang, D.; Jiang, H. Iron Concentration Does Not Differ in Blood but Tends to Decrease in Cerebrospinal Fluid in Parkinson's Disease. *Front. Neurosci.* **2019**, *13*, 939. [CrossRef]
233. Xing, Y.; Sapuan, A.; Dineen, R.A.; Auer, D.P. Life Span Pigmentation Changes of the Substantia Nigra Detected by Neuromelanin-Sensitive MRI. *Mov. Disord.* **2018**, *33*, 1792–1799. [CrossRef] [PubMed]
234. Sohrabji, F. Guarding the Blood–Brain Barrier: A Role for Estrogen in the Etiology of Neurodegenerative Disease. *Gene Expr. J. Liver Res.* **2006**, *13*, 311–319. [CrossRef]
235. Wang, L.F.; Yokoyama, K.K.; Chen, T.Y.; Hsiao, H.W.; Chiang, P.C.; Hsieh, Y.C.; Lo, S.; Hsu, C. Male-Specific Alleviation of Iron-Induced Striatal Injury by Inhibition of Autophagy. *PLoS ONE* **2015**, *10*, e0131224. [CrossRef]
236. Mariani, S.; Ventriglia, M.; Simonelli, I.; Bucossi, S.; Siotto, M.; Donno, S.; Vernieri, F.; Squitti, R. Association between Sex, Systemic Iron Variation and Probability of Parkinson's Disease. *Int. J. Neurosci.* **2016**, *126*, 354–360. [CrossRef]
237. Chen, T.Y.; Lin, C.L.; Wang, L.F.; Tsai, K.L.; Lin, J.Y.; Hsu, C. Targeting GPER1 to Suppress Autophagy as a Male-Specific Therapeutic Strategy for Iron-Induced Striatal Injury. *Sci. Rep.* **2019**, *9*, 6661. [CrossRef]

238. Xu, M.; Tan, X.; Li, N.; Wu, H.; Wang, Y.; Xie, J.; Wang, J. Differential Regulation of Estrogen in Iron Metabolism in Astrocytes and Neurons. *J. Cell. Physiol.* **2019**, *234*, 4232–4242. [CrossRef] [PubMed]
239. Sääksjärvi, K.; Knekt, P.; Lundqvist, A.; Männistö, S.; Heliövaara, M.; Rissanen, H.; Järvinen, R. A Cohort Study on Diet and the Risk of Parkinson's Disease: The Role of Food Groups and Diet Quality. *Br. J. Nutr.* **2013**, *109*, 329–337. [CrossRef] [PubMed]
240. Micha, R.; Wallace, S.K.; Mozaffarian, D. Red and Processed Meat Consumption and Risk of Incident Coronary Heart Disease, Stroke, and Diabetes: A Systematic Review and Meta-Analysis. *Circulation* **2010**, *121*, 2271–2283. [CrossRef] [PubMed]
241. Rohrmann, S.; Overvad, K.; Bueno-de-Mesquita, H.B.; Jakobsen, M.U.; Egeberg, R.; Tjønneland, A.; Nailler, L.; Boutron-Ruault, M.C.; Clavel-Chapelon, F.; Krogh, V.; et al. Meat Consumption and Mortality—Results from the European Prospective Investigation into Cancer and Nutrition. *BMC Med.* **2013**, *11*, 63. [CrossRef]
242. Hare, D.J.; Cardoso, B.R.; Raven, E.P.; Double, K.L.; Finkelstein, D.I.; Szymlek-Gay, E.A.; Biggs, B.A. Excessive Early-Life Dietary Exposure: A Potential Source of Elevated Brain Iron and a Risk Factor for Parkinson's disease. *NPJ Parkinsons Dis.* **2017**, *3*, 1. [CrossRef] [PubMed]
243. Logroscino, G.; Chen, H.; Wing, A.; Ascherio, A. Blood Donations Iron, Stores, and Risk of Parkinson's Disease. *Mov. Disord.* **2006**, *21*, 835–838. [CrossRef] [PubMed]
244. Miyake, Y.; Tanaka, K.; Fukushima, W.; Sasaki, S.; Kiyohara, C.; Tsuboi, Y.; Yamada, T.; Oeda, T.; Miki, T.; Kawamura, N. Dietary Intake of Metals and Risk of Parkinson's Disease: A Case-Control Study in Japan. *J. Neurol. Sci.* **2011**, *306*, 98–102. [CrossRef]
245. Deng, Q.; Zhou, X.; Chen, J.; Pan, M.; Gao, H.; Zhou, J.; Wang, D.; Chen, Q.; Zhang, X.; Wang, Q. Lower Hemoglobin Levels in Patients with Parkinson's Disease Are Associated with Disease Severity and Iron Metabolism. *Brain Res.* **2017**, *1655*, 145–151. [CrossRef]
246. Hong, C.T.; Huang, Y.H.; Liu, H.Y.; Chiou, H.Y.; Chan, L.; Chien, L.N. Newly Diagnosed Anemia Increases Risk of Parkinson's disease: A Population-Based Cohort Study. *Sci. Rep.* **2016**, *6*, 29651. [CrossRef]
247. Santiago, J.A.; Bottero, V.; Potashkin, J.A. Biological and Clinical Implications of Comorbidities in Parkinson's Disease. *Front. Aging Neurosci.* **2017**, *9*, 394. [CrossRef]
248. Mariani, S.; Ventriglia, M.; Simonelli, I.; Donno, S.; Bucossi, S.; Vernieri, F.; Melgari, J.M.; Pasqualetti, P.; Rossini, P.M.; Squitti, R. Fe and Cu do not Differ in Parkinson's Disease: A Replication Study Plus Meta-Analysis. *Neurobiol. Aging* **2013**, *34*, 632–633. [CrossRef] [PubMed]
249. Sian-Hülsmann, J.; Mandel, S.; Youdim, M.B.H.; Riederer, P. The Relevance of Iron in the Pathogenesis of Parkinson's Disease. *J. Neurochem.* **2011**, *118*, 939–957. [CrossRef] [PubMed]
250. Savica, R.; Grossardt, B.R.; Bower, J.H.; Ahlskog, J.E.; Rocca, W.A. Risk Factors for Parkinson's Disease May Differ in Men and Women: An Exploratory Study. *Horm. Behav.* **2013**, *63*, 308–314. [CrossRef] [PubMed]
251. Seidl, S.E.; Santiago, J.A.; Bilyk, H.; Potashkin, J.A. The Emerging Role of Nutrition in Parkinson's Disease. *Front. Aging Neurosci.* **2014**, *6*, 36. [CrossRef] [PubMed]
252. Du, X.; Wang, X.; Geng, M. Alzheimer's Disease Hypothesis and Related Therapies. *Transl. Neurodegener.* **2018**, *7*, 1–7. [CrossRef]
253. Chen, M.; Zheng, J.; Liu, G.; Zeng, C.; Xu, E.; Zhu, W.; Anderson, G.J.; Chen, H. High Dietary Iron Disrupts Iron Homeostasis and Induces Amyloid-β and Phospho-τ Expression in the Hippocampus of Adult Wild-Type and APP/PS1 Transgenic Mice. *J. Nutr.* **2019**, *149*, 2247–2254. [CrossRef]
254. Perry, G.; Cash, A.D.; Smith, M.A. Alzheimer Disease and Oxidative Stress. *J. Biomed. Biotechnol.* **2002**, *2*, 120–123. [CrossRef]
255. Xu, J.; Jia, Z.; Knutson, M.D.; Leeuwenburgh, C. Impaired Iron Status in Aging Research. *Int. J. Mol. Sci.* **2012**, *13*, 2368–2386. [CrossRef]
256. Ayton, S.; Faux, N.G.; Bush, A.I. Association of cerebrospinal fluid ferritin level with preclinical cognitive decline in APOE-epsilon4 carriers. *JAMA Neurol.* **2017**, *74*, 122–125. [CrossRef]
257. Ayton, S.; Diouf, I.; Bush, A.I. Alzheimer's Disease Neuroimaging, Evidence that Iron Accelerates Alzheimer's Pathology: A CSF Biomarker Study. *J. Neurol. Neurosurg. Psychiatry* **2018**, *89*, 456–460. [CrossRef]
258. Bartzokis, G.; Lu, P.H.; Tishler, T.A.; Peters, D.G.; Kosenko, A.; Barrall, K.A.; Finn, J.P.; Villablanca, P.; Laub, G.; Altshuler, L.L. Prevalent Iron Metabolism Gene Variants Associated with Increased Brain Ferritin Iron in Healthy Older Men. *J. Alzheimers Dis.* **2010**, *20*, 333–341. [CrossRef] [PubMed]

259. Burger, A.; Kotze, M.J.; Stein, D.J.; van Rensburg, S.J.; Howells, F.M. The Relationship between Measurement of vice versa Brain Glutamate and Markers of Iron Metabolism: A Proton Magnetic Resonance Spectroscopy Study in Healthy Adults. *Eur. J. Neurosci.* **2020**, *51*, 984–990. [CrossRef] [PubMed]
260. Simpkins, J.W.; Perez, E.; Wang, X.; Yang, S.; Wen, Y.; Singh, M. The Potential for Estrogens in Preventing Alzheimer's Disease and Vascular Dementia. *Ther. Adv. Neurol. Disord.* **2009**, *2*, 31–49. [CrossRef] [PubMed]
261. Wahjoepramono, E.J.; Asih, P.R.; Aniwiyanti, V.; Taddei, K.; Dhaliwal, S.S.; Fuller, S.J.; Foster, J.; Carruthers, M.; Verdile, G.; Sohrabi, H.R.; et al. The Effects of Testosterone Supplementation on Cognitive Functioning in Older Men. *CNS Neurol. Disord. Drug Targets* **2016**, *15*, 337–343. [CrossRef]
262. Lei, Y.; Renyuan, Z. Effects of Androgens on the Amyloid-β Protein in Alzheimer's Disease. *Endocrinology* **2018**, *159*, 3885–3894. [CrossRef]
263. Ruiz-Larrea, B.; Leal, A.; Martín, C.; Martínez, R.; Lacort, M. Effects of Estrogens on the Redox Chemistry of Iron: A Possible Mechanism of the Antioxidant Action of Estrogens. *Steroids* **1995**, *60*, 780–783. [CrossRef]
264. Requintina, P.J.; Oxenkrug, G.F. The in Vitro Effect of Estradiol and Testosterone on Iron-Induced Lipid Peroxidation in Rat Brain and Kidney Tissues. *Ann. N. Y. Acad. Sci.* **2005**, *1053*, 400–404. [CrossRef]
265. Wolters, F.J.; HZonneveld, H.I.; Licher, S.; Cremers, L.G.M.; Heart Brain Connection Collaborative Research Group; Ikram, M.K.; Koudstaal, P.J.; Vernooij, M.W.; Ikram, M.A. Hemoglobin and Anemia in Relation to Dementia Risk and Accompanying Changes on Brain MRI. *Neurology* **2019**, *93*, e917–e926. [CrossRef]
266. Atti, A.R.; Palmer, K.; Volpato, S.; Zuliani, G.; Winblad, B.; Fratiglioni, L. Anaemia Increases the Risk of Dementia in Cognitively Intact Elderly. *Neurobiol. Aging* **2006**, *27*, 278–284. [CrossRef]
267. Shah, R.C.; Buchman, A.S.; Wilson, R.S.; Leurgans, S.E.; Bennett, D.A. Hemoglobin Level in Older Persons and Incident Alzheimer Disease: Prospective Cohort Analysis. *Neurology* **2011**, *77*, 219–226. [CrossRef]
268. Carlson, E.S.; Magid, R.; Petryk, A.; Georgieff, M.K. Iron Deficiency Alters Expression of Genes Implicated in Alzheimer Disease Pathogenesis. *Brain Res.* **2008**, *1237*, 75–83. [CrossRef] [PubMed]
269. Falkingham, M.; Abdelhamid, A.; Curtis, P.; Fairweather-Tait, S.; Dye, L.; Hooper, L. The Effects of Oral Iron Supplementation on Cognition in Older Children and Adults: A Systematic Review and Meta-Analysis. *Nutr. J.* **2010**, *9*, 4. [CrossRef] [PubMed]
270. Garry, P.J.; Hunt, W.C.; Baumgartner, R.N. Effects of Iron Intake on Iron Stores in Elderly Men and Women: Longitudinal and Cross-Sectional Results. *J. Am. Coll. Nutr.* **2000**, *19*, 262–269. [CrossRef] [PubMed]
271. Rutten, B.P.F.; Schmitz, C.; Gerlach, O.H.H.; Oyen, H.M.; de Mesquita, E.B.; Steinbusch, H.W.M.; Korr, H. The Aging Brain: Accumulation of DNA Damage or Neuron Loss? *Neurobiol. Aging* **2007**, *28*, 91–98. [CrossRef] [PubMed]

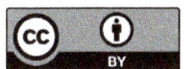

© 2020 by the authors. Licensee MDPI, Basel, Switzerland. This article is an open access article distributed under the terms and conditions of the Creative Commons Attribution (CC BY) license (http://creativecommons.org/licenses/by/4.0/).

MDPI
St. Alban-Anlage 66
4052 Basel
Switzerland
Tel. +41 61 683 77 34
Fax +41 61 302 89 18
www.mdpi.com

Nutrients Editorial Office
E-mail: nutrients@mdpi.com
www.mdpi.com/journal/nutrients

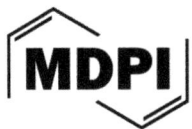

www.ingramcontent.com/pod-product-compliance
Lightning Source LLC
LaVergne TN
LVHW070628100526
838202LV00012B/757